Nursing care of
THE CANCER PATIENT

Nursing care of
THE CANCER PATIENT

Rosemary Bouchard, A.B., A.M., Ed.D., R.N.

Assistant Professor, Department of Nursing Education,
Queensborough Community College of the City University
of New York; formerly Instructor, Department of Nursing
Education, Hunter College of the City University of New
York; formerly Assistant Professor, Department of Nurse
Education, School of Education, New York University;
formerly Science Instructor, The Roosevelt Hospital
School of Nursing, New York

With 134 illustrations

4 6 1 6

The C. V. Mosby Company

Saint Louis   1967

First printing, December, 1967

Printed in the United States of America

Library of Congress Catalog Card Number 67-27961

Distributed in Great Britain by Henry Kimpton, London

Preface

This book is designed primarily for nurses who care for patients with the diagnosis of cancer—the nurse in the hospital, in the outpatient department, in the public health service, or in the doctor's office.

Regardless of where she works, the nurse should have an understanding of all aspects of the care such patients are receiving. Thus, this text discusses prevention, detection, diagnosis, therapy, and rehabilitation as they relate to total care and management of the patient. Pathology is presented so that the nurse can understand how this alters normal physiologic processes and how nursing measures can be adapted to meet the needs of each individual. Since the discussions presented are in no way meant to replace the need for special reference books in the various areas, suggested references will be found at the end of each chapter.

General aspects of cancer are presented in the first chapters of the book, including historical highlights, pathology, psychological impact, prevention and detection, and modes of therapy, including surgery, radiation, and chemotherapy. These are followed by chapters devoted to management and care of the patient with cancer in specific body sites.

This book could never have been completed without the assistance and encouragement of many people. Special thanks go to Miss Pauline Vaillancourt and her staff at the Lee Coombs Memorial Library of Memorial–Sloan Kettering Cancer Center for their assistance in obtaining books that were not available to me from other sources. Thanks are also extended to Inga Thornblad (a former colleague), Ethel Kistler, and Emma Svoboda, each of whom reviewed parts of the manuscript and offered helpful suggestions.

In addition, I wish to acknowledge the assistance and cooperation of Virginia Barckley, Nurse Consultant of the American Cancer Society, Inc.; Sandra Munsell, Photographic Department of the American Cancer Society, Inc.; and Herbert Schwartz, Statistical Department of the American Cancer Society, Inc.

To Leo Bouchard and Janet Martinez, who typed the manuscript, and Maureen Jones, who provided the medical illustrations, I am deeply indebted. Special thanks go, too, to my family and friends, who have been most understanding and encouraging when everything seemed impossible.

Rosemary E. Bouchard

Contents

Nursing care of
THE CANCER PATIENT

Chapter 1

Historical highlights

During the last quarter of a century tremendous strides have been made by all disciplines of the health team to bring under control one of the major health problems affecting society today—*CANCER*. Physicists, chemists, virologists, epidemiologists, medical doctors, laboratory technicians, psychologists, sociologists, and nurses have all waged an out-and-out war against this dread disease. What is there about it that produces such phenomenal reactions in man? Why is it that the mere mention of the word elicits strange behavior among many members of society? Where did this malady first arise? When will it be conquered? These are only the beginning in a series of questions and events that have led to the present-day awareness of the magnitude of the problems arising from the group of abnormal conditions clustered under the heading *CANCER*.

According to Heller*: "Man's attempt to understand cancer and to find ways of preventing, controlling, and curing it began in ancient times. Yet not until the late nineteenth century did science produce the kind of knowledge that will ultimately lead to the elimination of this threat to health and life."

Sixty years ago, an individual with cancer had only a remote chance of being cured; between 1935 and 1940, the survival rate was one in four. Currently one person in three is being saved, and many experts believe that the rate could be improved to one in two if all cancers were diagnosed at the earliest moment and if the individuals were treated promptly by means now available.

In 1900, cancer held seventh place among the major causes of disease in the United States. Today, it ranks second only to heart disease as a cause of death. Approximately 580,000 new cases will be diagnosed this year (1967), while about 890,000 patients will be under medical care for cancer.*†

---

*Heller, John: Trends in cancer research, Mod. Med. 28:68, 1960.

†1967 Cancer facts and figures, New York, October, 1966, American Cancer Society, Inc., p. 3.

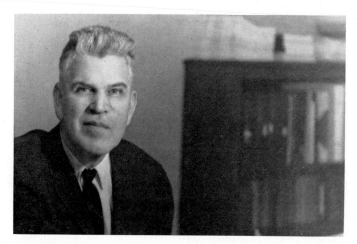

Fig. 1-1. Dr. John R. Heller, Former Director, National Cancer Institute, Bethesda, Md.; Former President, American Cancer Society, Inc. (Courtesy American Cancer Society, Inc., New York, N. Y.)

The malignant neoplastic diseases are older than man, and they affect not only the animal kingdom but also plant life. Evidence of cancer has been found and recorded since ancient times, and the general trend in theories relating to cancer has developed consistently since then. Much evidence and data have been accumulated, and recording of such data was first made as long ago as 2500 B.C., in the Hindu epic, the Ramayana, in which there are descriptions of tumors and their treatment.

Hippocrates (C. 460-375 B.C.), from available recorded medical literature, was the first to classify neoplasms, internal and external, into superficial and deep-seated lesions. He differentiated between indolent ulcers and progressive lesions, which he termed carcinomas. Celsus (C. 30 B.C.-A.D. 38), a nonmedical patrician who has given us the best history of Roman medicine, was the first to record his achievements in the treatment of cancer. Galen (C. A.D. 130-200) was a Greek physician whose doctrines, all based on theory, dominated medical thought for more than 1,000 years. His restricted humoral theory that cancer was caused by "black bile" led him to advocate such treatments as vegetable diets, colonic irrigations, and nutrient enemas, and these regimens are still used by the uninformed today. Leonides of Alexandria (C. A.D. 180) is said to be the first to have used thermal cautery in the destruction of cancer of the breast. He also advocated removal of tumors, by cautery and excision, which included healthy tissues.

The Renaissance (C. A.D. 1453-1700), highlighted by such epochal discoveries as the printing press, the circulation of the blood by Harvey in 1628 and of the red blood cells by Malpighi in 1661, produced little advance in the field of cancer. Surgery, however, was improving, and benign and malignant tumors were given separate classifications by Marco Aurelio Severino (1580-1656).

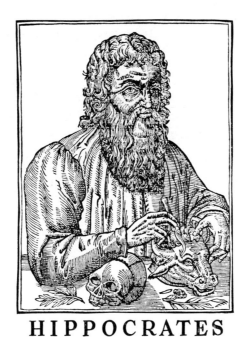

HIPPOCRATES

Fig. 1-2. Hippocrates. (Courtesy American Cancer Society, Inc., New York, N. Y.)

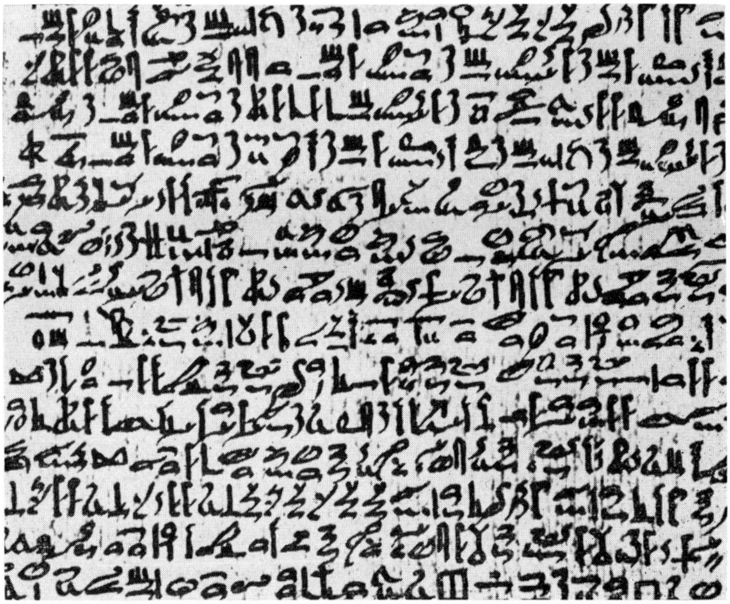

Fig. 1-3. Papyrus papers. (Courtesy American Cancer Society, Inc., New York, N. Y.)

Knowledge concerning cancer proceeded at a slow pace for many centuries. Early concepts of the histologic structure of cancer awaited the improvement of the microscope by van Leeuwenhoek, who is credited with perfecting the first simple instrument in 1683. Prior to this, Hooke in 1665 used the term "cell" in describing minute cavities in cork.

Descartes,* the philosopher, introduced the sour lymph theory. This theory assumed "that extravascular lymph coagulated through some process and became hard, and that then scirrhus arose, which was mild; if the lymph, however, fermented, or became sour, or otherwise contained some acid substance, severe cancer developed." This theory was a subject for investigation for well over 100 years.

Morgagni, the Italian pathologic anatomist, initiated the scientific study of morbid anatomy and led the way in the study of the gross pathology of tumors. Others who followed him in this field included Le Dran, Bayle, and Laennec of France, as well as John Hunter, Wardrop, Hodgkin, and Cooper of England. Although Morgagni was the first to begin opposition to the Descartian theory, he offered nothing as a substitute.

Boerhaave, a contemporary of Morgagni in Holland, introduced the theory that inflammation resulting from mechanical injury played a large part in the pathology of cancer. He believed that the seat of the inflammation was in the lymph vessels. Sylvius proposed a theory based on the chemical constituents of the body as the disturbance resulting in cancer. This theory was a natural outgrowth of humoral pathology.

In 1718, Friedrich Hoffmann, a German physician, introduced his theory, which was actually a combination of the three most popular concepts following the black bile era, namely, the Descartian theory of sour lymph, the Boerhaave theory of mechanical injury resulting in inflammation, and the chemical theory proposed by Sylvius. In essence, he believed strongly in the heredity of cancer.

In 1775, Sir Percival Potts described the classical chimney sweep scrotal cancer. He was the first to suggest cancer as an industrial disease as well as the first to indicate an external causative agent. Johannes Müller, in 1838, established cellular differences in tumors, and in 1839 Schwann established the cell theory of animal structure. Before this, in 1827, Meckel traced the origin of buccal carcinoma to the oral epithelium. Volkmann, in 1875, recognized tar and paraffin as external and/or irritative causes of cancer. In 1877, Cohnheim (one of Virchow's students) presented the embryonal theory of the origin of cancer in his textbook on pathology.

During the nineteenth century, the therapy for cancer was progressing along surgical lines. Roux, in 1839, reported the first major surgical operation for the removal of carcinoma of the tongue. In 1884, Sédillot first described the modern technique of dividing the lower lip and mandible for removal of the tongue.

---

*American Cancer Society (Mass. Div.), Inc.: Cancer: a manual for practitioners, ed. 3, Boston, 1956, p. 1.

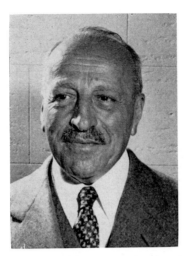

Fig. 1-4. Dr. George N. Papanicolaou. (Courtesy American Cancer Society, Inc., New York, N. Y.)

While many theories are available as to the cause or causes of cancer, no one of them is wholly acceptable to any one group of investigators, and periodically distinguished scientists and cancer specialists meet to consider new approaches that might lead to major advances in human cancer. Major areas of research are being explored intensively in an effort to learn more about the causes, diagnosis, and treatment of the malignant neoplastic diseases.

Progress in cancer knowledge has been made largely as a result of new techniques developed in other fields and through the application of concepts from other disciplines to the over-all problem. For example, the science of optics led to the development of the microscope, which today is one of the most essential instruments used in cancer diagnosis. Roentgen's discovery of the x-ray in 1895 was one of the great milestones in medical history. This was followed by the work of the Curies and Becquerel with the discovery of radium and radioactivity. Needless to say, the impact of these findings on cancer diagnosis and treatment is phenomenal.

Inasmuch as early detection of cancer is of vital importance if cures are to be effected and lives saved, numerous investigations have been carried out to adapt the cytologic method for detection of cancer in various body sites, including the lung, stomach, large bowel, and prostate. The method itself, originally used as a means for detecting cancer of the uterus, is now well established as a means for discovering this form of cancer long before symptoms appear.

Many scientists have been in agreement for years that chemotherapy represents the best way to provide lasting control of, or possible cure for, cancers that do not respond to other established forms of therapy, namely, surgery or radiation. Working on the assumption that cancer is a cellular biochemical abnormality, researchers in this field are hopeful that a drug will be discovered that will destroy the abnormal cancer tissue but prove unharmful to normal tissue. To this end, new chemotherapeutic agents are constantly under investigation in research institutions throughout the world.

In recent years, sufficient evidence has been accumulated to convince many of the most skeptical investigators that viruses may be a causative factor in human cancer. As a result, numerous studies and investigations are in progress in this area.

It is impossible to discuss the numerous trends in the diagnosis and treatment of cancer without mentioning the progress that has been made in the fields of surgery, radiology, and nursing.

Surgery, in its broadest sense, has been known since early times, with excellent descriptions of operations for cancer of the lip having been recorded by Celsus in the first century. Hildanus, late in the sixteenth century, performed the first axillary dissection for breast cancer. John C. Warren, Professor of Anatomy and Surgery at Harvard University, published the first American work on cancer in 1837.*

Enormous strides in surgical techniques have been made since the development of general anesthesia following Morton's introduction in 1846 of ether as an anesthetic agent and, more recently, since Lundy's introduction of pentothal sodium with intratracheal oxygen in 1933. Furthermore, the discovery of aseptic technique, antibiotics, and the means of repair of the nutritionally depleted patient have offered much assistance for more extensive surgical procedures. With greater knowledge of physiology and biochemical status of the patient, organs and anatomical areas formerly considered inaccessible to the surgeon have now become relatively frequent sites for radical extirpation.

Many articles were published during the early part of the nineteenth century dealing with operations for cancer in various organs. An important article published in 1867 by Moore† of London had a profound influence on subsequent surgical technique. Much more has been written in the twentieth century that has had even greater impact on surgical procedures today. Through the efforts of capable surgeons who were and are willing to experiment, many radical and ultraradical surgical procedures are being utilized in the treatment and "cure" of cancer. The ever-decreasing morbidity and mortality rates are indeed rewarding.

Radiology as a major field in the treatment and diagnosis of cancer opened up in the twentieth century following the development of the x-ray and the discovery of radium. It has now achieved the status of a medical specialty. Sjögren, in 1899, reported the use of x-ray in the treatment of an epithelioma of the skin.

Since that time, its use in diagnostic and therapeutic procedures has greatly expanded. Today, it is used extensively in therapy when surgery

---

*Warren, John C.: Surgical observations on tumors, with cases and observations, Boston, 1837, Crocker & Brewster.

†Moore, Charles H.: On the influence of inadequate operations on the theory of cancer, 1867.

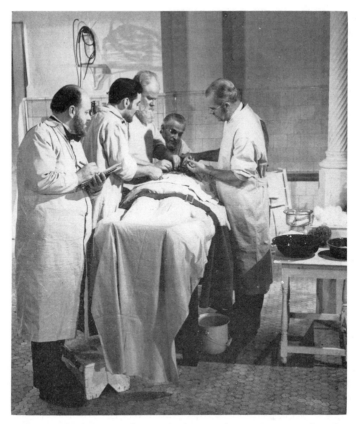

Fig. 1-5. Picture depicting early surgical procedure. (Courtesy American Cancer Society, Inc., New York, N. Y.)

is contraindicated, as well as in conjunction with surgery when metastasis has already occurred. Furthermore, radiology plays a large part in diagnosis not only of cancer but also of other diseases associated with internal organs. Currently, radioactive isotopes present a new method for exploration into the biology, diagnosis, and treatment of cancer.

The challenge of increasingly effective forms of therapy for neoplastic diseases and of the prolongation of life for so many individuals with cancer requires that all members of the health team be well informed in order to assist these patients to adjust to the physiological alterations and difficulties resulting from therapy. The nursing profession has long been cognizant of the multiplicity of problems presented both by the person with cancer and by his family, and nurse educators have constantly been evaluating and revising the curricula in an effort to increase content knowledge related to cancer. This, in turn, will provide the increased competence essential in the care of cancer patients. With the newer knowledge and techniques in the medical field, it is of utmost importance that the nurse have a complete understanding of the disease and of its treatment in order to make an accurate nursing diagnosis and in order to formulate the best plan possible for the care of the patient and his family.

Knowledge of anatomy and physiology is essential to understanding the nursing problems that arise from extensive surgical procedures and the resulting physiological alterations. Maintenance of adequate and normal fluid electrolyte balance is an important area that, if not thoroughly understood by the nurse, can frequently lead to a stormy recovery period for these individuals. Alert, accurate observations based upon scientific knowledge and recognition of symptoms will greatly enhance the early and uncomplicated recovery of cancer patients.

With the ever-increasing use of radiation therapy in its varying forms, the nurse of today must have some understanding of what radiation therapy is and what can be achieved by its use. It is essential to understand when and how to protect oneself from exposure to radiation. Both the patient receiving radiation therapy and his family are extremely anxious and filled with fears regarding the treatment. The thoughtful and knowledgeable nurse can do much to allay such apprehension by explaining the form of therapy to be utilized. She should understand that the patient receiving x-ray therapy, for example, is not radioactive—this is a question frequently asked by both the patient and the family. Another question frequently asked is whether the treatments are painful, and here the nurse should be able to assure the patient that there is no pain involved in the therapy. She must also be able to teach the patient the appropriate measures for good skin care when therapy is being given. This varies tremendously in many instances, and the nurse must, therefore, be familiar with the method that is to be used. The nurse must also be able to explain the reason for the skin markings that are applied painlessly but do not look very attractive. Further, the nurse must observe the skin for signs of local irritation, avoiding the use of the word "burns," and must report any change since severe reactions may require cancellation of therapy.

Chemotherapy points up the need for the nurse to have a sound knowledge of drugs in current use and their symptoms of toxicity. She must understand their mechanism of action (if known). She must also be fully aware of symptoms of toxicity that can be expected from experimental drugs so that these symptoms can be reported immediately upon occurrence to the physician in charge.

Some methods whereby the nurse can assist in prevention and detection of cancer are through a more thorough knowledge of the epidemiologic factors related to it. Case-finding in the home can be accomplished through knowledge and utilization of interviewing skills whereby the nurse can elicit significant symptoms pertaining to other members of the family. Knowledge and understanding on the part of the industrial nurses of industrial carcinogens as well as industrial hazards and how they may be lessened will also be helpful in preventing cancer in the United States.

Since cancer is a disease greatly feared by our society, the nurse must be able to analyze her own feelings about it in order to utilize her skills intelligently based on the present knowledge of the disease, its prevention, control, and treatment.

From the prerequisites discussed, it is obvious that the nurse of today must have a liberal arts education in which the physical, biological, and social sciences are predominant. Furthermore, the nurse must be competent in observing and recording pertinent information as well as in being able to accomplish the technical skills essential in the treatment of the individual with cancer.

Briefly, in summary, cancer is not one but many diseases. It produces biological, physiological, and chemical alterations that provide many implications for nursing. Surgery and radiation are the accepted methods of treatment for "cure" or palliation. Chemotherapy (while in its infancy) is still considered only palliative, but in conjunction with the other modes of therapy it can be considered acceptable for treatment. Furthermore, nurses can assist in prevention and detection through knowledge of epidemiologic factors related to cancer, use of interviewing methods, and knowledge and understanding of industrial carcinogens and industrial hazards.

The present era marks the convergence of all the trends in cancer to a concentration on the subject unprecedented in history. The search for new knowledge to meet the mounting challenge of the cancer problem is ongoing in research centers and special cancer hospitals and clinics in many countries of the world. While cancer is the problem of every individual and every small community, it is also international in scope.

Chapter 2

Cancer: what is it?

In order to recognize and understand the underlying pathology that results from disease, it is essential to have a basic knowledge of the normal processes involved in life itself. The cell is the unit of structure of all plant and animal life, and while many of the simpler forms of life consist of only a single cell, man, a highly complex organism, has billions of these units.

Each cell in the human body is thought to have a definite function that it performs in conjunction with other cells to form a useful machine (that is, epithelial cells protect the body surface, muscle cells produce movement, etc.). In the normal processes involved in daily living, cells are constantly growing and degenerating, sustaining injury and repairing the damage, and adapting to variations in the environment. As a result, millions of cells are destroyed daily, while new cells are formed through the organized process of cell growth in order to maintain life.

Occasionally, a cell or group of cells does not conform to the normal growth pattern but develops in a disorganized manner. In most instances these masses of cells serve no useful purpose, interfere with normal bodily functions, and are referred to as neoplasms or tumors. More specifically, neoplasm or tumor is the term applied to cellular proliferation of parenchymal, stromal, or supportive cells of the body without regard to the function of the tissue of origin. It is an autonomous new growth. Neoplasms, in turn, may be classified as either benign or malignant.

CHARACTERISTICS OF BENIGN AND MALIGNANT TUMORS

A benign tumor or neoplasm is a cell growth without a definite purpose. A malignant tumor or neoplasm is one in which there is an uncontrolled growth of cells, destructive in nature. Any malignant tumor is frequently referred to as cancer. The term cancer is further broken down according to the type of tissue from which the lesion arises. Carcinoma refers specifically to a malignant tumor arising in epithelial tissue, while sarcoma is the term applied to malignant tumors arising from connective tissues, muscle tissues, or any tissue other than that of epithelial origin.

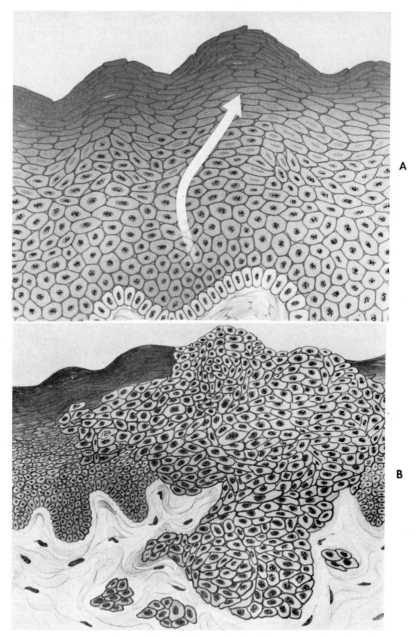

Fig. 2-1. A, Normal cell growth (skin). **B,** Growth of cancer cells (skin). (Courtesy American Cancer Society, Inc., New York, N. Y.)

Table 2-1. Classification of neoplasms

Parent tissue	Benign	Malignant
I. Epithelium		
Skin and mucous membrane	Papilloma	Squamous cell carcinoma
Glands	Polyp	Basal cell carcinoma
		Transitional cell carcinoma
	Adenoma	Adenocarcinoma
	Cystadenoma	
II. Endothelium		Endothelioma
Blood vessels	Hemangioma	Hemangioendothelioma
		Angiosarcoma
Lymph vessels	Lymphangioma	Lymphangiosarcoma
		Lymphangioendothelioma
Bone marrow		Multiple myeloma
		Ewing's sarcoma
		Leukemia
Lymphoid tissue		Malignant lymphoma
		Lymphosarcoma
		Reticulum cell sarcoma
		Lymphatic leukemia
III. Connective tissues		
Embryonic fibrous tissue	Myxoma	Myxosarcoma
Fibrous tissue	Fibroma	Fibrosarcoma
Adipose tissue	Lipoma	Liposarcoma
Cartilage	Ghondroma	Chondrosarcoma
Bone	Osteoma	Osteogenic sarcoma
Synovial membrane	Synovioma	Synovial sarcoma
IV. Muscle tissue		
Smooth muscle	Leiomyoma	Leiomyosarcoma
Striated muscle	Rhabdomyoma	Rhabdomyosarcoma
V. Nerve tissue		
Nerve fibers and sheaths	Neuroma	Neurogenic sarcoma
	Neurinoma	
	(Neurilemoma)	
	Neurofibroma	(Neurofibrosarcoma)
Ganglion cells	Ganglioneuroma	Neuroblastoma
Glia cells	Glioma	Glioblastoma
		Spongioblastoma
Meninges	Meningioma	
VI. Pigmented neoplasms		
Melanoblasts	Pigmented nevus	Malignant melanoma
		Melanocarcinoma
VII. Miscellaneous		
Placenta	Hydatidiform mole	Chorionepithelioma
		(Choriocarcinoma)
Gonads	Dermoid cyst	Embryonal carcinoma
		Embryonal sarcoma
		Teratocarcinoma

PHYSIOLOGY OF BENIGN TUMORS

Some neoplasms tend to grow slowly and to remain localized at the site of origin. These are referred to as benign tumors (Table 2-1). In general, these tumors are relatively harmless to the host, although if the tumor causes pressure on a vital organ, it can become a serious threat to life. Physiologically, benign tumors are independent of all regulatory influences of the parent organism. They are usually less capable of functioning than the cells from which they arise. Symptoms resulting from such tumors will vary depending on the location of the neoplasm. A benign tumor may cause obstruction of a lumen, such as a bronchus, thereby producing some respiratory embarrassment. Such a tumor may produce pressure on adjacent nerves, thereby causing pain. If it is a cranial tumor, there may be evidence of increased intracranial pressure. On occasion, the tumor may become inflamed or infected. This can result in spread of the infection into surrounding tissues, producing characteristic symptoms of any inflammatory or infectious process. Certain types of benign tumors may undergo malignant degeneration, in which case they become rapidly destructive neoplasms. Those benign lesions and tumors that have a tendency toward malignant transformation are usually referred to as precancerous lesions.

PRECANCEROUS LESIONS

Precancerous lesions or conditions are diverse structural and metabolic states that, either because of their location or because of the fact that they are subject to repeated injury, give rise to an increased incidence of malignant neoplasms. Among the numerous conditions characterized as precancerous lesions are benign lesions and tumors such as leukoplakia of the oral cavity, senile keratosis, burn scars, arsenical keratosis, radiation dermatitis, pigmented moles, Plummer-Vinson syndrome, portal cirrhosis, polypoid tumors of the stomach, intestine, and rectum, solitary adenoma of the thyroid, cystadenoma of the ovary, tumors of the bladder, Paget's disease of bone, pernicious anemia, and many others.

PHYSIOLOGIC PATHOLOGY OF MALIGNANT TUMORS

While benign tumors tend to grow slowly and are usually encapsulated, malignant tumors are characterized by an uncontrolled growth of cells destructive in nature. These tumors generally have young, immature types of cells that grow rapidly. Since they are rarely, if ever, encapsulated, they tend to invade the surrounding tissue by infiltration. Furthermore, they tend to form secondary growths at distant sites, spreading by means of the blood or lymphatics. These secondary growths are termed metastases.

It is believed that malignant neoplasms develop and continue to grow due to a faulty mechanism within the nucleus. DNA, or deoxyribonucleic acid, is one of the basic constituents of the nucleus. It has been shown that the molecule of DNA consists of a long, unbranched chain and is made up of alternate five carbon-sugar (deoxyribose) and phosphate groups. A nitrogen base is attached to each sugar. There are four such bases in most DNA

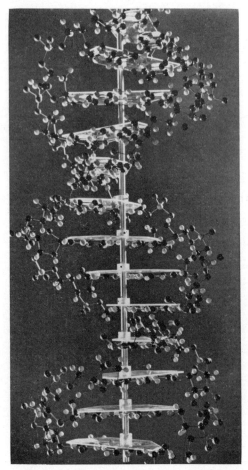

Fig. 2-2. Watson Crick model of DNA. (Courtesy American Cancer Society, Inc., New York, N. Y.)

molecules: adenine, guanine, thymine, and cytosine. The unit in the chain is called a nucleotide and consists of phosphate-sugar-base. Two such chains make up a DNA molecule. In chains made up of all four bases, the sequence of bases in one chain will govern the sequence in the other chain. Thus, this is the information necessary for replication or, in other words, it is the chemical code for cell growth and development. In order to convey this information to the site of most protein synthesis in the cytoplasm, RNA (ribonucleic acid) serves as the messenger. This polynucleotide differs from DNA in that the sugar is ribose and the main bases are adenine, guanine, cytosine, and uracil. Any slight change in the structure of DNA (mutation), sometimes referred to as a typographical error in the molecular code, produces a distortion of the biological information that directs the cell machinery. Therefore, affected cells run wild and a malignant neoplasm or cancer results.

Table 2-2. Characteristics of neoplasms

Benign	*Malignant*
1. Grow slowly	1. Grow rapidly
2. Usually encapsulated	2. Rarely encapsulated
3. Grow by expansion; do not infiltrate surrounding tissues	3. Infiltrate surrounding tissues; tumor process extended out in all directions; poorly differentiated from normal tissue
4. Do not spread but remain localized	4. Spread via lymph stream and/or blood and set up secondary tumors in distant sites
5. Do not tend to recur when removed surgically	5. Frequently tend to recur after surgical removal as a result of infiltration into surrounding tissues
6. Cells usually closely resemble those of the normal tissue from which they arise	6. Cells usually do not resemble those of the normal tissue from which they arise
7. Produce minimal tissue destruction	7. Produce extensive tissue destruction as a result of infiltration and metastatic lesion
8. Do not produce typical cachexia	8. Produce typical "cancer" cachexia-anemia, weakness, weight loss, etc.
9. Do not cause death to host except when located in areas where they produce pressure or obstruction to vital organs	9. Always cause death unless removed surgically before they metastasize

Morphologically, malignant tumors are characterized by growth of undifferentiated and often atypical cells that show many changes in the cytoplasm or nucleus. On gross examination, such a tumor appears as an ill-defined mass showing a different color and consistency than the host organ. These tumors are usually firmly embedded in and attached to the surrounding tissue and, for this reason, are not easily removed. Microscopically, they vary in size from the normal cell and contain vacuoles and inclusions not usually found in normal cells. The nuclei tend to be enlarged and contain much more chromatin than usual. The chromatin is frequently arranged in irregular patterns, and mitotic figures are more numerous and atypical.

Metastasis can occur as a result of direct invasion, lymphatic spread, blood spread, or serosal spread. Spread by direct invasion occurs as a result of infiltration by the tumor process into the surrounding tissues extending out in all directions. When tumor cells invade the lymphatic vessels, they tend to spread in a regular pattern along these vessels. The lymph nodes, which are located at various regions in the lymphatic system, serve as a deterrent to the early dissemination of the malignant cells. Malignant neoplasms of epithelial tissue origin metastasize characteristically via the lymphatic system (Table 2-3).

Table 2-3. Cancer spread*

Main features	Data on incidence			Prevention attempts
Invasion				
1. Frequent along tissue spaces, veins and nerve sheaths, and into veins	Great variation between different cancer types even in same location, e.g., in skin, basal cell carcinoma shows stubborn tendency of direct invasion, but rarely metastasizes			Radiotherapy to supplement excision
2. Rare across capsules and into arteries	Willis, R. A.: The spread of tumours in the human body; this book contains many interesting data			

Lymphatic spread	*Cancer*	*Early stages*	*Late stages*	
1. Regular pattern (important for radical surgery and radiation therapy)	Cervix	Stage I 18% Stage II 22%	Stage III 59% Stage IV 90%	1. Prophylactic node dissection 2. Radiotherapy to lymph node drainage area
	Breast	Operable 62% Outer half 67% Inner half 59%		3. Interstitial or intralymphatic injection of radiocolloids or chemotherapeutic drugs
2. Lymph nodes prevent early dissemination	Tongue	2 cm. 22%	4 cm. 92%	

		Periph. blood		*Local blood*		
Blood spread	*Cancer*	*Early*	*Late*	*Early*	*Late*	
1. Probably quite common even in early stages	Digestive	0%	23%	8%	21%	1. Systemic or intravascular chemotherapy or radiation therapy
	Genitourinary	27%	57%	50%	100%	
2. Single cancer cells probably harmless; only cancer cell clusters grow into metastases	Breast	24%	23%	27%	—	
	Gynecol.	14%	32%	100%	100%	2. Heparin or fibrinolysin
	Miscellaneous	30%	28%	29%	38%	3. Radiation therapy to lungs and liver
3. Irregular pattern	Total	20%	29%	28%	37%	
	Long, Roberts, McGrath, McGrew, and Cole, 1960					

Serosal spread	*Cancer*	*Early*	*Late*	
1. Early seeding throughout cavity	Ovary	50%	96%	1. Intraperitoneal or intrapleural radiocolloids (gold 198, phosphorus 32, yttrium 90
	Colon	15%	30%	
2. Predilection for dependent portions of cavity	Stomach	40%		2. Intraperitoneal or intrapleural chemotherapeutic drugs
	Uterus	20%		
	Rectum	10%		
	Moore, Burke, Skjorten, Badillo, and Kondo, 1960			

*Henschke, U. K.: Radiation Therapy Lecture Series, 1966, p. 2.

Table 2-3. Cancer spread—cont'd

Wound spread	Authors	Year	No. patients	% wound washings with cancer cells	
1. Sometimes long delayed	Smith et al.	1955	36	28%	1. Protection of wound
	Moore et al.	1957	155	36%	
2. Incidence high with poor technique	Smith et al.	1958	120	26%	2. Wound washing with saline or chemotherapeutic drugs
	Sako et al.	1961	279	6%	
	Thomas et al.	1961	125	20%	
	Smith et al.	1963	98	23%	
	Smith and Malmgren: Ca 14:90, 1964				3. Preoperative or postoperative radiation therapy

When cancer spreads via the bloodstream, it would appear that the cancer cells invade the venous system first. From here, these cells are carried to the liver and/or the lungs; eventually they enter the arterial system and may be distributed to all other organs in the body.

Serosal spread is characterized by early seeding through the cavity, intraperitoneal or intrapleural, with a predilection for the dependent portions of the cavity.

The specific location of eventual metastasis varies with the type of cancer and the type of tissue from which the lesion arises. For example, breast cancers tend to metastasize first to the axillary lymph nodes or to the internal chain of mammary nodes and later to the mediastinal nodes and lung or bone. Carcinoma of the prostate, however, usually metastasizes first to the lymphatics throughout the pelvis and later to the bones in the pelvic region. This is frequently referred to as selective metastases.

SYSTEMIC EFFECTS OF MALIGNANT TUMORS

Since a malignant neoplasm is one in which there is an uncontrolled growth of cells destructive in nature, it is obvious then that as the lesion continues to grow and enlarge it will not obtain sufficient nutrition, thus resulting in a devitalization of a portion of the lesion and in consequent necrosis. This in turn gives rise to ulceration and bleeding. Pain may or may not be present at this time, depending on whether or not there is involvement of the regional sensory nerves.

Many other symptoms may occur concurrently with those mentioned. These are frequently referred to as the syndrome of "cancer cachexia." Typically, one can observe in the patient a gradual or rapid weight loss, signs of muscular weakness, anorexia, insomnia, pain, and an attitude of hopelessness. Frequently, severe terminal toxemia will result, accompanied by acidosis and a rapid rise of waste products in the blood. Deep coma or death will ensue due to one or more of the following symptoms: severe hemorrhage, asphyxia, intestinal obstruction, involvement of the brain by metastases, or uremia caused by compression of the ureters.

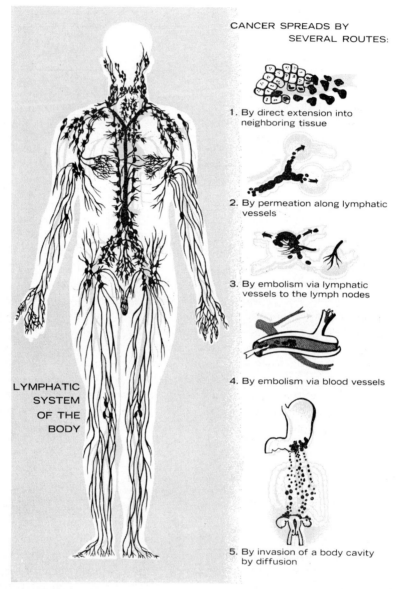

CANCER SPREADS BY
SEVERAL ROUTES:

1. By direct extension into neighboring tissue

2. By permeation along lymphatic vessels

3. By embolism via lymphatic vessels to the lymph nodes

4. By embolism via blood vessels

5. By invasion of a body cavity by diffusion

LYMPHATIC SYSTEM OF THE BODY

Fig. 2-3. Modes of dissemination of cancer. (Courtesy American Cancer Society, Inc., New York, N. Y.)

Many of the symptoms observed in neoplastic disease result from excessive function of an enlarged organ, pressure exerted by the abnormal-sized tumor on adjoining organs, or because the cancer cells act more or less as parasites, drawing on the rest of the body for their nutrition but contributing nothing to the well-being of the body.

Pain is probably the most common symptom considered in terms of the patient with cancer; however, it is frequently one of the latest symptoms to be presented. There are numerous mechanisms involved whereby a cancer will produce pain. In invading surrounding structures, cancer may cause distortion and destruction of tissue. This may serve as the stimulus for activating pain fibers. Infiltration, compression, and/or destruction of nerves may result from direct extension of the lesion, thereby affecting adjacent nerves, nerve roots, and nerve trunks. Infiltration and occlusion of arteries, veins, and lymphatics may cause obstruction, thereby producing pain by distention and distortion of the vessels and the surrounding pain-sensitive structures. Partial or complete occlusion or thrombosis of an artery may give rise to ischemia or gangrene, which secondarily gives rise to pain. Inflammation is known to lower the threshold for pain, and, moreover, inflammatory changes may render certain organs such as the stomach, urinary bladder, and bowel sensitive to stimuli that normally are not painful. Infection and necrosis produce a similar effect. Pathologic fractures due to primary or metastatic disease in bone may produce pain due to injury to the periosteum and/or invasion of adjacent pain-sensitive structures. As is to be expected, any one or all of the factors mentioned may contribute to the onset of pain in a patient with cancer.

The nurse who is caring for the cancer patient is a very important member of the health team. Whether in the hospital, in the clinic, in the home, in industry, or in the doctor's office, directly or indirectly, her knowledge and influence can supplement the doctor's plan of action for the diagnosis, treatment, rehabilitation, and/or terminal care of these patients. What may be even more important is her ability to assist in preventive teaching for the patient or his family. The nurse, therefore, needs to know the nature of the tumor, how it grows and metastasizes, in order to interpret for the patient and his family the information provided by the physician.

Bibliography

Ackerman, L. V., and del Regato, J. A.: Cancer: diagnosis, treatment, and prognosis, ed. 3, St. Louis, 1962, The C. V. Mosby Co.

Anderson, W. A. D.: Pathology, ed. 3, St. Louis, 1957, The C. V. Mosby Co.

Bacon, H. E.: Cancer of the colon, rectum, and anal canal, Philadelphia, 1964, J. B. Lippincott Co., chap. 3, pp. 54-68.

Breslow, L.: Epidemiology of cancer, Ca 12:215, 1962.

Butler, F. S.: The complete nature of cancer, J. Amer. Geriat. Soc. 8:689, 1960.

Crick, F. H.: Nucleic acids, Sci. Amer. 197:188, 1957.

Dalldorf, G.: Viruses and cancer, Med. Clin. N. Amer. 45:753, 1961.

Foulds, L.: The natural history of cancer, J. Chron. Dis. 8:2, 1958.

Furth, J., and Metcalf, D.: An appraisal of tumor-virus problems, J. Chron. Dis. 8:88, 1958.

Goldthwait, D. A.: Nucleic acids and cancer, Amer. J. Med. 29:1034, 1960.

Green, H. N.: The immunologic theory of cancer. Some implications in human pathology, J. Chron. Dis. 8:123, 1958.

Harris, R. J. C.: Cancer: the nature of the problem, Baltimore, 1962, Penguin Books.

Hedge, A. R.: Can a single injury cause cancer? Calif. Med. 90:55, 1959.

Heller, J. R.: Research on cancer viruses, Public Health Rep. 75:501, 1960.

Kit, S.: Nucleic acid synthesis in the neoplastic cell and impact of nuclear changes on the biochemistry of tumor tissue, a review, Cancer Res. 20:1121, 1960.

Lee, M. M.: The nurse in cancer epidemiology, Nurs. Outlook 6:160, 1958.

Moore, G. E.: The significance of cancer cells in the blood, Surg., Gynec. Obstet. **110:** 360, 1960.

Mueller, C. B.: Of cancer and viruses, Ca **11:**30, 1961.

Reimann, S. P.: Cancer control in view of its present background, J. Amer. Geriat. Soc. **8:**30, 1960.

Rigdon, R. H.: Trauma and cancer: a review of the problem, Southern Med. J. **51:** 1105, 1958.

Shimkin, M. B.: The epidemiology of cancer, Modern Med. **28:**81, 1960.

Shimkin, M. B.: On the etiology of cancer, J. Chron. Dis. **8:**38, 1958.

Southam, C. M.: Viruses in the field of cancer, Modern Med. **28:**74, 1960.

Southam, C. M.: Relationship of immunology to cancer: a review, Cancer Res. **20:**271, 1960.

Wynder, E. L.: Environmental causes of cancer in man, Med. Clin. N. Amer. **40:**629, 1956.

Chapter 3

Psychological impact of cancer

In providing patient care today, nursing has accepted a major responsibility for assisting the patient to meet his emotional needs while undergoing physiological therapy. Each individual patient is considered to be a person with his own unique problems and needs. These must be met if he is to become rehabilitated and take his place with his family in the community with a minimum of stress.

To the layman, cancer is one of the most dreaded diseases. Society is conscious of the potential danger associated with it. Many people are convinced that once a diagnosis of cancer has been made, "a death warrant has been signed."

The manner in which any individual will react to a diagnosis of cancer will depend upon his ability to adapt to a situation of threat. In large measure, it is also dependent upon his chronological age, emotional maturity, general pattern of behavior, normal reactions to stress, family relationships, economic situation, and what he knows about cancer in general. As a result, the individual may employ any one of a variety of techniques in his attempt to cope with the situation. It is of utmost importance, therefore, that the nurse understand these various techniques and be able to recognize the approach the individual is using to handle the situation.

In most instances, when a person becomes ill, the recognition that something is wrong produces a state of anxiety. The course of action he pursues is usually determined by his perception of the magnitude of the problem. He may respond by utilizing the mechanism of avoidance. This type of reaction often indicates his awareness that something is wrong and that he does not want it confirmed. On the other hand, it may indicate that he is attempting to integrate and handle the threat presented by the symptoms in his own way before being able to cope with such confirmation. In some cases, the perception of the disease is so frightening that the person cannot accept it and reacts as though nothing is wrong. This is the technique often referred to as denial, which actually is a forceful rejection of the threatening situation. Some people will rush for help at the first sign of illness. This is often an attempt to hide a panic reaction.

The nurse needs to recognize that awareness of any threat to health is accompanied by anxiety and that people respond differently to the situation according to their individual ability to adapt to it. As a member of a community she may be called upon even before the person consults a physician. What she says, and perhaps, even more vital, how she says it, is extremely important as it may determine the course of action the individual may take—face reality and seek medical advice or feel more threatened and deny his symptoms. It must also be remembered that how the nurse perceives the diagnosis of cancer may be projected to the person, so that she needs to analyze thoroughly her own reactions to this disease.

If the person consults a physician and a diagnosis of cancer is confirmed, what course of action should be taken? Whether the patient should be told he has cancer or not is still debatable. The consensus is that this is an individual matter to be decided between the doctor, the patient, and the family. It is agreed that if the patient is not told, some member of the family must be told. Bard* states that "the primary purpose for telling an individual he has cancer is to create in the patient a state of mind that enables him to cooperate fully with a minimum of anxiety during therapy and to resume functioning with a modicum of comfort."

The nurse needs to be aware of what the patient and the family have been told in order to help them build constructively for the future. Being the person closest to the patient for more hours of the day, listening to and watching the patient and/or his family will frequently provide appropriate clues in determining the need for further information. Close interdisciplinary relationships become very important in order to create a supportive atmosphere and not one of confusion.

The nurse must recognize that there is no blueprint to be followed in dealing with or avoiding the psychological problems involved in the nursing care of a patient with cancer. Each patient is unique and must be regarded as someone reacting to his disease with feelings, attitudes, concerns, and fears specifically his own. With this in mind, it will be recognized readily that no care is routine. All the skill, understanding, support, and empathy the patient can receive from the time of admission through his therapy and to his discharge will greatly facilitate a more rapid rehabilitation for him.

The nurse who is knowledgeable and has an adequate understanding and empathy for "what the patient is going through" can provide much assistance for his rehabilitation. First, understanding the patient is of utmost importance—what he knows or does not know, as well as what he really wants to hear. Knowing him as a person and not as a "case" is essential. This means

---

*Bard, Morton: The psychologic impact of cancer, Illinois Med. J., vol. 118, no. 3, September, 1960.

having respect for the dignity of the human being, eliciting his likes and dislikes, determining what his hopes and plans were prior to his illness as well as what his fears and worries are now. Many patients fear the loss of money a long illness brings and the possible loss of their job due to the lengthy illness. Others fear pain, mutilation, death, rejection by family and friends, and becoming dependent on others.

The decision to submit to surgery is often a difficult one. The patient is afraid to have the operation and is equally afraid to risk the consequences of not having it. Here, if the nurse is a good listener and can allow the patient to articulate his fears, he can usually arrive at a decision that nobody can make except himself. Following the surgery, the nurse can be most helpful if she recognizes how the patient has accepted the procedure. Acceptance of and adjustment to one's altered physiology and anatomy are not automatic or easy. The nurse who approaches the care of the patient with positive attitudes will transmit these feelings to the patient by the way she carries out nursing procedures as well as by her expressions of empathy.

Teaching the patient and his family concerning the care needed is very important for the impact it has on satisfactory rehabilitation. This should be a continuous part of the care given by the nurse and should begin at the time the patient is admitted. Explanations should accompany the various therapeutic procedures, and as the patient gains strength he should be encouraged to participate in his own care. By the time the patient is ready to be discharged, he should be able to feel independent in terms of his own care.

Teaching the family is also important. Oftentimes the problem of adjustment is greatly increased when the family rejects the patient or lacks sufficient understanding to cooperate with the necessary routines.

To provide the best possible assistance for meeting the patient's total needs, the nurse needs to be familiar with all available resources to the patient. This includes where he can get assistance in paying his hospital bill, how he can get assistance (if needed) to provide help with his care when he goes home, where he can obtain necessary dressings, drugs, or special equipment needed, and so forth.

When patients have problems, their families cannot escape involvement. Some families react by being overly solicitous while others reject the person involved with his illness. Both types of reactions can be considered normal, and if the nurse recognizes this she can be helpful to the families by merely accepting their feelings and supporting those of the patient. This can be extremely frustrating at times, but when the nurse understands why the members of the family do what they do, she can move ahead in giving the necessary support and help so sorely needed in a period of stress. Many authorities in the fields of psychiatry and clinical psychology have pointed up the fact that where there have been true love and affection and a closely knit family association, this same attitude prevails, and the patient continues to receive the necessary support essential to a full rehabilitation. However, where there have been feelings of ambivalence or outright hostility prior to diagnosis and therapy, there is an out-and-out rejection of the patient, and his rehabilitation will be greatly hampered. As with the patient himself, in many instances the extensiveness of the surgery is too threatening for the family, and for this reason they reject him. The alert, understanding, and knowledgeable nurse can frequently elicit these fears and help the family adjust to a difficult situation so that the patient is supported in his time of greatest need, when he returns home.

The nurse frequently faces a much more difficult and frustrating situation when death is imminent. In our society, emphasis is placed on physical fitness, and there is no room for dying. For the most part nurses do not know what to say or how to handle the situation when a patient asks, "Nurse, am I going to die?" The answer, of course, is that there is no standard reply. Needless to say, if the nurse is sure of her own feelings and has a sound philosophy, the exact words she uses do not matter—her manner, her voice, the expression on her face, and her empathy for the patient are all that matter. This applies as well for the family. However, it is of utmost importance, especially in relation to the family, that the nurse observe and evaluate just what their goals are. In some instances, they are anxious to see the patient die because they never liked him anyway; or because his illness cost a lot in terms of time, energy, and money; or because they could use his insurance. On the other hand, the family may truly feel that the patient has suffered so much that death would be welcomed so that his suffering is not prolonged. Either way, the nurse is placed in a position of having to understand, work within the framework of what she feels is right, and still maintain a position of neutrality so that neither side is hurt irreparably.

With the extensive and ultraradical surgery of today, both the patient and his family have many complex problems that must be faced. The patient himself faces not only the disease but also the surgical procedure that frequently constitutes the only definitive treatment available. Sutherland and his associates have stated that the specific site affected by cancer and its treatment introduces very special problems, since different body parts acquire special meaning in the emotional life of each individual. Thus, the problems associated with radical mastectomy will vary according to the value placed on the breast by the individual. In like manner, the problems of laryngectomy will be quite different from those associated with loss of the genital organs, loss of the rectum, or loss of a limb. The nurse, therefore, needs to recognize that the problems created by surgery will never be exactly the same for any two people. An individualized care plan is essential for each patient if his needs are to be met adequately and his personal problems resolved.

The fact that patients are people who have families, relatives, and friends poses still other problems with which the nurse will be faced. In many instances, how the patient responds to his therapy will be determined in large part by how his family and others react to his illness. With some families, fear and apprehension may prove so overwhelming that the families seem to "completely fall apart." This may lead to multiple problems that often the nurse will be called upon to help in resolving. Her ability to understand and recognize what some of these situations are and what measures are most appropriate in assisting the family to overcome them is of extreme value. This calls for adequate knowledge of the patient's condition as well as the ability to answer his questions and those of the family. It is frequently her responsibility to interpret and clarify information that has been provided by the physician. She needs to know about the various community resources that can be of assistance to both patient and family, since many times the mere fact that such agencies are available to offer help will provide the assurance needed in allaying apprehension and fear.

The nurse needs to create an atmosphere in which the patient (or his family) can feel free to talk about his (or their) problems without feeling that they are causing too much trouble. This also calls for full communication between the nurse, other nursing personnel, and the medical team and will greatly enhance easier communication with both patient and family and will avoid contradicting statements.

It should be emphasized here, too, that the nurse must know and be sympathetic with the philosophy of the treatment program since her attitudes are all too readily communicated to the patient and family, even when not expressed verbally.

Clinical psychologists have studied the reactions of patients with respect to the impact of cancer, and they have observed six clinical types of reactions that may occur following extensive surgery. Almost all patients will show one or more of these reactions to some degree. Anxiety is often still present. This may or may not be accompanied by depression. The anxiety is often due to concern over family acceptance and finances, as well as to whether they will be able to participate in community activities without being rejected.

Dependency and depression often accompany one another and may be referred to as regressive behavior. This usually occurs early in the postoperative period when the patient is overwhelmed by the results of the surgery and feels he cannot handle all his problems and needs alone. Assistance and support from the nurse are essential at this time in meeting the patient's physical and emotional needs. When not offered, the patient may become increasingly anxious and feel that no one wants to help him, or that he is no longer worthy of help.

Late reactions, usually noted after discharge from the hospital, include hypochondriasis, paranoid reactions, and obsessive-compulsive reactions. The patient who demonstrates hypochondriacal tendencies is the one who has often faced surgery expecting serious injury and irreparable damage. Thus, even though he is discharged, he no longer feels he can carry on normal life activities. The patient who exhibits paranoid reactions may have guilt feelings and blame the disease on himself because of some forbidden activity. He frequently considers that his disease was a form of punishment. An obsessive-compulsive response usually is noted in the patient whose surgery involved loss of sphincter control. This is apparently an effort to gain some control on his own and thereby replace the lost sphincter.

The nurse must be aware that the patient with cancer is subject to recurrences, all kinds of complications, altered anatomy and physiology, emotional upsets, and prejudices of others. Any or all of the reactions mentioned may be noted, and the nurse must recognize these as the approach that the patient is using to handle the stressful situation. With intelligent understanding and constructive help, she should be able to advise, counsel, and teach the patient ways of adapting that will be compatible with life and with full rehabilitation.

The nurse, like the patient, is a person. She will have her own ideas, feelings, attitudes, and concepts concerning cancer and the current modes of therapy. It is essential, therefore, that she look objectively at herself concerning these attitudes and beliefs since they can easily be projected to the patient, who is already overwhelmed with his own problems. Unless she is convinced that she is in agreement with the philosophy of the modes of therapy carried out in the agency where she is employed, she can do more harm than good for the patient and his family. She must realize, too, that she cannot take upon her shoulders the total burden of rehabilitation and problem solving for the patient and the family. She needs to recognize that this requires an interdisciplinary approach with consultation, communication, and assistance from all members of the health team.

Cancer offers a challenge to the physician, the surgeon, the radiologist, the scientist, and the nurse. That she is doing her part as an intelligent, efficient member of an interdisciplinary health team offers one of the greatest challenges that nursing provides. For the nurse who has an honest, sincere interest in the welfare of the patient and his family, cancer nursing can offer many deeply rewarding experiences.

Bibliography

Barckley, Virginia: What can I say to the cancer patient? Nurs. Outlook 6:316, 1958.
Bard, Morton: The psychologic impact of cancer, Illinois Med. J., vol. 118, no. 3, September, 1960.
Bard, Morton, and Dyk, Ruth: The psychodynamic significance of beliefs regarding the cause of serious illness, Psychoanalyt. Rev. 43:146, 1956.
Bard, Morton: Psychological reactions to oral cancer, O. Surg., O. Med., & O. Path., vol. 12, no. 8, August, 1959.
Bard, Morton, and Sutherland, A. M.: Psychological impact of cancer and its treatment. IV. Adaptation to radical mastectomy, Cancer 8:656, 1955.
Braceland, Francis: The role of the psychiatrist in rehabilitation, J.A.M.A. 165:211, September 21, 1957.
Brauer, P. H.: Should the patient be told the truth? Nurs. Outlook 8:672, 1960.
Campbell, Emily, and Ingles, Thelma: The patient with a colostomy, Amer. J. Nurs. 58:1544, 1958.
Connolly, M. G.: What acceptance means to patients, Amer. J. Nurs. 60:1754, December, 1960.
Drellich, M. G., Bieber, Irving, and Sutherland, A. M.: The psychological impact of cancer and cancer surgery. VI. Adaptation to hysterectomy, Cancer 9:1120, 1956.
Dyk, R. B., and Sutherland, A. M.: Adaptation of the spouse and other family members to the colostomy patient, Cancer 9:123, 1956.
Eldred, S. H.: Improving nurse-patient communication, Amer. J. Nurs. 60:1600, November, 1960.
Ficarra, B. J.: Psychologic management of the aged surgical patient, J. Amer. Geriat. Soc. 8:55, 1960.

Gerle, B., Luden, G., and Sandblom, P.: The patient with inoperable cancer from the psychiatric and social standpoints, Cancer **13:**1206, 1960.

Gregg, D. E.: Anxiety—a factor in nursing care, Amer. J. Nurs. **52:**1363, November, 1952.

Holmes, Marguerite: The need to be recognized, Amer. J. Nurs. **61:**86, 1961.

Neylan, M. P.: Anxiety, Amer. J. Nurs. **62:**110, 1962.

Norris, Catherine: The nurse and the dying patient, Amer. J. Nurs. **55:**1214, 1955.

Norris, Catherine: The nurse and the crying patient, Amer. J. Nurs. **57:**323, 1957.

Oken, D.: What to tell cancer patients, a study of medical attitudes, J.A.M.A. **175:** 1128, 1961.

Perrin, G. M., and Pierce, I. R.: Psychosomatic aspects of cancer, Psychosomat. Med. **21:**397, 1959.

Schmahl, Jane: The price of recovery, Amer. J. Nurs. **58:** 88, 1958.

Sopchak, A. L., and Sutherland, A. M.: Psychological impact of cancer and its treatment. VII. Exogenous sex hormones and their relation to lifelong adaptations in women with metastatic cancer of the breast, Cancer **13:**528, 1960.

Sutherland, A. M.: Psychological impact of cancer and its therapy, Med. Clin. N. Amer. **40:**705, 1956.

Sutherland, A. M., and Orbach, C. E.: Psychological impact of cancer and cancer surgery. II. Depressive reactions associated with surgery for cancer, Cancer **6:**958, 1953.

Titchener, James, and Levine, Maurice: Surgery as a human experience, New York, 1960, Oxford University Press.

Watkins, C.: The emotional response to tumors of the breast, Amer. Assoc. Industr. Nurses J. **9:**27, February, 1961.

Chapter 4

Prevention and detection of cancer

Second only to heart disease as a cause of death in this country, cancer is truly one of the major health problems of our times. Statistics show that approximately 50 million Americans now living will eventually develop cancer. This means about one out of every four. About 890,000 Americans will be under medical care for cancer in 1967, while an estimated 580,000 new cases will be diagnosed in the same year. Deaths from cancer by the end of 1966 were estimated at 300,000. This is 5,000 more deaths than in 1965 and 10,423 more than in 1964. For 1967, it is expected that 305,000 Americans will die of this disease, or 835 persons a day—more than one every two minutes. Somewhat on the brighter side, it is anticipated that about 193,000 Americans will be saved from cancer this year, although nearly 97,000 cancer patients who might have been saved by earlier diagnosis and better treatment will probably die in 1967.

These startling statistics provide grim evidence that a concerted effort must be made by medical and health teams to develop programs that will lead to prevention and early detection. According to several authorities in the field, cancer detection can be defined as "the search for and identification of cancer or its precursors in the asymptomatic, presumably healthy individual by means of a standardized routine examination." This is in contrast to cancer diagnosis that "usually refers to the identification of the disease in an individual as a result of physical, laboratory, or other examinations prompted by specific symptoms or complaints."*

The importance of controlling cancer by every possible means is obvious. Cancer control implies actual prevention of cancer whenever possible and discovery of the disease in its earliest stages while it is still localized and susceptible to cure by surgery or radiation therapy (Table 4-1).

---

*O'Donnell, W. E., Day, E., and Venet, L.: Early detection and diagnosis of cancer, St. Louis, 1962, The C. V. Mosby Co.

Table 4-1. Cancer control commandments*

1. Circumcise at birth to prevent cancer of the penis and to reduce incidence of cancer of the cervix and prostate.
2. Eliminate smoking to reduce the incidence of cancer of the respiratory tract.
3. Biopsy every persistent ulcerated lesion.
4. Do not cut into a nonulcerated tumor for a biopsy specimen unless the entire tumor is subsequently to be removed.
5. Regard every lump in the breast as malignant until proved benign.
6. Suspect an altering nevus.
7. Think of cancer first, if blood appears in the sputum or urine or comes from the rectum.
8. Exclude malignancy before treating hoarseness, cough, indigestion, and constipation.
9. Treat endocervicitis to prevent cancer of the cervix.
10. Prepare to treat for cancer if vaginal bleeding occurs after menopause.
11. Include a "Pap" smear of the vaginal secretions when doing a physical examination of women.
12. Complete the physical with digital, rectal, and proctoscopic examinations.

*From Goldman, L. B.: Early cancer, New York, 1963, Grune & Stratton, Inc., p. 10.

Every nurse has the opportunity, as well as the obligation, to participate in a community program for cancer control. She has a responsibility to help inform the public about cancer and of the importance of regular periodic health examinations regardless of age. This involves the hospital nurse, the public health nurse, the industrial nurse, the private duty nurse, the office nurse, the school nurse teacher, and the nurse educator. To be fully effective in such a program, however, the nurse must have a thorough knowledge concerning the pathology of cancer and the present methods of diagnosis and treatment, as well as an awareness of the early signs and symptoms that may be indicative of a possible early cancer (Table 4-2). Needless to say, the nurse must apply this knowledge to herself and carry out the health practice measures she advocates to others, if she is to be effective.

At the present time there are relatively few sites for which actual preventive measures can be applied in the control of cancer. For this reason, more and more emphasis is being placed on the earliest possible detection of cancer, preferably in the asymptomatic, presumably healthy adult. It is in this area that the nurse can participate in a variety of ways and can contribute effectively to cancer control.

The nurse in industry has a key role in contributing to cancer control. Her understanding of the principles of modern cancer control can be invaluable in saving many lives each year. Her role is literally threefold. First, at the time of preemployment physical examination or annual checkup, she can be most helpful if she recognizes what constitutes a "good physical" with emphasis on cancer detection. With knowledge of the major sites considered as "high incidence areas" for both males and females, the nurse can frequently win cooperation and overcome resistance to such examinations through a kindly word of explanation to the individual. These sites include the breast, cervix, rectum, and prostate. Next, an educational program is needed that will provide all

Table 4-2. Leading cancer sites, 1967*

Site	Estimated new cases 1967	Estimated deaths 1967	Warning signal When lasting longer than 2 weeks see your doctor	Safeguards	Comment
Breast	64,000	27,000	Lump or thickening in the breast	Annual checkup; monthly breast self-examination	The leading cause of cancer death in women
Colon and rectum	73,000	44,000	Change in bowel habits; bleeding	Annual checkup, including proctoscopy	Considered a highly curable disease when digital and proctoscopic examinations are included in routine checkups
Kidney and bladder	31,000	15,000	Urinary difficulty; bleeding, in which case consult your doctor at once	Annual checkup with urinalysis	Protective measures for workers in high-risk industries are helping to eliminate one of the important causes of these cancers
Larynx	6,000	3,000	Hoarseness; difficulty in swallowing	Annual checkup, including mirror laryngoscopy	Readily curable if caught early
Lung	59,000	52,000	Persistent cough, or lingering respiratory ailment	Prevention: heed facts about smoking, annual checkup; chest x-ray	The leading cause of cancer death among men, this form of cancer is largely preventable
Oral (including pharynx)	15,000	7,000	Sore that does not heal; difficulty in swallowing	Annual checkup	Many more lives should be saved because the mouth is easily accessible to visual examination by physicians and dentists

Prostate	34,000	16,000	Urinary difficulty	Annual checkup, including palpation	Occurs mainly in men over 60; the disease can be detected by palpation and urinalysis at annual checkup
Skin	90,000	5,000	Sore that does not heal, or change in wart or mole	Annual checkup; avoidance of overexposure to sun	Skin cancer is readily detected by observation, and diagnosed by simple biopsy
Stomach	20,000	18,000	Indigestion	Annual checkup	A 40% decline in mortality in 20 years, for reasons yet unknown
Uterus	44,000	14,000	Unusual bleeding or discharge	Annual checkup including pelvic examination and Papanicolaou smear	Uterine cancer mortality has declined 50% during the last 25 years; with wider application of the "Pap" smear, many thousand more lives can be saved
Leukemia	18,000	14,000	Leukemia is a cancer of blood-forming tissues and is characterized by the abnormal production of immature white blood cells. Acute leukemia strikes mainly children and is treated by drugs which have extended life from a few months to as much as three years. Chronic leukemia strikes usually after age 25 and progresses less rapidly		Cancer experts believe that if drugs or vaccines are found which can cure or prevent cancers they will be successful first for leukemia and the lymphomas
Lymphomas	21,000	16,000	These diseases arise in the lymph system and include Hodgkin's and lymphosarcoma; some patients with lymphatic cancers can lead normal lives for many years		

*From 1967 Cancer facts and figures, New York, 1966, American Cancer Society, Inc., p. 5.

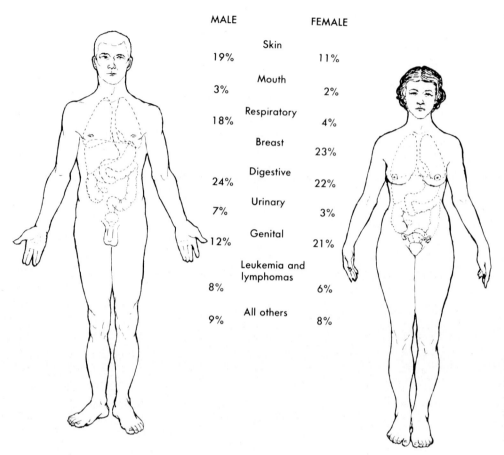

MALE   FEMALE

Skin
19%   11%

Mouth
3%   2%

Respiratory
18%   4%

Breast
23%

Digestive
24%   22%

Urinary
7%   3%

Genital
12%   21%

Leukemia and
lymphomas
8%   6%

All others
9%   8%

Fig. 4-1. Cancer incidence by site and sex

employees with a high level of understanding of the cancer problem. This can best be accomplished by having materials available to employees, utilizing films available for lay education, and securing guest speakers either in conjunction with the films or at different times. This type program can supplant ignorance and fear and will reinforce the need for regular physical examinations as a means of early detection.

Finally, counseling of the employee and his family will provide the essential knowledge for dealing with this disease. Hopefully this will keep the patient in appropriate channels of adequate treatment and will prevent him from seeking advice of quacks who prey upon the confused, the ignorant, or those abandoned as "hopeless."

Perhaps a fourth area should be included in relation to the services available for the person with cancer. Contacts with social service agencies in specific communities will provide the nurse with such necessary information. In many communities, services offered by the local division of the American

Cancer Society are available to the individual with cancer: (1) nursing services to the medically indigent, (2) loan closets, offering sickroom necessities such as hospital beds, wheelchairs, commodes, and so forth, (3) surgical dressings, (4) patient transportation, (5) homemaker services, such as help with housework, cooking, and care of children, (6) rehabilitation, including occupational and recreational therapy, (7) personal hospital needs, and (8) personal terminal care needs. It should be emphasized that not all divisions provide all of these services, while some divisions may provide all of these and more, including cost of certain drugs and equipment, speech therapy, and so forth. Although this has been specifically stated as the responsibility of the nurse in industry, it is obvious that every nurse in every field should function in this same manner.

The nurse needs to have a knowledge of the various agencies within the community where the asymptomatic individual as well as the one with symptoms can obtain the most effective advice or treatment. In cases in which an individual has no private physician or feels he cannot afford one, the nurse can recommend that he report to or call the local health department where referral can be made to a local cancer detection clinic or suitable hospital; or that he call the local division of the American Cancer Society where similar information can be secured. *1967 Cancer facts and figures** indicates that all fifty states have cancer control measures and that there are 1,000 cancer clinics and registries approved by the American College of Surgeons plus expansion of teaching, research, and treatment centers.

O'Donnell and Day† have indicated that: "Efforts at cancer control take many forms and call upon many medical disciplines, but immediate practical measures can be identified as having the following simple objectives:

"1. To identify, detect, and remove premalignant lesions.

"2. To detect or diagnose cancer in the earliest possible stage.

"3. To give patients the benefit of speedy application of the most advanced methods of treatment—surgery, x-ray, or chemotherapy."

These objectives can best be accomplished by the complete physical examination. The most useful procedures employed in the cancer detection examination are outlined in Fig. 4-2. The physical examination involves a thorough inspection and palpation of all accessible sites. Other examinations may be performed on the basis of clinical suspicion aroused by findings encountered (Fig. 4-3).

As was stated previously, there are relatively few sites for which actual preventive measures can be applied in the control of cancer at present; however, there are numerous measures available whereby certain forms of cancer can be decreased, and others can be found in a very early stage when the possibility of cure is greatest. Everyone should know cancer's seven danger signals.‡ If any

---

*1967 Cancer facts and figures, New York, 1966, American Cancer Society, Inc., p. 11.

†O'Donnell, W. E., and Day, E.: Early cancer—its detection, diagnosis and management, Med. Clin. N. Amer. **40**:591, 1956.

‡1967 Cancer facts and figures, New York, 1966, American Cancer Society, Inc., p. 19.

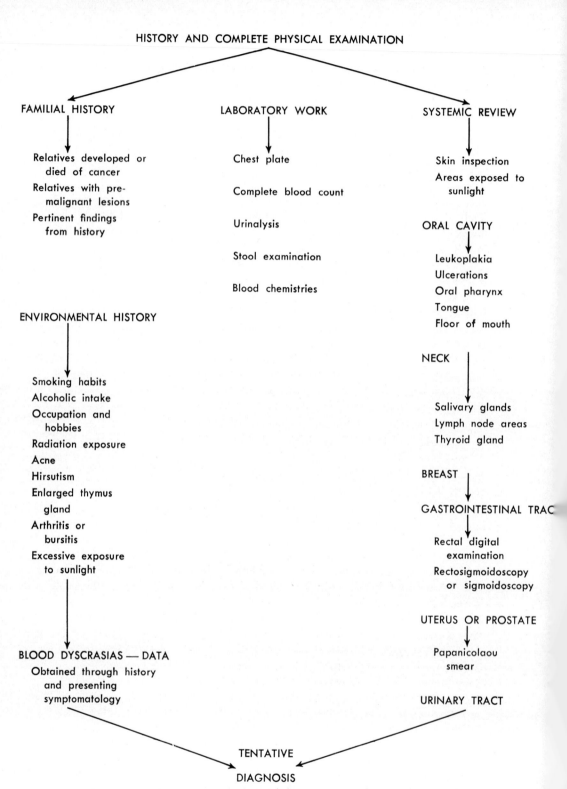

HISTORY AND COMPLETE PHYSICAL EXAMINATION

FAMILIAL HISTORY

Relatives developed or
died of cancer

Relatives with pre-
malignant lesions

Pertinent findings
from history

LABORATORY WORK

Chest plate

Complete blood count

Urinalysis

Stool examination

Blood chemistries

SYSTEMIC REVIEW

Skin inspection
Areas exposed to
sunlight

ORAL CAVITY

Leukoplakia
Ulcerations
Oral pharynx
Tongue
Floor of mouth

NECK

Salivary glands
Lymph node areas
Thyroid gland

BREAST

GASTROINTESTINAL TRAC

Rectal digital
examination
Rectosigmoidoscopy
or sigmoidoscopy

UTERUS OR PROSTATE

Papanicolaou
smear

URINARY TRACT

ENVIRONMENTAL HISTORY

Smoking habits
Alcoholic intake
Occupation and
hobbies
Radiation exposure
Acne
Hirsutism
Enlarged thymus
gland
Arthritis or
bursitis
Excessive exposure
to sunlight

BLOOD DYSCRASIAS — DATA
Obtained through history
and presenting
symptomatology

**TENTATIVE
DIAGNOSIS**

Fig. 4-2. Initial interview with physician

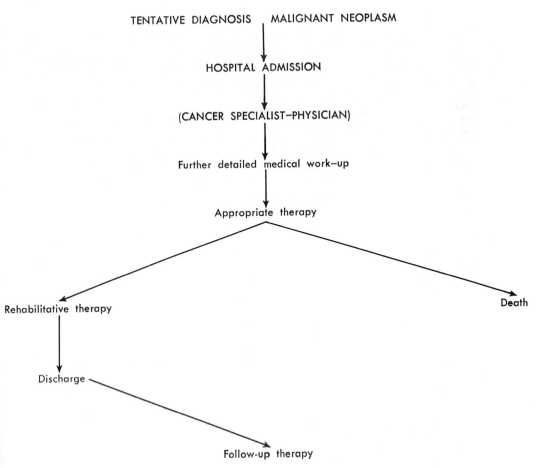

TENTATIVE DIAGNOSIS   MALIGNANT NEOPLASM

HOSPITAL ADMISSION

(CANCER SPECIALIST–PHYSICIAN)

Further detailed medical work–up

Appropriate therapy

Rehabilitative therapy   Death

Discharge

Follow-up therapy

Fig. 4-3. Clinical course of cancer therapy

sign lasts longer than two weeks, it should be called to the attention of a physician immediately for adequate evaluation:

1. Unusual bleeding or discharge.
2. A lump or thickening in the breast or elsewhere.
3. A sore that does not heal.
4. Change in bowel or bladder habits.
5. Hoarseness or cough.
6. Indigestion or difficulty in swallowing.
7. Change in a wart or mole.

Any source of chronic irritation that may lead to cancer should be avoided. The nurse can actively participate in teaching what measures can be effective to minimize such hazards. The person who has a fair complexion should avoid prolonged exposure to sun, wind, and dirt, which may lead to cancer of the skin. The presence of moles in locations where clothing may cause chronic irritation should be considered a possible hazard, and, for this reason, moles

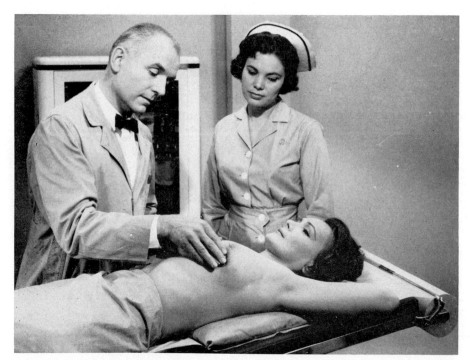

Fig. 4-4. Dr. Emerson Day of Strang Clinic examining the breast of a female patient. (Courtesy American Cancer Society, Inc., New York, N. Y.)

present in such locations should be removed. Girdles, brassieres, and shirt collars are examples of clothing that may produce such chronic irritation. Rough, jagged teeth are a constant source of irritation to the mucous membrane in the mouth. These should be extracted to avoid cancer of the mouth. Likewise, ill-fitting dentures may produce the same effect.

Breast cancer is the leading cause of cancer in women today. The American Cancer Society has estimated that there will be approximately 62,000 cases of breast cancer in 1967, with an estimated 26,000 deaths. Effective health teaching by the nurse in terms of breast self-examination could serve as a measure whereby the mortality rate from this disease could be cut nearly in half. Further discussion will not be included here because, through the local divisions of the American Cancer Society, there are available pamphlets describing this procedure in detail, as well as a film entitled "Breast—self-examination."

It should be emphasized, however, that when the nurse does teach individuals or groups the technique of breast self-examination, she must reinforce the fact that this is carried out only once a month following the menstrual period—temporary changes in breast tissue normally occur at the time of menstruation. Women should be instructed to make an appointment immediately with their physician if any abnormal condition arises. The nurse needs to recognize that if an abnormal condition does arise, she may be called upon to assist the individual in this period of stress.

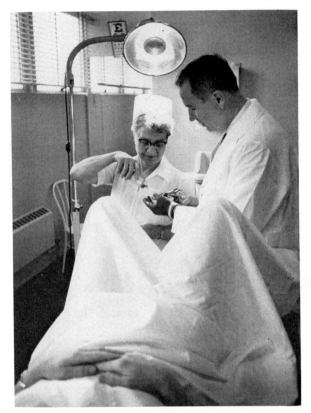

Fig. 4-5. Vaginal smear taken during annual checkup. (Courtesy American Cancer Society, Inc., New York, N. Y.)

Any unusual "bleeding or discharge" has been cited as one of the seven danger signals of cancer. The nurse can participate actively in detection of early cervical or uterine cancer by interpreting the importance of periodic pelvic examination including the Papanicolaou smear (cytologic examination) or "Pap" test for all women past 35 years of age. She should explain that this test is a simple, quick, painless procedure whereby cancer of the cervix can frequently be diagnosed before symptoms are apparent, thereby almost guaranteeing eradication of this condition. Women of all ages should be taught the importance of reporting any abnormal vaginal bleeding or discharge between menstrual periods or after the menopause has occurred.

Other facts that the nurse must transmit to women about such an examination include: (1) a vaginal douche should not be taken for at least 24 hours prior to the examination; (2) their physician should be consulted regarding a tub bath on the day of examination, since many doctors are against such a procedure; (3) their physician should be consulted regarding intercourse during the 24-hour period prior to examination; (4) they should avoid going for the examination during a menstrual period; and (5) annual smears are important as a preventive measure. Other sites from which bleeding may be a cardinal sign of cancer include the urinary bladder and the rectum. Specific procedures, such as cystoscopy and proctoscopy, may be carried out to determine whether or not a neoplasm is present, and whether it is benign or malignant. The nurse can allay fear, apprehension, and anxiety for the individual if she is able to interpret the importance of such tests as well as to explain in appropriate terminology what the patient might expect when such procedures are required.

Regardless of the way in which one classifies precancerous lesions, it is generally agreed that certain lesions warrant medical evaluation since some of them may become malignant. These include: dark, blue-black, or pigmented moles that suddenly change in size; dry, scaly, brown patches (senile keratoses) that change in size or color, which can develop into skin cancer, especially in individuals who are exposed to the sun and wind; whitish areas (leukoplakia), which cannot be dislodged from the mucous membrane; polyps that show increased activity; and some benign breast conditions. With any or all of these lesions, the nurse needs to reinforce the importance of early and accurate diagnosis and prompt treatment. In this way, and only in this way, can the lesion be eradicated and provide the greatest opportunity for cure.

Control of cancer can be accomplished only by a concerted effort on the part of all members of the health team. Knowledge of the disease must be disseminated at all levels to all people in order to eliminate the erroneous ideas and misconceptions that prevail. The nurse, who has a sound personal philosophy and an objective positive attitude toward the disease based on scientific knowledge, is in a key position to provide encouragement, support, and hope to those with whom she is in daily contact.

Bibliography

Aide, G. C.: The simplest test for making the diagnosis in bronchogenic carcinoma, Ca **10**:60, 1960.

1967 Cancer facts and figures, New York, October, 1966, American Cancer Society, Inc.

Arnold, W. T., Hampton, J., Olin, W., Glass, H., and Carruth, C.: Gastric lesions, including exfoliative cytology. A diagnostic approach, J.A.M.A. **173**:1117, 1960.

Ayre, J. E : A simple office test for diagnosis of throat and lung cancer, GP, **21**:108, 1960.

Bangle, R., Jr.: Appraisal of needle biopsy, Postgrad. Med. **29**:138, 1961.

Cabaud, P. G., De Veer, J. A., and Flinckinger, E.: Diagnostic cytology, Amer. J. Surg. **101**:761, 1961.

Cameron, A. B.: A cytologic method of diagnosis of carcinoma of the colon, Dis. Colon Rectum 3:230, 1960.

Cameron, A. B., and Thabet, R. J.: Sigmoidoscopy as part of routine cancer clinic examinations with correlated fecal chemistry and colon cytologic studies, Surgery 48:344, 1960.

Day, E.: Practical aspects of cancer detection: selection of patients, Med. Clin. N. Amer. 45:503, 1961.

Day, E.: What is an adequate cancer checkup? Postgrad. Med. **27**:274, 1960.

Evang, K., and Pederson, E.: Public health aspects of cancer control, J. Chronic Dis. **11**:149, 1960.

Farber, S. M.: Clinical appraisal of pulmonary cytology, J.A.M.A. **175**:345, 1961.

Goldman, L. B.: Early cancer, New York, 1963, Grune & Stratton, Inc.

Hertz, R. E. L., Deddish, M. R., and Day, E.: Value of periodic examinations in detecting cancer of the rectum and colon, Postgrad. Med. **27:**290, 1960.

Jablon, R., and Volk, H.: Revealing diagnosis and prognosis to cancer patients, Social Work **5:**51, 1960.

Kaiser, R. F., Bouser, M. M., Ingraham, S. C., and Hilberg, A. W.: Uterine cytology, Public Health Rep. **75:**423, 1960.

Lilly, T. E.: Cancer an industrial health problem, J. Amer. Assoc. Industr. Nurses, p. 39, September, 1957.

New York City Division, American Cancer Society, Inc.: Services for cancer patients. (Pamphlet, Patient Service Department.)

O'Donnell, W. E., and Day, E.: Early cancer—its detection, diagnosis and management, Med. Clin. N. Amer. **40:**591, 1956.

O'Donnell, W. E., Day, E., and Venet, L.: Early detection and diagnosis of cancer, St. Louis, 1962, The C. V. Mosby Co.

Rhoads, C. P.: Cancer control—present and future, Am. J. Nurs., vol. 58, No. 4, April, 1958.

Shafer, K. N., Sawyer, J. R., McCluskey, A. M., and Beck, E. L.: Medical-surgical nursing, ed. 3, St. Louis, 1964, The C. V. Mosby Co.

Slaughter D. B.: What is early cancer? Postgrad. Med. **27:**271, 1960.

Stewart, F. W.: The problems of the precancerous lesion, Postgrad. Med. **27:**317, 1960.

Turner, T. E., and Isaac, J. R.: Office endometrial biopsies, Obstet. Gynec. **17:**644, 1961.

U. S. Department of Health, Education, and Welfare, Public Health Service, Cancer manual for public health nurses, Publication No. 1007, 1963.

Wynder, E. L.: Some thoughts on the epidemiology of cancer, Cancer Res. **21:**858, 1961.

Chapter 5

Modalities of therapy

The main therapeutic approaches to malignancy at the present time are surgery, radiation therapy, and chemotherapy. Of these, only surgery and radiation therapy can provide a long-term survival or "cure." Chemotherapy has much to offer, but, as yet, is considered only palliative for the patient with advanced disease.

As was implied in the discussion of cancer pathology, cells, tissues, and organs affected by cancer (whatever form) show biochemical, physiological, and physical alterations from the normal. It is the result of these changes within the individual that provides the nurse with the signs and symptoms essential to making a nursing diagnosis and initiating nursing therapy.

The challenge of increasingly effective forms of therapy for neoplastic diseases and the prolongation of life for so many people with cancer requires that all members of the health team be well informed in order to assist the patient in his adjustment to the physiological alterations as well as the other difficulties resulting from therapy.

SURGERY

Surgery is not only the most widely used of the three methods employed in cancer therapy, but it is also the oldest. Surgery for cancer today differs somewhat from surgery for other types of lesions in that the operative approach is a radical one—excision of the local lesion as well as a generous margin of normal-appearing tissues along with the regional lymph nodes. This usually entails extensive and prolonged surgery, and for this reason the preoperative care is of utmost importance. The nurse needs to provide for good skin care and oral hygiene. She must be aware of the importance of maintaining normal fluid and electrolyte balance in those patients who are to undergo surgery because they are prone to dehydration, which can be a serious problem.

Dehydration results in water loss as well as loss of electrolytes that govern the activity of the body, assist in maintenance of osmotic pressure, and assist

Table 5-1. Electrolyte structure of plasma and intracellular fluid*

	Plasma mEq./L.	I.C.F. mEq./L. I.C. water
Cations		
Sodium (Na)	142	8
Potassium (K)	5	151
Calcium (Ca)	5	2
Magnesium (Mg)	3	28
Anions		
Chloride (Cl)	103	—
Bicarbonate (HCO₃)	27	10
Phosphate (PO₄)	2	100
Sulfate (SO₄)	1	10
Protein	16	65
Organic acids	6	4

*From Black, D. A. K.: Essentials of fluid balance, ed. 2, Springfield, Ill., 1960, Charles C Thomas, Publisher, p. 7.

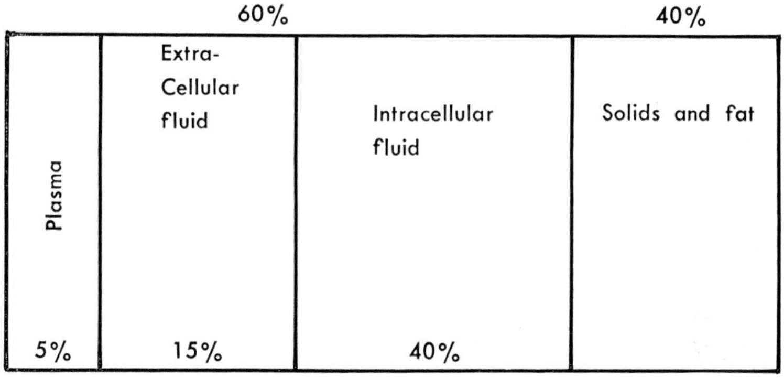

Fig. 5-1. Average chemical anatomy of the body. Percentages vary slightly according to sex. (Adapted from Statland, H.: Fluids and electrolytes in practice, ed. 3, Philadelphia, 1963, J. B. Lippincott Co., p. 13.)

in maintenance of a normal acid-base balance. The individual who is dehydrated will frequently complain that he feels weak and thirsty. His mucous membranes usually appear dry, and skin turgor is lost. In most instances, urinary output is greatly decreased.

Sodium and potassium are the most important electrolytes to be considered, since sodium is the major electrolyte found in extracellular fluid while potassium is of major importance in intracellular fluid. Severe depletion of sodium results in collapse, while an excess may produce increased edema and loss of proteins and potassium. Severe depletion of potassium, on the other hand, results in muscular weakness, lassitude, and paralysis. An excess of potassium produces myocardial hyperirritability that in turn may lead to heart block and death.

Maintenance of normal fluid and electrolyte balance is greatly enhanced when the nurse keeps an accurate record of oral and parenteral intake and urinary output.

Preoperative preparation of the patient about to undergo major surgery for cancer does not differ drastically from that required by any patient who faces a surgical procedure. At this time, in order for the health team to provide adequate care, it is important that all members understand how much the patient knows and how much the physician has told him and his family. Nurses' notes, doctors' progress notes, and interdisciplinary conferences are helpful in maintaining open channels of communication and in providing continuity of care preoperatively, postoperatively, and after discharge from the hospital. Lines of communication must also be maintained by the nurse with the patient and his family. Listening to the patient and the family will provide clues as to what they need to have explained in terms they will understand. This will provide a feeling of security and psychological support as each will know what to expect.

Postoperatively, the patient who has undergone radical surgery for cancer needs the same type of alert nursing care as any other patient. Depending on the operative site, the needs of these patients may be very great indeed and may entail the most involved and most complex forms of therapy. These measures will be discussed in subsequent chapters as each operative site is considered.

The nurse is the person who has the closest contact with the patient while he is hospitalized. She must be observing and evaluating him constantly for symptoms or warning signs produced by his illness and treatment and for any complications that may arise. Alert, accurate observation based on scientific knowledge, recognition of symptoms resulting from altered physiological processes, and reporting such signs to the physician will greatly enhance the early uncomplicated recovery for the patient who has undergone radical surgery for cancer.

RADIATION THERAPY

Radiation is a term used to describe many natural phenomena. Only a few forms of radiation are considered harmful to man. Major emphasis is given to x-rays, gamma rays, beta rays, and alpha rays when one considers those forms hazardous to man. The amount of damage or destruction to human tissue is due, in great measure, to the variation in dosage, intensity of irradiation, and the particular site irradiated.

The primary purpose of radiation therapy is to destroy or contain tumor cells in vivo without producing excessive destruction of surrounding normal tissues. The most common forms of irradiation utilized in the treatment of cancer include: cobalt[60] teletherapy, or its equivalent, supervoltage roentgentherapy; high-voltage roentgentherapy (200-250 kv.); low-voltage roentgentherapy (100-125 kv.); locally applied radium; and/or radioisotopes. Any or all of these forms of therapy have a definite place in the treatment of cancer.

Subsurface growths and certain deep-seated cancers (brain, head and neck, esophagus, lung, and bladder) are treated preferably with cobalt[60] tele-therapy. This form of therapy has several advantages over conventional high-voltage therapy: (1) it provides increased depth dose; (2) it has a skin-sparing effect; (3) it is absorbed in bone as it is in soft tissues; and (4) it produces less radiation sickness since the high-energy gamma rays scatter less than the high-voltage roentgen rays.

Therapeutic ratio is the term used to determine the relationship between the sensitivity of the tumor and that of the surrounding nonneoplastic tissue. The formula for expressing this ratio is as follows:

$$\text{T.R.} = \frac{\text{Damage of cancer cells*}}{\text{Damage of normal cells}}$$

With this in mind, most tumors can be grouped under three main headings: (1) those that are radiosensitive, (2) those that are radioresponsive, and (3) those that are radioresistant.

There are various factors that influence the radiosensitivity of cells and tissues. These include:

1. Mitotic activity: cells that actively divide are generally more sensitive than cells that do not divide.

2. Stage of mitosis: the rise of sensitivity commences in prophase; in-creases during segmentation and migration of the segmented nucleus and attains a first maximum before division; radiosensitivity then falls again and reaches a second maximum in the gastrula stage; the increased radiosensitivity during mitosis could be explained by the fact that chromatin exposes a larger surface to the action of rays during mitosis.

3. Degree of differentiation: embryonic and immature cells are in general more radiosensitive than adult cells to which they give rise.

4. Metabolism: increased cellular metabolism is accompanied by an in-crease in radiosensitivity.

Clinical and experimental evidence has brought to light not only the variation of radiosensitivity of cells of the same type but also considerable differences in the response of cells of different types in their reaction to irradiation.

Radiation therapy has a definite place in the treatment of malignant disease. It may be used as the primary form of treatment in some instances or it may be used in conjunction with surgery (either preoperatively or post-operatively or both) or chemotherapy. Various forms of therapy may be em-ployed depending upon the type of tumor to be treated and its location. Ex-ternal radiation therapy is provided by various types of machines such as x-ray (low voltage), betatron, cobalt teletherapy, and cesium teletherapy (high voltage).

Another method of delivering a destructive dose of radiation to a tumor is by means of topical and internal applications. This can be accomplished

*Henschke, Ulrich K.: Primer on radiation therapy, Memorial Center, New York, N. Y., July-August, 1966, p. 2.

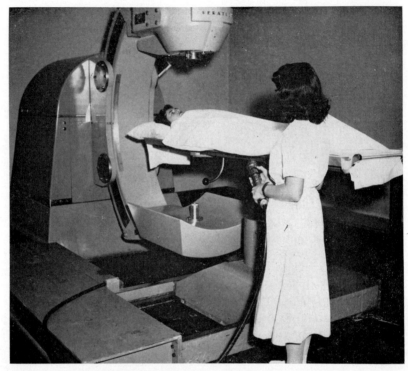

Fig. 5-2. The cobalt irradiator. (Courtesy American Cancer Society, Inc., New York, N. Y.)

by the use of: (1) surface application of the radioactive material directly on the affected area (such as the skin); (2) interstitial implantation of needles, seeds, wires, ribbons, or catheters containing the radioactive material directly into the tumor; (3) intracavitary applications that may be introduced directly into a body cavity (radium applicators into the uterus and vagina and/or radioactive materials in colloidal form into the thoracic or abdominal cavity in cases of pleural effusions or abdominal ascites due to metastatic disease); and (4) systemic administration of radioactive isotopes as a means of diagnosis of a specific lesion, or as treatment in specific conditions.

In caring for the patient who is receiving radiation therapy in any form, the nurse has some very specific obligations for herself as well as for the patient. Since the nurse is an essential part of the professional team required, she should have a basic understanding of the fundamentals and techniques of radiation protection in order to deal intelligently with the problems encountered in her work and in order to alleviate apprehension of patients and other uninformed personnel concerning radioisotopes and ionizing radiation. The nurse needs to know and observe the cardinal rule for radiation protection at all times. In other words, she needs to know how to utilize distance, shielding, and time in relation to planning care so that minimal time is spent

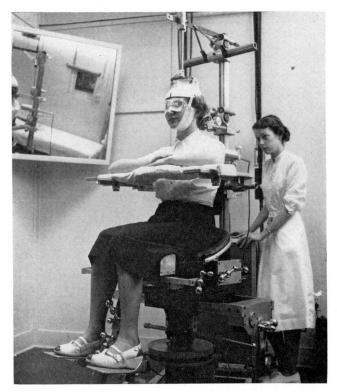

Fig. 5-3. Rotation radiation, a method for treating deep-seated cancer. (Courtesy American Cancer Society, Inc., New York, N. Y.)

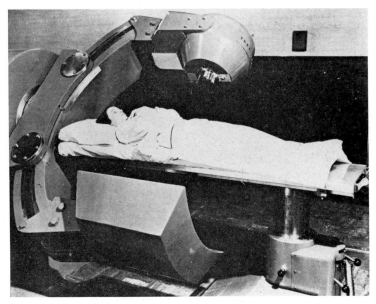

Fig. 5-4. Cobalt[60] rotation therapy. (Courtesy American Cancer Society, Inc., New York, N. Y.)

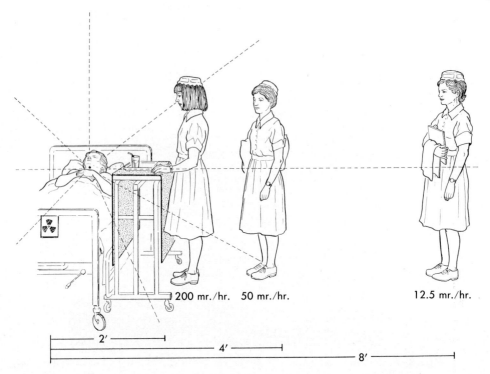

200 mr./hr.   50 mr./hr.   12.5 mr./hr.

2'

4'

8'

Fig. 5-5. Nurse nearest source of radioactivity (the patient) is more exposed.

at the bedside; she must maintain a safe distance from the patient (who is the source of radiation). It is essential, however, that the patient receive adequate information and explanation as to the reasons for limiting the time spent with him.

The nurse should have some understanding of what radiation therapy is and what can be achieved by its use. She should have visited the department so that she will be able to describe it to the patient. This will help to allay fears of large machines and of being alone in the treatment room. She should understand that the patient receiving x-ray therapy is not radioactive—this question is frequently asked by both the patient and the family. The nurse should be able to assure the patient that there is no pain involved in the therapy.

The patient should be given adequate explanation concerning (1) the mode of transportation to the Radiology Department; (2) the reasons for the skin markings that are applied painlessly but do not look very attractive; and (3) care of the skin during therapy. Some institutions require the use of special soap or bland or medicated ointments, while others recommend that ointments be used only if prescribed; otherwise, keep the skin dry and apply cornstarch.

The nurse needs to be familiar with the techniques used to control con-

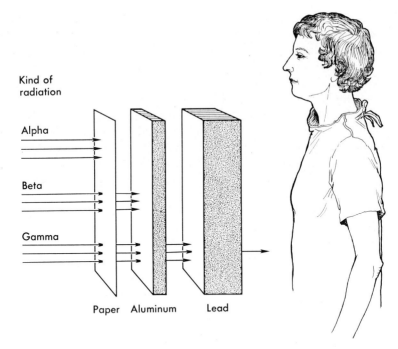

Kind of
radiation

Alpha

Beta

Gamma

Paper   Aluminum   Lead

Fig. 5-6. Relative penetrating power of various types of radiation.

tamination and internal hazards from radioisotopes: (1) how to prevent ingestion, inhalation, or absorption of radioisotopes; (2) how to handle items
such as needles, syringes, tubing, bedside equipment when contamination is
suspected; (3) how to handle, store, and dispose of excreta; and (4) how to
dispose of contaminated items such as bed linen, clothing, and towels both
before and after they have been checked by the radiological safety officer.

The patient who is undergoing daily x-ray therapy is usually rather
lethargic and complains of general malaise. Nausea and vomiting are also
common systemic reactions. The nurse should plan to spend extra time with
this patient in order to reassure him. In planning his care, time should be
provided for a quiet rest period following therapy. Special attention should
be given to diet and medications. The diet should provide small frequent
feedings of a high-caloric, high-protein nature. Citrus juices should be forced.
This is of great importance since x-ray destroys tissues, and the kidneys tend
to retain uric acid. Accurate intake and output should be maintained since
the patient is frequently dehydrated and has a moderate to severe anorexia
due to the therapy. This will also be of value in preventing the onset of
uremia.

With the advent of tranquilizers and antiemetic drugs, the problems of
postirradiation nausea, vomiting, and anorexia have been lessened. Many
patients receiving therapy are placed on such drugs routinely.

Radiation therapy sometimes results in a systemic reactions known as "radiation sickness" or "radiation syndrome," the usual manifestations being anorexia, nausea, vomiting, and severe weakness. The appearance and intensity of the symptoms usually depend on the site being irradiated, the volume of tissue being irradiated, the rate of administration of the radiation, and the radiosensitivity of the tumor. Patients in whom these symptoms develop should have a light diet, ample fluid intake, bed rest with sedation as needed, and should be kept as free from infection as possible. Complete blood count and hemoglobin level should be obtained prior to starting therapy and should be repeated at least once a week thereafter to determine the degree of leukopenia that develops, since radiation depresses bone marrow. Thus production of white blood cells, red blood cells, and thrombocytes is depressed as well, often resulting in anemia and thrombocytopenia along with the leukopenia. These all may require symptomatic therapy such as blood transfusion for the anemia and antibiotic therapy to prevent infection. Therapy may even have to be discontinued if leukopenia is too severe.

Other local effects such as epilation and skin erythema may occur, and these must be treated accordingly. Impotence, sterility, and amenorrhea may result from therapy. These can probably not be materially affected by treatment but should be investigated by a competent clinical consultant.

Henschke* has summarized the radiobiological effects on skin according to the types occurring during or immediately following therapy, as well as long-term reactions.

Radiobiological effects on skin*

Types of skin effects

A. Early reactions (during or immediately after radiation exposure):
  1. *Erythema* by capillary dilatation, probably caused by the local release of histamine from injured cells. Similar to erythema from ultraviolet rays. Followed by pigmentation.
  2. *Desquamation* caused by destruction of the rapidly multiplying basal columnar cells of the germinal layer of the epidermis. In the normal life cycle of epidermal cells, the basal cells change in 3 to 4 weeks first into squamous and then into the superficial cornified cells. The latter are constantly shed off or rubbed off. If their supply is completely halted (6,000 R in 6 weeks), moist desquamation occurs, since without the epidermis cover the serum oozes out from the dermis. Healing (covering with new epidermis) starts from epidermis growing in from the edges of the field as well as from undamaged islands of basal cells within the field. With lower doses (4,000 R) or with longer treatment times (6,000 R in 12 weeks) only dry desquamation (peeling and flaking of the upper epidermal layers) occurs, since enough cells are produced to keep the dermis covered.
  3. *Pigmentation* (1) by increased melanin formation in basal cells of

---

*Henschke, Ulrich K.: Primer on radiation therapy, Memorial Center, New York, N. Y., 1966, p. 17.

epidermis following erythema and (2) by darkening of the melanin already present in the epidermis. Pigmentation protects the basal layers against ultraviolet rays, but not against x-rays.

B. Late reactions (months to years after radiation exposure):

    1. Atrophy by thinning of the epidermal layer; usually only after high doses, which produce moist desquamation, but smaller doses given over long periods of time, such as formerly widely used for treatment of acne, can have the same effect.

    2. *Telangiectasis* by damage of capillaries and small vessels.

    3. *Depigmentation* by damage of pigment-forming elements.

    4. *Subcutaneous fibrosis* by damage of deeper dermal layer; more frequently seen with supervoltage, which spares the epidermal layer but gives the same dosage in deeper layers.

C. Occasional late sequelae (years after therapy):

    1. *Ulceration* and necrosis often precipitated by mechanical, thermal, or chemical trauma.

    2. *Skin cancer:* Good statistics on threshold doses and incidence are lacking, but skin cancer after irradiation for benign dermatoses (especially acne) has occurred frequently enough to make at least doses over 500 R inadvisable for benign conditions.

It should be evident from the foregoing discussion that the nurse must have a thorough knowledge of what radiation therapy means, the forms whereby it can be administered, the reasons for use, whether diagnostic or therapeutic, the potential hazards for the patient as well as for herself, and appropriate measures of interpreting this information to the patient and his family. She needs to be familiar with procedures relating to use of radioactive isotopes within the agency where she is employed and to know whom to contact in the event of contamination of the room, bed linen, clothing, and so forth. What she knows and how well she can interpret this is of great importance in order to allay fear in the patient who is undergoing treatment.

CHEMOTHERAPY

Many authorities in the field of oncology are in agreement that both surgery and radiation therapy have developed as far as possible for the treatment of cancer at the present time. Chemotherapy, while still in its infancy, is undergoing extensive study and research and shows considerable promise for palliation in metastatic disease.

Although chemotherapy has been recognized since the early days of medicine, it has only been within the last fifteen to twenty years that newer agents have been found effective in the treatment of disseminated disease. This came about during World War II when a ship carrying 100 tons of mustard gas was sunk during a bombing in Bari Harbor. A United States medical officer on board ship recognized and reported on those members who had survived the initial shock of blast and immersion, indicating that all survivors had a profound depression of leukocyte formation. This led Rhoads, in 1947, to investigate the potential of the nitrogen mustard in use against neoplastic disorders of the leukopoietic tissues.

Since then, a program of nationwide, even worldwide, scope has been established as a means of accelerating the search for new agents to treat cancer. Sponsored by the National Cancer Institute and coordinated by the Cancer Chemotherapy National Service Center, many independent research centers, colleges, universities, and private industry have joined forces in an all-out effort to develop these new agents. Funds are appropriated by Congress to assist in financing this program. It is an extremely complex program but a most worthwhile one in terms of its ultimate objective, to provide drugs that will cure cancer either alone or in combination with other forms of treatment.

Chemotherapeutic agents utilized in the treatment of cancer have been classified by various authorities in the field. Today, drugs are available in the following categories: polyfunctional alkylating agents, antimetabolites, steroid compounds and ACTH, and miscellaneous drugs.

The polyfunctional alkylating agents represent a large group of chemically reactive compounds generally considered to be cell poisons. It is believed that the "alkyl group" reacts with deoxyribonucleic acid in the nucleus so that cell growth and division are impaired. The changes produced are similar to those seen following radiation therapy, and for this reason they are frequently referred to as being radiomimetic.

The most common alkylating agents in use are the following: nitrogen mustard (Mustargen), chlorambucil (Leukeran), cyclophosphamide (Endoxan or Cytoxan), triethylenemelamine (TEM), triethylenethiophosphoramide (TSPA or Thio-TEPA), and busulfan or Myleran. For further clarity, these drugs have been subclassified according to their chemical composition and properties. The subclassifications include:

1. *Nitrogen mustards,* of which nitrogen mustard, chlorambucil, and cyclophosphamide, are considered. These drugs have been used in treating cases of chronic leukemia, Hodgkin's disease, and lymphosarcoma and have shown some success in treating solid tumors of the lung, ovary, and breast.

2. *Ethylenemines,* or compounds that appear to have similar effects on cell division and tumor growth, of which triethylenemelamine and triethylenethiophosphoramide are considered. These, too, have been found useful in the treatment of chronic leukemia as well as carcinoma of the breast and ovary.

3. *Sulfonic acid esters,* such as busulfan or Myleran, have shown considerable promise in treating patients with chronic myelocytic leukemia.

Major toxic manifestations from this class of chemotherapeutic agents consist of severe bone marrow depression with leukopenia, thrombocytopenia, and anemia. Others include stomatitis, nausea and vomiting, and diarrhea.

The second important category of drugs effective in treating cancer is the antimetabolites, substances similar in structure to vitamins, coenzymes, or normal intermediary metabolic products. They differ sufficiently, however, that essential metabolic processes are inhibited. Like the polyfunctional alkylating agents, the antimetabolites have been classified into three major groups of drugs that are of value in cancer chemotherapy: the antifolic compounds, the purine analogs, and the pyrimidine analogs. These drugs interfere with the metabolic pathways normally used in synthesizing certain chemicals (metabolites) essential to the normal cell. The antimetabolites that have proved effective against cancer act by affecting cell nucleic acid synthesis (DNA and RNA). They may affect the biosynthesis of DNA or RNA by altering the rates of synthesis of the purines or pyrimidines. They may also produce their effect by substituting abnormal components for those essential to biosynthesis.

The folic acid antagonists (aminopterin, Amethoperin, or methotrexate) produce their effect by interfering with the conversion of folic acid to its active form (folonic acid):

Folic acid $\longrightarrow$ Dihydrofolic acid $\longrightarrow$ Tetrahydrofolic acid $\longrightarrow$ Folonic acid
  (enzyme)   (enzyme)   (enzyme)

This then brings about interference with purine and pyrimidine metabolism, the essential components of the nucleic acids.

Purine analogs act as antagonists to certain purines that are constituents of nucleic acids, thus interfering with their formation and thereby inhibiting growth and division of cells; 6-mercaptopurine is the best known and most useful drug in this group.

Pyrimidine analogs are believed to affect specific steps in pyrimidine metabolism by inhibiting the synthesis of thymine, an essential component of DNA. They also interfere with the synthesis of RNA by inhibiting protein synthesis. Drugs in this category that have been effective in cancer chemotherapy are 5-fluorouracil (5-Fu) and 5-fluorodeoxyuridine (5-FUDR).

These three groups of drugs have similar toxic manifestations including stomatitis (with oral and digestive tract ulcerations), nausea and vomiting, diarrhea, and bone marrow depression, accompanied by leukopenia, thrombocytopenia, and anemia.

Since these symptoms and signs are common occurrences in patients receiving polyfunctional alkylating agents and/or antimetabolites, the nurse caring for them must be alert to the early onset of toxic manifestations because she can do much to assist the patient in overcoming these problems.

Stomatitis is a generalized inflammatory involvement of the oral mucosa. A line of erythema and edema along the mucocutaneous junction of the lip with dryness of the mouth and burning sensation of the lips are usually the initial symptoms noted. Ulceration may occur and may be extensive, including buccal and palatal lesions. Severe dysphagia and secondary infection may result. Prior to therapy, the nurse should determine the patient's state of oral hygiene, that is, presence of inflammatory process, whether dentures are used, how well they fit, and so forth. Nursing care during therapy will consist of daily inspection of the patient's mouth and the inner margins of the lips. She should be alert to signs of dryness of the mouth, burning sensations from acid foods, irritation of the lips, and painful mastication. The nurse needs to teach the patient the importance of correct oral hygiene. This will include the importance of not using self-prescribed mouthwashes or oral medications as well as the reasons for eating warm rather than very hot food or fluids. When stomatitis is observed, the nurse needs to provide supportive care. Topical anesthetics, analgesics, and mild alkaline mouthwashes may be utilized. In some instances both local and systemic antibiotics may be ordered. Diet should be carefully considered, and highly seasoned or highly acid foods should be avoided. In severe cases, it may be necessary to discontinue oral feeding and administer intravenous preparations to provide adequate protein, vitamin, and fluid intake.

Nausea and vomiting may occur for numerous physiological reasons. Irritability and increased tension upon the walls of the stomach and/or duodenum may be the cause. Irritation of either the gastric or the intestinal mucosa will possibly lead to nausea by stimulation of the vomiting center in the medulla, with subsequent anorexia. Anorexia and nausea can usually be tolerated by the patient, and no severe side effects are produced. Vomiting, on the other hand, can lead to fluid and electrolyte imbalance, since fluid is depleted from loss of gastric secretion and loss of water content of food. This is accompanied by a deficiency of hydrogen and chloride ions and may lead to hypochloremic alkalosis. Other electrolyte imbalances may ensue if the condition continues. Thus, the nurse who is caring for the patient with nausea and vomiting needs to be aware of measures she can utilize to overcome this problem. Needless to say, the patient should be assisted to a comfortable sitting position, should be given good mouth care before eating, should be offered small, more frequent meals, and should have a pleasant environment free of sights, sounds, and odors that may contribute to the condition. Nausea can be minimized by encouraging the patient to take deep breaths and to take small sips of effervescent fluids or warm tea or ice chips. Those measures taken for any patient who is vomiting can be followed in this instance: proper positioning to prevent aspiration, accurate reporting of nature of vomitus, time of onset in relation to intake of food, and frequency of episodes. The nurse needs to maintain an accurate record of intake and output and to be alert for signs of electrolyte imbalance and dehydration. Accurate and prompt reporting of such signs is essential to minimize these complications.

Diarrhea, like vomiting, may lead to electrolyte imbalance and dehydration. With diarrhea, large amounts of water are lost in the stool. This is almost always accompanied by loss of sodium, potassium, chloride, and bicarbonate and usually leads to acidosis. Observations, similar to those described with vomiting, are essential in minimizing this complication. The diet should be low residue or bland, and antidiarrheal drugs may be required.

Bone marrow depression leading to leukopenia, thrombocytopenia, and anemia is perhaps the most severe toxic manifestation of drug therapy. Since this occurs most often in the patient with leukemia or one of the lymphomas, the physiological alterations and nurse's responsibilities will be discussed in that chapter.

Steroid therapy is based upon the principle of hormonal alteration. These

drugs possibly act by interfering with pituitary activity, by inhibiting androgenic or estrogenic hormone activity, or by direct action of the androgens or
estrogens, thereby producing a hormonal imbalance that may interfere, in
turn, with growth of hormone-dependent tumors. Androgens most commonly
used in cancer chemotherapy include testosterone proprionate, 17-methyltes-
tosterone, and dihydrotestosterone. Estrogens in common use include diethyl-
stilbestrol (stilbestrol), ethinyl estradiol (Estinyl), sodium estrone sulfate
(Premarin), and estradiol benzoate.

Steroids are used primarily in the treatment of carcinoma of the breast
and carcinoma of the prostate since, in many instances, these tumors are
hormone dependent. The patients who are receiving androgen therapy must
be observed closely for signs of toxicity such as fluid retention, hirsutism,
lowered pitch of voice, and increased libido. Congestive heart failure may
result, especially in arteriosclerotic individuals, due to pulmonary edema from
fluid retention. With estrogen therapy, signs of toxicity include fluid retention,
enlargement of the breasts, and uterine bleeding. Nausea and vomiting are
not uncommon with estrogen therapy.

Another complication that may occur as a result of androgen and estrogen

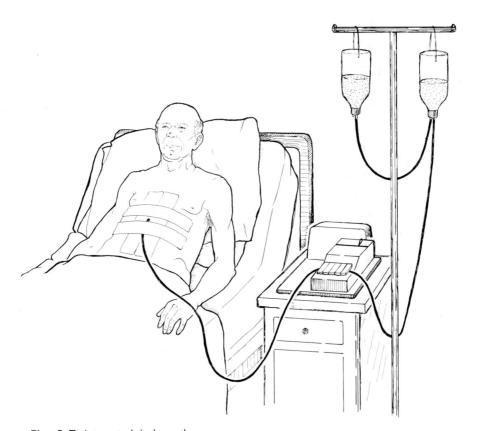

Fig. 5-7. Intraarterial chemotherapy.

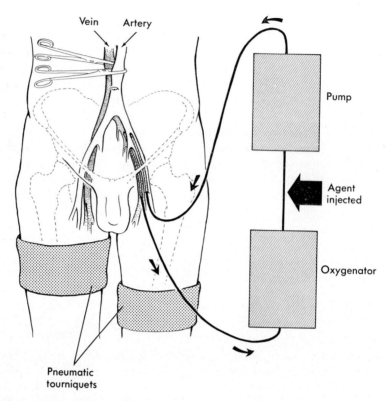

Vein   Artery

Pump

Agent
injected

Oxygenator

Pneumatic
tourniquets

Fig. 5-8. Schematic drawing showing regional perfusion for a pelvic tumor.

therapy is neuromuscular hypoexcitability. This condition gives rise to weakness, anorexia, constipation, and generalized pain from hypercalcemia, especially if the patient is not ambulatory.

Adrenocortical hormones and ACTH are useful agents in the treatment of cancer, especially with leukemias, lymphomas, breast cancer, undifferentiated cancer of the lung, and prostatic cancer. Patients undergoing corticosteroid therapy must be observed closely for signs of general toxicity. These include fluid retention, hypertension and coma, diabetes mellitus, Cushing's syndrome, and increased susceptibility to infection. In most instances, patients should be placed on a low salt diet in order to minimize fluid retention. Usually additional potassium is given in order to control hypokalemia. Patients who have a history of duodenal ulcer, diabetes, or heart disease must be observed closely, since toxicity gives rise to these conditions.

Miscellaneous drugs that have proved useful in cancer chemotherapy include actinomycin D (an antibiotic), urethane, and Fowler's solution. At the present time, actinomycin D is being used in the treatment of Wilms' tumor. It is believed that it potentiates the effects of roentgentherapy. Urethane and Fowler's solution are being replaced by the polyfunctional alkylating agents.

Intraarterial chemotherapy (Fig. 5-7) was initiated in 1950 by Klopp*
and his associates in order to increase the effectiveness of cytotoxic agents
against solid tumors located in the area of the injected artery. This is a
method whereby an antimetabolite in supralethal dosage is infused in the
accessible blood supply of an inoperable localized cancer. The purpose of this
technique is to augment the tumoricidal effect of the drug in the tumor site,
meanwhile protecting the rest of the body by intermittent intramuscular
administration of the corresponding metabolite. This requires exact and secure
placement of the catheters in the desired artery to be infused and that the tips
of the catheters be sufficiently close to the origin of the artery that the drug
will be mixed adequately in the bloodstream and carried to all branches of
the artery. Once it has been accurately established that the catheters are
properly positioned, either a Bowman pump or a Sigmamotor is used to pump
the drug through the artery into the tumor. A flow rate of 1 to 1.5 liters in
24 hours is usually employed. The infusion may be continued 5 to 6 days or
longer depending on dosage of drug being infused.

Regional perfusion was first introduced by Creech and Krementz and their
associates in 1957. This procedure requires the temporary exclusion of the
tumor-bearing area of the body from the general circulation with establishment of an extracorporeal circulation to the isolated part, which can then
be perfused with drugs in concentrations otherwise dangerously toxic to the
hematopoietic tissues and gastrointestinal organs.

With both intraarterial infusion and regional perfusion, the type and
intensity of nursing care needed will vary according to the area being treated.
The nurse needs to understand what these procedures involve as she will need
to be able to reinterpret what the physician has told the patient and his
family. She needs to understand the local and systemic effects resulting from
the chemotherapeutic agent given and will need the technical skill essential
to operating the special equipment utilized. She needs to be able to provide
emotional support to the patient and family throughout the entire course of
therapy. Patients undergoing these forms of therapy present a tremendous
challenge to the nurse, since she will utilize all her skills, medical, surgical,
and psychological, in providing care to the patient and the family.

---

*Klopp, C. T., et al.: Fractionated intra-arterial cancer; chemotherapy with methyl
bisamine hydrochloride; preliminary report, Ann. Surg. **132:**811, 1950.

Bibliography

A cancer source book for nurses, New York, 1963, American Cancer Society, Inc.

Abatt, J. D., Lakey, J. R. A., and Mathias, D. J.: Protection against radiation. A
    practical handbook, Springfield, Ill., 1961, Charles C Thomas, Publisher.

Ackerman, L. V., and del Regato, J. A.: Cancer: diagnosis, treatment, and prognosis,
    ed. 3, St. Louis, 1962, The C. V. Mosby Co.

Alston, F., Hilkemeyer, R., White, M., and Schmolke, H.: Perfusion, Amer. J. Nurs.
    60:1603, 1960.

Baker, W. H., Kelley, R. M., and Sobier, W. D.: Hormonal treatment of metastatic
    carcinoma of the breast, Amer. J. Surg. **99:**538, 1960.

Black, D. A. K.: Essentials of fluid balance, ed. 3, Springfield, Ill., 1964, Charles C Thomas, Publisher.

Blakemore, W. S., and Ravdin, I. S., editors: Current perspectives in cancer therapy, New York, 1966, Hoeber Medical Division, Harper & Row Publishers, Inc.

Braestrup, C. B., and Wycoff, H. O.: Radiation protection, Springfield, Ill., 1958, Charles C Thomas, Publisher.

Brookhaven National Laboratory: ABC's of radiation, Upton, N. Y., 1957, Associated Universities, Inc.

Burchenal, J. H.: Chemotherapy of cancer, Modern Med. **28:**145, 1960.

Buschke, F.: Progress in radiation therapy, New York, 1965, Grune & Stratton, Inc., vol. 3.

Cancer manual for public health nurses, Washington, D. C., 1963, U. S. Department of Health, Education, and Welfare, Public Health Division of Chronic Diseases Cancer Control Branch.

Clark, R. L., editor: Cancer chemotherapy, Springfield, Ill., 1961, Charles C Thomas, Publisher.

Clarkson, B., and Lawrence, W.: Perfusion and infusion techniques in cancer chemotherapy, Med. Clin. N. Amer. **45:**689, 1961.

Clarkson, B., Young, C., Dierick, W., Kuehn, P., Kim, M., Berrett, A., Clapp, P., and Lawrence, W.: Effects of continuous hepatic artery infusion of antimetabolites on primary and metastatic cancer of the liver, Cancer **15:**472, 1962.

Cole, W. H.: Recent advances in treatment of the cancer patient, J.A.M.A. **174:**1287, 1960.

Creech, O., Jr., Krementz, E. T., Ryan, A. F., and Winblad, J. N.: Chemotherapy of cancer: regional perfusion utilizing an extracorporeal circuit, Ann. Surg. **148:**616, 1958.

Cripp, W. E., and Ullery, J. C.: Preparation and maintenance of the patient receiving irradiation for gynecologic cancer, Ca **11:**88, 1961.

Davis, C. M.: Nursing knowledge and functions directly related to patients receiving 5-fluorouracil, New York, 1964, American Nurses Association, No. 1 Clinical Sessions.

Diemath, H. E., Heppner, F., and Walker, A. E.: Anterolateral chordotomy for relief of pain, Postgrad. Med. **29:**485, 1961.

Eckert, C.: Extended operations for the treatment of cancer, Arch. Surg. **82:**526, 1961.

Ellison, R. R.: Treating cancer with antimetabolites, Amer. J. Nurs. **62:**79, November, 1962.

Ellison, R. R.: Clinical applications of the fluorinated pyrimidines, Med. Clin. N. Amer. **45:**677, 1961.

Essentials of Cancer Nursing, New York, 1963, American Cancer Society, Inc.

Field, J. B., editor: Cancer: diagnosis and treatment, Boston, 1959, Little, Brown & Co.

Golbey, R. B.: Chemotherapy of cancer, Amer. J. Nurs. **60:**521, 1960.

Goldman, L. B.: Early cancer, New York, 1963, Grune & Stratton, Inc.

Haut, A., Abbott, W. S., Wintrobe, M. M., and Cartwright, G. E.: Busulfan in the treatment of chronic myelocytic leukemia. The effect of long term intermittent therapy, J. Hemat., vol. 17, no. 1, January, 1961.

Karnofsky, D. A.: Cancer chemotherapeutic agents, Ca **11:**58, 1961.

Kautz, H. D., Storey, R. H., and Zimmerman, A. J.: Radioactive drugs, Amer. J. Nurs. **64:**124, 1964.

Knock, F. E.: Newer anticancer agents, Med. Clin. N. Amer. **48:**501, 1964.

Mrazek, R., Strehl, F., and Southwick, H.: Chemotherapy for cancer, Surg. Clin. N. Amer. **44:**113, 1964.

Nora, P., and Preston, F. W.: Chemotherapy as an adjunct to surgery in the treatment of cancer, Surg. Clin. N. Amer. **43:**39, 1963.

Of water, salt, and life: an atlas of fluid and electrolyte balance in health and disease, Lakeside Laboratories, Inc., 1955.

Perlia, C. P., and Taylor, S. G., III: Hormonal treatment of breast cancer, Med. Clin. N. Amer. **47:**159, 1963.

Ravdin, R. G., and Elkins, W. L.: Chemotherapy of solid tumors, Surg. Clin. N. Amer. **40:**1641, 1960.

Shanbrom, E.: Advances in cancer chemotherapy, J. Chron. Dis. **13:**69, 1961.

Sinclair, W. K.: Handbook of rules for administration of radioactive material to patients, Houston, Texas, 1959, M. D. Anderson Hospital and Tumor Institute. (Reproduced for distribution by E. R. Squibb & Sons.)

Snively, W. D., Jr.: Sea within, the story of our body fluid, Philadelphia, 1961, J. B. Lippincott Co.

Statland, H.: Fluids and electrolytes in practice, ed. 3, Philadelphia, 1963, J. B. Lippincott Co.

Stehlin, J. S., Jr., and Clark, R. L., Jr.: Chemotherapy for cancer by regional perfusion, Arch. Surg. **83:**196, 1961.

Stehlin, J. S., Jr., Clark, R. L., Jr., and Dewey, W. C.: Continuous monitoring of leakage during regional perfusion, Arch. Surg. **83:**943, 1961.

Stehlin, J. S., Jr., Clark, R. L., Jr., Vickers, W. E., and Monges, A.: Perfusion for malignant melanoma of the extremities, Amer. J. Surg. **105:**607, 1963.

Stehlin, J. S., Jr., Clark, R. L., Jr., White, E. C., Healey, J. E., Jr., Dewey, W. C., and Beerstecher, S.: The leakage factor in regional perfusion with chemotherapeutic agents, Arch. Surg. **80:**934, 1960.

Sullivan, R. D., Miller, E., Zurek, W. Z., and Rodriguez, F. R.: Clinical effects of prolonged (continuous) infusion of Streptonigrin (NSC-45383) in advanced cancer, Cancer Chemother. Rep. **33:**27, 1963.

Sullivan, R. D., Watkins, E., Jr., and Bibb, S. P.: Advances in chemotherapy of solid tumors, Surg. Clin. N. Amer. **42:**807, 1962.

Sullivan, R. D., Young, C. W., Miller, E., Glatstein, N., Clarkson, B., and Burchenal, J. H.: The clinical effects of the continuous administration of fluorinated pyrimidines (5-fluorouracil and 5-fluoro-2-deoxyuridine), Cancer Chemother. Rep. **8:** 77, 1960.

Tucker, J. L., and Talley, R. W.: Prolonged intra-arterial chemotherapy for inoperable cancer. A technique, Cancer **14:**493, 1961.

Wasserman, L. R., and Nussbaum, M.: The chemotherapy of leukemia, Seminar Rep. **5:**16, 1960.

Wright, J. C.: Clinical cancer chemotherapy, New York J. Med. **61:**249, 1961.

Zubord, C. G.: Useful drugs in the treatment of cancer, Arch. Intern. Med. **106:**663, 1960.

Chapter 6

Management of the patient with a disorder of the blood and blood-forming organs

Many disease conditions affect the blood and blood-forming organs. The major neoplastic diseases associated with the blood, blood-forming organs, and lymphatics include polycythemia vera, the leukemias, and the lymphomas. In order to provide optimum care for the patient with any of these conditions, it is essential for the nurse to have a thorough knowledge of normal physiology as well as how the disease process affects the individual.

GENERAL FUNCTIONS OF THE BLOOD

The blood is a circulating tissue of the body that is comparable to a transportation system in a community, since its chief function is that of providing the millions of body cells with the materials essential for life.

The average-sized individual has approximately five quarts of blood or about 6% to 8% of his body weight circulating through the blood vessels at all times. The pumping action of the heart is responsible for propelling the blood through the vessels.

The blood has many important functions, including maintenance of nutrition, acid-base balance, fluid and electrolyte balance, and so forth. The major functions may be summarized as follows:

1. Serves as a medium for maintaining a suitable and nearly constant environment for the growth and function of the innumerable cells of the body.

2. Serves as a medium for exchange between the external environment and the various tissues of the body.

3. Provides the delicate adjustment of the circulation to the local needs of various organs.

4. Provides specialized mechanisms for controlling the functions of such

organs as the lungs, kidneys, liver, bone marrow, spleen, and endocrine glands that in various ways maintain the relative constancy of the volume and composition of the blood with respect to both its formed and liquid components.

5. Transports oxygen to the cells and tissues and removes carbon dioxide from them, thus maintaining respiration.

6. Serves to neutralize acids and bases through its buffer systems, thereby maintaining normal acid-base balance.

7. Assists in maintaining and regulating body temperature.

8. Assists in the production and delivery of antibodies in the circulating blood.

9. Carries the secretions of the endocrine glands (hormones) to the various parts of the body where they are needed.

10. Serves to protect the body against infection through the action of the phagocytes.

Undoubtedly, many other functions of the blood could be mentioned. The preceding functions, however, are the ones of major concern in terms of any discussion of diseases of the blood and blood-forming organs.

MORPHOLOGY, PHYSIOLOGY, AND BIOCHEMISTRY OF THE PRODUCTION OF BLOOD CELLS

Soon after the formation of the germ layers in the embryo, the blood and the blood vessels begin to appear. Both are derived from the mesodermal layer. Blood islands are seen to appear in the wall of the yolk sac. These are connected by means of endothelial tubes lined with endothelial cells. Blood plasma is secreted by the endothelial cells. This same process occurs within the embryo, and its vascular structures connect with those of the yolk sac.

Blood is an opaque, viscous fluid composed of a liquid portion, the plasma, and formed elements, namely, the erythrocytes, leukocytes, and thrombocytes. The plasma portion comprises between 53% and 58% of the blood with the formed elements being between 42% and 47%. Depending on the degree of oxygenation, the blood varies in color from bright red to dark red. It is slightly alkaline in reaction.

The plasma contains a little over 90% water, the remainder being proteins, carbohydrates, lipids, inorganic constituents and waste products. Of these solids, the proteins are the most abundant, comprising between 6% and 8% of the total plasma content. They include fibrinogen, serum albumins, and serum globulins. The primary site for formation of the plasma proteins is the liver. There is some evidence indicating that they may also be formed in the lymphocytes.

Plasma proteins have a variety of functions. Those of major importance include:

1. Fibrinogen and prothrombin are essential to the clotting process and the prevention of excessive hemorrhage from small wounds.

2. Albumin has an important role in the osmotic regulation of blood volume and is used in the treatment of hypoproteinemia, shock, and burns.

3. Antihemophilic globulin is useful in the treatment of hemophilia.

4. Beta globulin is combined with cholesterol, carotenoids, phosphatases, and phosphatids, and it is important in the transportation of fats.
5. Gamma globulin, the antibody protein, is important for immunity. It is essential in epidemics of measles and infectious hepatitis.
6. Agglutinins and complement are needed in the laboratory for blood typing.

The erythrocytes are nonnucleated biconcave discs containing hematin and globulin. The amount of hemoglobin in the erythrocytes varies slightly according to sex. Normally, there is approximately 14.0 Gm. per 100 ml. of blood in the female and 16.0 Gm. per 100 ml. in the male. Likewise, the red cell blood count ranges between 4.5 and 5.4 million per cubic millimeter.

The red blood cells are produced by a process called hemopoiesis. This occurs primarily in the bone marrow following birth; however, in the fetus

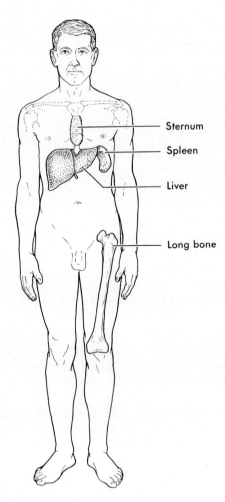

Fig. 6-1. Sites of red blood cell formation.

it is the red bone marrow, liver, and spleen that are responsible for erythrocyte formation. During childhood, the red bone marrow is the major vehicle for red blood cell formation. In the adult, these cells are formed in the red marrow of the vertebrae, ribs, sternum, diploë of cranial bones, and in the proximal epiphyses of the femur and humerus. In an emergency, the spleen may take over this function.

Hemoglobin-containing cells resembling megaloblasts of bone marrow appear early in the blood islands of the yolk sac of the human embryo. By the end of the second month, extravascular erythroblasts appear in the liver and later in the spleen. About the fifth month, foci of blood formation appear in the centers of bone, and soon thereafter the expanding bone marrow cavities take over almost entirely. The cavities of all bones are filled with red marrow at birth, but as life progresses the red marrow of the long bones is gradually replaced by fatty marrow. This process also occurs in other bones but to a lesser extent. Erythropoiesis is, in part, dependent upon the oxygen-carrying capacity of the cells. Newly formed mature cells leave the bone marrow by way of the veins. This process within the marrow probably takes 4 to 6 days. The life of the reticulocyte in the bloodstream is 5 days or less while that of the erythrocyte has been estimated to be 100 to 120 days. These same cells are destroyed by the phagocytes of the liver and the spleen. The hematin is retained and reused; the remainder of the hemoglobin molecule is transformed to bile pigments and eliminated through the large intestines.

The leukocytes comprise a second portion of the formed elements of the blood. They are classified, according to type, into the granulocytes (neutro-

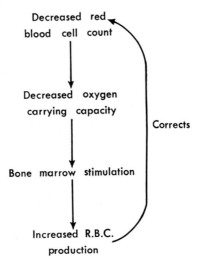

Fig. 6-2. The homeostatic regulation of the red cell concentration in the blood. (After Langley, L. L., Cheraskin, E., and Sleeper, R.: Dynamic anatomy and physiology, New York, 1958, McGraw-Hill Book Co., Inc.)

phils, eosinophils, and basophils) and the nongranulocytes (lymphocytes and monocytes). The granulocytes, like the erythrocytes, are formed in the red bone marrow, while the nongranulocytes are derived from lymphoid tissue, specifically from the lymph nodes, tonsils, Peyer's patches, the spleen, and the thymus. Normally, there are between 5,000 and 9,000 cells per cubic millimeter of blood. When infection is present, there is a temporary increase in the number of leukocytes, and this is referred to as leukocytosis, while a decrease in the number of white blood cells is referred to as leukopenia. While the life cycle of the erythrocytes has been fairly accurately determined, this has not been the case with the leukocytes. Many investigators have estimated a life-span somewhere in the vicinity of 12 or 13 days, although many leukocytes are probably disintegrated within as short a time as 12 hours after they have appeared in the circulating blood. The granulocytes, especially the neutrophils, are of major importance in the repair of injured tissues through the process of phagocytosis. The lymphocytes are a major source of the gamma globulin in the plasma. They also play an important part in assisting the body in chronic infectious diseases such as tuberculosis.

The blood platelets, or thrombocytes, normally vary between 300,000 and 600,000 per cubic millimeter of blood. They contain specific substances essential to the process of blood clot formation. These cells are much smaller than either the red blood cells or the leukocytes. They are round discs 1.5 to 3m. in diameter. Their life-span has never really actually been defined, since they quickly disintegrate and disappear entirely when blood is removed from the circulatory system.

DISORDERS OF THE BLOOD

Disorders of the blood and blood-forming organs result in various abnormalities and are classified according to the tissue of origin affected. Abnormalities in corpuscular composition result in such disease entities as the anemias, leukemias, agranulocytosis, and erythrocytosis. Prothrombin deficiency and hemophilia result from abnormalities in coagulating ability of the blood, and purpuras result because of spontaneous lesions of small blood vessels.

Anemias and polycythemias

Anemia is a term used to describe any condition in which the concentration of hemoglobin in the peripheral blood falls below the normal range, thereby resulting in a reduction of oxygen-carrying capacity. There may or may not be a decrease in the number of red blood cells.

Numerous factors are responsible for the production of the anemias. When the body lacks the essential materials for red cell production, the condition is referred to as a deficiency anemia. When there is faulty maturation of the red blood cells, pernicious anemia ensues. Where there is a severe disease involving the bone marrow with destruction of the bone marrow, aplastic anemia results. A positive diagnosis can be made only by microscopic study of tissue obtained from bone marrow aspiration.

Since none of the anemias are classified as being neoplastic in origin, the modes of therapy and problems associated with nursing care will not be discussed here.

Polycythemia may result from an abnormal increase in concentration of hemoglobin or from an abnormal increase in the number of red blood cells in the peripheral blood. This condition is categorized by some investigators into three forms, namely, relative polycythemia, secondary polycythemia, and polycythemia vera or primary polycythemia. Other investigators have suggested two forms, namely, physiologic polycythemia (comparable to the type referred to as secondary polycythemia) and polycythemia vera.

Relative polycythemia is a temporary condition resulting from loss of plasma or its diffusible constituents so that red blood cells become more concentrated. Restricted fluid intake over a period of days can lead to this condition. With an increased loss of fluids and electrolytes from profuse diaphoresis, vomiting, or diarrhea, this condition may develop. Likewise, in the individual with extensive burns, there is considerable plasma loss resulting in a higher concentration of red blood cells. The treatment of choice involves determination of the underlying cause and utilization of both symptomatic and supportive therapeutic measures.

Secondary polycythemia may result from reduced oxygen tension in the cells controlling erythropoiesis, thereby stimulating bone marrow. This causes an absolute increase in erythrocytes within the vascular system. It may occur as a result of residing in a high altitude over a long period of time, or it may occur in a variety of disorders. Certain cardiac and respiratory disorders such as defective septum, dextroposition of the aorta, emphysema, or silicosis may be present. These conditions interfere with normal oxygenation of the blood and may produce secondary polycythemia. Massive obesity, abdominal tumors, or ascites may impede ventilation, and chronic exposure to certain chemicals, such as aniline or nitrobenzol, may be exciting factors leading to secondary polycythemia.

Symptomatology may vary according to the etiology. Frequently it is observed that the individual has had a long-standing history of recurrent bronchitis and laryngitis accompanied with headache, tinnitus, dyspnea, anorexia, vomiting, and lethargy. Often there is a picture of reduced vital capacity, cyanosis, or clubbing of the fingers. Pulmonary hypertension, diffuse fibrosis with accompanying emphysema, and enlargement of the liver are also observed in the individual with secondary polycythemia.

In many instances phlebotomy will be the treatment of choice. In other cases treatment of the underlying cause or causes will eliminate the condition.

Primary polycythemia or polycythemia vera is considered to be a neoplastic condition of the erythropoietic tissue. It is a disease of unknown etiology that is manifested by an increase in all of the formed elements in peripheral blood. Individuals with this condition show a persistent granulocytic leukocytosis and elevated platelet level in the peripheral blood accompanied with a prominence of megakaryocytes. There is a decreased velocity of blood flow resulting from thickened blood. Due to the increased mass of blood cells, they present a history of bleeding freely as a result of a minor injury or a minor surgical procedure. These individuals have a ruddy color to their skin observed as a blue-red tint on the skin of the face, lips, oral cavity, neck, hands, and feet. Enlargement of the spleen is a common occurrence, and increased size of the liver is present in about 50% of the cases.

Various methods of treatment for this condition have been utilized. They are generally aimed at inhibiting red blood cell production, reduction of blood volume, and depression of bone marrow activity. Many authorities in the field recommend phlebotomy or venesection in order to reduce the blood volume to produce a rapid relief of symptoms. Other authorities, however, believe that the serious disadvantages of producing a gross iron deficiency and stimulation of bone marrow activity without an appreciable reduction in platelets and white blood cells may lead to thrombotic complications of the disease. In many instances, however, phlebotomies are carried out at 2-day to 3-day intervals until the hematocrit is less than 55%. Before this type procedure is carried out, each patient must be screened carefully for any active infectious process, such as tuberculosis, and treatment for any such infection must precede treatment for polycythemia vera. Once all infections have been cleared up and dental repair completed, phlebotomy may be carried out.

Frequently, today, P^{32} is used in the treatment of polycythemia vera following phlebotomy. This may be given orally or intravenously, and the dosage will be determined by the therapist (5 to 7 mc.) depending on the severity of the condition. Nitrogen mustard (HN_2) or triethylenemelamine (TEM) may be used if the P^{32} has not brought the cell counts down to normal. More recently, however, busulfan (Myleran) has been used to inhibit bone marrow activity in these patients. In order to secure adequate control, the original dose may be repeated in 3 months.

When busulfan (Myleran) is used, 2 to 10 mg. per day has been employed as an initial dose. This is commonly followed by a maintenance dose of between 2 and 8 mg. per week.

The incidence of peptic ulcer among individuals who have polycythemia vera is significantly higher than in the general population. In many instances, the first symptom will be massive hemorrhage with no previous history of ulcer pain.

While primary polycythemia is an unrestricted, apparently purposeless reaction to maximal bone marrow stimulation, secondary polycythemia represents a physiologic bone marrow response well beyond the point of optimal function. In this instance, phlebotomy must be done in order to reduce the red blood cell mass to reach this level.

Erythropoiesis is accelerated often as a result of reduced arterial oxygen tension due to cardiopulmonary abnormalities. For this reason, all efforts must be directed toward relief of the primary disorder.

Agranulocytosis

Agranulocytosis is a disorder involving the leukocytes. It is characterized by severe sore throat, marked prostration, and extreme reduction or even complete disappearance of granulocytes from the blood.

This condition most frequently occurs when coal tar derivatives are used as therapeutic agents. Apparently the individual develops a sensitivity to the drug used (aminopyrine, sulfonamides, etc.). Generally, the person develops agranulocytopenia followed by a loss of resistance to infection, resulting in a sore throat. Due to the agranulocytosis, an overwhelming infection ensues that may lead to death. Treatment consists of discontinuance of the offending drug and the use of antibiotics until leukocyte formation returns to normal.

Leukemia

Leukemia can be defined as a neoplastic disorder. It is manifested by widespread and abnormal proliferation of the white blood cells and their precursors throughout the body. This is evidenced in the bone marrow, spleen, and lymph nodes. Leukemias may be classified according to the predominating type of cell (myelocyte, lymphocyte, and monocyte) as well as according to the acute or chronic form.

It has been estimated* that there will be approximately 18,000 newly diagnosed cases of leukemia, with over 14,000 deaths occurring due to this disease. Of these, about 1 in 6 will be children under the age of 15. Males are affected more than females, with the ratio being 3 males : 2 females. The disease has a higher incidence among white persons than among Negroes.

Acute leukemia is observed more frequently among children than among adults. Treatment with chemotherapy has extended the life of the child from a few months to as much as 3 years. After the age of 25 years, chronic leukemia is diagnosed more frequently. Chronic leukemia progresses far less rapidly than acute leukemia.

The diagnosis of leukemia is on the rise. In the past 20 years there has been an increase of 50% in the mortality rate from this disease. With the possible exception of congenital malformations, it is the leading cause of death among children between the ages of 4 and 14 years.

Leukemia occurs occasionally as a congenital defect, although this is rare. If it does occur as a congenital condition, it is grouped together with other congenital defects such as mongolism and cardiac defects; this is suggestive of an intrauterine disturbance between the sixth and ninth weeks of gestation. There is no direct evidence that leukemia is transmitted from the mother to the child.

There is a peak incidence in this disease between the ages of 3 and 4 years that drops between the ages of 5 and 9 years and is still lower in the 10 to 14 year age group. After 35 years of age, the incidence remains at about the same level but then gradually increases the remainder of the life-span. Chronic forms of the disease have their highest incidence after 40 years of age—for example, chronic granulocytic leukemia between 40 and 50 years, and chronic lymphocytic leukemia over 50 years of age.

It is known that human leukemia can occur as the result of exposure to ionizing radiation and to certain chemicals; it is also known that the number

---

*1967 Cancer facts and figures, New York, 1966, American Cancer Society, Inc., p. 22.

of cases of leukemia in survivors from the atomic bomb explosion in Japan is nearly twenty times the number anticipated. There is also a somewhat higher incidence of leukemia reported for radiologists.

There is a strong argument that viruses or a virus will soon be proved to be the major etiologic factor in the cause of human leukemia.

Leukemia, in its earliest stage, is most often detected by a routine physical examination that includes blood work. Early symptoms that might make a physician suspicious of leukemia include: easy fatigability, pallor, anemia, or hemorrhagic diathesis. If abnormal cells appear in either the peripheral blood or the bone marrow, this is usually suggestive of a diagnosis of leukemia. The symptoms of leukemia will vary somewhat according to the type of leukocyte predominating.

When the myelocytic form of leukemia is present, this condition is characterized by enormous proliferation of the neutrophils, eosinophils, or basophils, all of which originate in the bone marrow. The leukocyte count may be 800,000 or higher per cubic millimeter. Myeloblasts, premyelocytes, and myelocytes will dominate the blood picture at different stages of the disease. Most organs and tissues of the body as well as the lymph nodes will show infiltration. Symptomatology will include: (1) bleeding tendencies in the mucous membranes leading to epistaxis, petechiae, ecchymoses, and hematuria; (2) anemia as evidenced by pallor, dyspnea, low-grade fever, weakness, and palpitation; (3) splenomegaly; (4) hepatomegaly; (5) weight loss; and (6) cachexia. The white blood cells produce rapidly until finally the metabolic drain is so great that death ensues.

Lymphatic leukemia is characterized by a lymphoid hyperplasia and infiltration anywhere in the body where lymphoid tissue is present. Painless enlargement of lymph nodes may be found in the neck, axilla, or groin. Nodular infiltrations may develop in the skin resulting in the appearance of yellow-brown, red, blue-red, or purple lesions that may itch or burn. Lymph nodes will vary in size, and in many instances their normal architecture will be destroyed completely so that they will appear as a homogeneous mass.

The least common form of leukemia is the monocytic type. It is assumed that this form is more likely either myelocytic or lymphocytic that has been incorrectly identified. Symptoms are almost identical to the other forms of leukemia previously discussed.

The acute leukemias represent a relatively undifferentiated form of white blood cell proliferation within the bone marrow, lymph nodes, or other tissues. Since this disorder is one that occurs primarily in childhood, it will be discussed in greater detail in Chapter 9.

Leukemia has many effects on the body. It causes a proliferation of cells in the bone marrow, lymphoid tissue, or within the reticuloendothelial system. As a result, these cells overgrow their normal bounds so that cells pour out into the bloodstream and are then transported to many different organs throughout the body. With proliferation of the cells, there is a resultant hyperplasia in the lymph nodes, spleen, and liver. This, then, produces an increase in cell numbers in the marrow, thereby causing crowding of cells in the marrow and

Table 6-1. Specific agents used to suppress leukemic cells*

I. Chronic myelocytic leukemia	II. Chronic lymphatic leukemia
A. Ionizing radiation	A. Ionizing radiation
1. Local x-ray therapy	1. Local x-ray therapy
2. Total-body irradiation	2. Total-body irradiation
3. Radioactive phosphorus	3. Radioactive phosphorus
B. Chemotherapeutic agents	B. Chemotherapeutic agents
1. Alkylating agents	1. Alkylating agents
a. Myleran	a. Chlorambucil
b. TEM	b. TEM
c. Nitrogen mustard	c. Nitrogen mustard
d. Cyclophosphamide	d. Cyclophosphamide
2. Antimetabolites	2. Hormones
a. 6-MP	a. ACTH
3. General cell poison	b. Corticosteroids
a. Demecolcine	3. General cell poisons
b. Arsenic	a. Urethane
c. Benzol	
d. Urethane	
4. Hormones	
a. Corticosteroids	

*From LaDue, J. S., and Molander, D. W.: In Pack, G. T., and Ariel, I. M.: Treatment of cancer and allied diseases, ed. 2, New York, 1964, Paul B. Hoeber, Inc., Medical Book Department of Harper & Row Publishers, vol. 9, p. 116.

leading to anemia and thrombocytopenia. Weakness, pallor, and weight loss result from excessive utilization of amino acids and vitamins occurring from rapid formation of white blood cells within the leukemic tissue.

Nonspecific skin lesions are often present. Patients may complain of pruritus, herpes zoster, erythema multiforme, acneform lesions, furuncles, and carbuncles. Later in the course of the disease, blood manifestations characterized by petechiae, purpura, and ecchymoses are common.

Treatment of chronic leukemia (whatever type) involves the suppression of overgrowth of leukocytes as well as management of the complications of the disease that include anemia, bleeding, and infection. Chemotherapy and ionizing radiation are the major modalities of therapy (Table 6-1).

Nursing care of patients with leukemia

Objectives. In caring for the patient with leukemia, the nurse needs to recognize that he may come from any age group and any walk of life—from the very young to the very old, or from the upper, middle, or lower income group. In many instances he will be unaware of the diagnosis, while in some cases he may know the diagnosis as well as the prognosis. He may be acutely ill and making preparations to die, or he may be having a remission of his symptoms and making preparations to go home. Whatever the situation, there are specific objectives for nursing care that must be taken into consideration in order to meet the needs of each individual patient.

One major objective is to give safe, effective care aimed at providing optimum comfort. The nurse will need to determine whether the patient is prone to bleeding tendencies because of a thrombocytopenia, whether he is likely to develop infections easily, and whether he is anemic due to blood loss or from the disease process itself.

When providing morning care, the nurse will need to use sound judgment as to whether the patient is able to bathe and feed himself, whether he will need some assistance, or whether he is too ill or too weak to do anything for himself. She will have to determine whether the patient can use a toothbrush without causing his gums to bleed, or whether cotton applicators will be necessary to prevent such trauma. Morning care should be planned so that the patient does not become overfatigued.

A second objective is to carry out the medical regime ordered for the patient. This may involve the administration of oral medications and intramuscular or subcutaneous injections, taking the patient to the radiation therapy department for treatment, administration of antileukemic drugs, assisting with specific diagnostic procedures, such as bone marrow aspiration, and so forth.

Much of what the nurse will need to tell the patient will depend upon whether this is his first hospital admission, in which case the diagnosis has not been firmly established, or whether he has had multiple admissions. His physical and emotional status will have to be evaluated carefully before any discussions concerning his present illness can be initiated. The nurse will need to know how much the patient understands about his illness, as well as whether he is aware of its diagnosis and prognosis.

The patient, whether he is being admitted to the hospital for the first time or not, may be fearful and apprehensive. The nurse, by showing an interest in him, by listening to him, and by attempting to answer his questions honestly, can do much to overcome this initial difficult experience. Being available to give emotional support when needed and to secure assistance from other sources (social service, dietary, clergy, etc.) in helping with problems are also important nursing responsibilities not only on admission but throughout his hospital stay. Introducing the patient to his roommates and personnel, as well as to the physical organization of the unit, may eliminate much of his feeling of insecurity and add to his comfort as well. Clarifying hospital "routines," such as hours when meals are served, how one receives mail, when visitors are permitted, and how a member of the clergy can be notified, will also add to the patient's well-being and sense of security.

Diagnostic procedures. It is more than likely that diagnostic procedures will be carried out during the first days following admission. The nurse will need to prepare the patient for the various tests and procedures, clarifying for him, at his level of comprehension, the reason and importance for these various tests and procedures. A considerable amount of blood work is essential. This will include a complete blood count and the gamut of blood chemistries to disclose other abnormalities or any electrolyte imbalance. Typing and cross-matching of blood is done in the event that transfusions are necessary to maintain the hemoglobin at as near normal a level as possible. Many times the patient may feel that he is giving so much blood for tests that he will become more ill than he now feels. Here, again, a careful explanation of the importance of knowing everything possible about him before initiating therapy may be all that is necessary to assure the patient that he is receiving adequate care.

Bone marrow aspirations may be extremely frightening for the patient. This procedure is essential for diagnosing hematological disorders. A calm, reassuring attitude on the part of the nurse and assurance that she will be with him throughout the procedure will help to allay his fear and apprehension.

Other diagnostic procedures may include a chest x-ray, in order to reveal or rule out any pathology, an electrocardiogram, to check for possible cardiac arrhythmias or evidence of cardiac decompensation, and a complete skeletal survey to determine whether there is involvement of the long bones of the spine. Needless to say, nursing care should be planned so that the patient has an opportunity to rest periodically between procedures.

Treatment. Once a diagnosis has been established, medical therapy will be initiated. The nurse will be responsible for the following: (1) observing the patient who is receiving a blood transfusion, recording and reporting any untoward effects; (2) administering chemotherapeutic agents, if ordered, and observing for early signs of toxicity that should be reported immediately; and (3) providing symptomatic care to the patient receiving radiation therapy. Whatever form of therapy is instituted, the nurse will need to understand the patient's response to his illness and to the therapy he is receiving. She is the one person who is with him most of the time, and for this reason she has an opportunity to gain his confidence and cooperation by helping him to understand that he is not alone with his problems.

In the treatment of leukemia, radiation therapy may involve the use of the x-ray or of the radioactive isotope, P^{32}. Radiotherapy is based on the property of radiation to destroy malignant cells in the tissues they penetrate.

In chronic myeloid leukemia, the treatment of choice is irradiation of the spleen. If the spleen is enlarged, treatment should be instituted immediately unless an acute crisis is present, in which case radiation therapy is contraindicated. Radioactive phosphorus (P^{32}) may also be used in treating this condition. It gives remissions equal to those obtained from deep x-ray therapy. It has the advantage that it is much more rapidly taken up by the nuclei of fast-growing malignant cells than it is by normal cells, and, therefore, selective irradiation can be maintained.

In early cases of chronic lymphatic leukemia with lymph node enlargement, x-ray treatment (small doses) may be given, and, in far-advanced cases, treatment to the liver and spleen may produce hemolytic improvement. While radioactive phosphorus (P^{32}) is of considerable value in chronic myeloid leukemia, it is of little value in chronic lymphatic leukemia. However, once the disease has become widespread and generalized, it may be effective in the destruction of the neoplastic cells.

Following radiation therapy, many patients are prone to experience anorexia, nausea, and vomiting. The nurse will want to plan care around the schedule for therapy in order to allow time for the patient to rest following his treatment. Small, frequent feedings may be necessary in order to provide the fluid and foods essential for maintaining adequate nutritional status. Many patients will find cold or frozen foods more palatable and easier to swallow at this time. The dietitian should be contacted to assist in planning for adequate nutritional intake. She is the person who can plan menus that will appeal most to the patient, taking into consideration his likes and dislikes as well as the time when the big meal might best be served in relation to therapy. In some instances, oral fluids may have to be withheld until the nausea has subsided. If there is a considerable lapse of time, the nurse may have to notify the physician so that intravenous fluids may be given to prevent an electrolyte imbalance or severe dehydration. Tranquilizers, barbiturates, or antiemetic drugs may be ordered to lessen the possibility of nausea and vomiting. These drugs should be administered as ordered. Keeping external noises and odors at a minimum can further reduce the patient's discomfort.

With the use of improved equipment that lessens scatter at the skin surface, there are fewer skin reactions observed following deep x-ray therapy. Nevertheless, the nurse needs to be alert to possible skin reactions. She will need to keep the skin dry, applying cornstarch whenever necessary. Ointments should be used only if prescribed by the physician.

The nurse will need to be alert to the development of symptoms that might be suggestive of the onset of radiation sickness. Nausea, anorexia, and weakness, in severe cases, with vomiting, diarrhea, and chills, are manifestations of this complication. They may appear as soon as one hour after therapy. Such symptoms should be accurately reported to the physician in order that modifications may be made when planning future therapy.

For some patients, chemotherapy will be the treatment of choice. Chemotherapy represents a serious nursing responsibility, and the nurse needs to understand its potential danger. She will also need to recognize early symptoms of toxicity and report them accurately as soon as they develop.

Chemotherapy involves the administration of chemical compounds selectively toxic to the neoplastic cells without damaging the normal cells seriously. These hormonal and chemical agents are not curative and do not control the disease indefinitely. They do, however, in most instances, prolong life, relieve discomfort, and temporarily produce remission of symptoms.

Complications that may result from chemotherapy pose many problems for the patient as well as for the nurse. Bleeding from the mouth and gums is common. The patient's lips may become cracked and will tend to bleed easily as well. Old blood may accumulate in the mouth. Mouthwashes or medicated solutions as prescribed by the physician may help in loosening crusts, and gentle swabbing of the teeth and gums with soft cotton applicators will be helpful in relieving foul breath and bad taste the patient has as a result of this accumulation.

Alkylating agents, such as nitrogen mustard or Myleran, may cause nausea and vomiting along with bone marrow depression resulting in anemia and thrombocytopenia. For these patients, the administration of intramuscular or

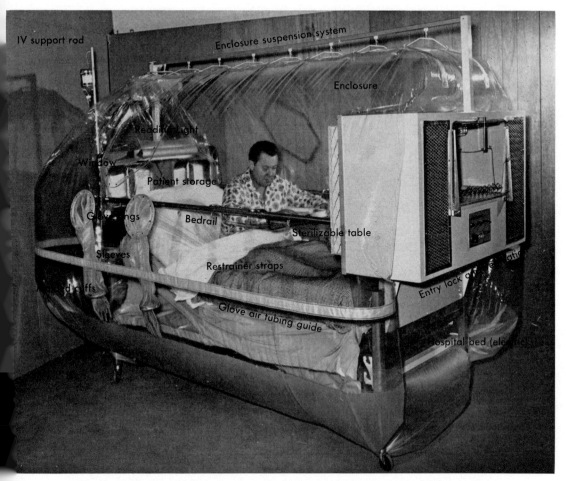

Fig. 6-3. Nomenclature of parts of basic Life Island. (Courtesy Matthews Research, Inc., Alexandria, Va., 1966.)

subcutaneous injections requires special consideration in order to minimize any chance of bleeding, infection, or maceration of tissues. Sites for injections should be rotated in order to lessen chances of tissue trauma. After an injection has been administered, bleeding and hematoma formation may be lessened if steady pressure is applied over the site for 3 to 5 minutes.

Patients who are receiving chemotherapy are prone to develop overwhelming infections due to the pancytopenia that results from therapy. Antibiotics, along with care in prevention of cross-infection, can aid in counteracting such infections. In some instances, the pancytopenia can become so severe that reverse isolation precaution measures may be necessary. In this case, the nurse will be required to wear a mask and gown and, on occasion, gloves. She will, of necessity, have to explain this to the patient—he must understand that he is being protected from contamination from the nurse, doctor, or visitors and

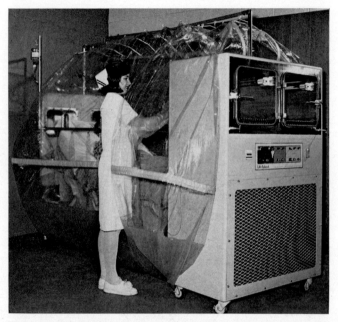

Fig. 6-4. The Life Island. Nurse has access to entire patient area using one pair of gloves. (Courtesy Matthews Research, Inc., Alexandria, Va., 1966.)

that he is not the one who is contaminating others. On occasion, the patient may be placed in the Life Island where he is completely protected from any form of contamination that might lead to overwhelming infection. Most hospitals today do not have this specialized form of equipment, but if it is available, it may be a lifesaving device. Nothing enters the Life Island before it has been completely sterilized and has been made germ-free, since everything (bedding, food, dishes, trays, etc.) passes through ultraviolet light.

The necessity for a blood transfusion is often frightening for the patient, since many people feel that blood transfusions are given only when someone is dying. This may call for explanation and clarification from the nurse. It should be remembered that with low red blood cell and hemoglobin levels, the patient is bound to experience fatigue. Transfusion plus frequent rest periods may often produce a favorable response in the patient's general condition.

When a blood transfusion has been started, whether it is whole fresh blood or resuspended red cells, the nurse needs to observe the patient closely for any signs of reaction. Sudden apprehensiveness, severe headache, restlessness, complaints of feeling chilly, or a frank chill occurring at any time during the transfusion is considered to be an indication of untoward reaction. The transfusion should be discontinued immediately and the physician notified promptly. Urticaria or itching may be considered to result from an allergic response to the blood and will necessitate discontinuing the procedure.

The nurse can be most supportive and reassuring if she will take her cues

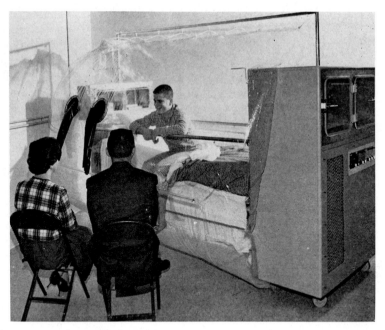

Fig. 6-5. The Life Island showing no restriction on visitors. (Courtesy Matthews Research, Inc., Alexandria, Va., 1966.)

from what the patient says, the way he looks, how he moves, and how he makes her feel. She must also remember that no two patients respond in the same way to their illness and that there is no "pat" answer or "set" routine for patients with leukemia.

Inherent in the nursing care plan is preparation and teaching with a view toward discharge in order to have the patient returned to his optimum health status and rehabilitated sufficiently to carry on as an active citizen in his community, either in business, a profession or at home. This may entail assistance from the social worker prior to discharge, teaching by the dietitian concerning his dietary regime, or referral to the visiting nurse service to follow the patient at home. It may also involve the need for securing assistance to pay for the much-needed antileukemic drugs, and referral to the local unit of the American Cancer Society in his community can be of value in averting this problem. The nurse will need to inform the patient of the importance of continued checkups at regular intervals, either in the clinic or in his physician's office, as well as adherence to medical instructions and the therapeutic program.

Caring for the patient with leukemia can be a challenging and rewarding experience providing the nurse assumes her responsibility for making accurate observations, reporting any changes in the patient's health status immediately, and initiating necessary interagency referrals whereby the patient can live at a maximum level of health.

DISORDERS INVOLVING THE LYMPHATIC SYSTEM— MALIGNANT LYMPHOMAS

Primary disease of the lymphatic system is practically unknown. Metastatic lesions are found but they all have characteristics of the primary site. If and when primary disease occurs in the lymph nodes, these are all malignant. Hodgkin's disease (paragranuloma, granuloma, or sarcoma) and lymphosarcoma (follicular lymphoma) may occur. Reticulum cell sarcoma may also occur. This condition arises from reticuloendothelial cells.

Hodgkin's disease

This is a chronic advancing disease of unknown etiology. Painless progressive enlargement of the lymph nodes as well as enlargement of the liver and the spleen are frequently observed. The disease is locally invasive and destructive and is capable of spreading to any area of the body. It affects males twice as frequently as females and has its highest incidence in young adults between the ages of 20 and 40 years.

Based on microscopic appearance, Hodgkin's disease has been classified into three categories: Hodgkin's paragranuloma, Hodgkin's granuloma, and Hodgkin's sarcoma.

Hodgkin's paragranuloma involves primarily the lymph nodes and is characterized by a diffuse lymphocytic infiltration. There may be alteration of the normal nodal architecture. Reed-Sternberg cells may be present in large numbers or may be sparse in quantity. On occasion, due to the predominating numbers of fully matured lymphocytes, an initial diagnosis of lymphocytic lymphosarcoma may be made. Other cells that may be present are plasma cells as well as eosinophils.

Hodgkin's granuloma is the most common form of the disease and is considered to be the classic form. In this condition, there is usually complete loss of normal node structure, and there is frequently extension of the process into the capsule. The disease may affect only the nodes, but in most instances it is extranodal as well. There is usually a predominance of Reed-Sternberg cells, but lymphocytes, eosinophils, and plasma cells are also found. There are areas of fibrosis and necrosis present in most patients.

Hodgkin's sarcoma is undoubtedly the most invasive and destructive form of the disease encountered. It may have its origin in the nodes as well as in extranodal structures. There is complete absence of normal nodal architecture with the predominating cell being the reticulum cell. Lymphocytes, eosinophils, and Reed-Sternberg cells are usually observed. There is a high incidence of mitotic activity, and necrosis is almost always present.

It is interesting to note that in some patients all three forms of the disease may be observed. It is also important to recognize that the primary tumor may arise in any structure of the body, although the lymph nodes, spleen, liver, bones, and lungs are the areas most frequently affected. Two areas seldom if ever affected are the brain and spinal cord although they may be compressed by surrounding tumor.

It has been stressed that every effort be expended to determine the extent of disease prior to initiating therapy since the stage of the disease will determine the most appropriate measures for treatment.

Lymphosarcoma

Like Hodgkin's disease, lymphosarcoma is a chronic disease of unknown etiology. Here again, the major organs involved are the lymph nodes, liver, and spleen, and any region of the body may be affected either as a primary site or as a result of metastases.

Lymphosarcoma has been classified into three types according to microscopic appearance: giant follicle lymphoma, follicular lymphosarcoma, and diffuse lymphosarcoma.

In giant follicle lymphoma, the predominant cells are lymphocytes. Follicular hyperplasia is prominent with an absolute increase in the general follicles in the lymph nodes and spleen. In many instances the microscopic appearance will be such that the diagnosis will be difficult to differentiate from hyperplasia only.

Follicular lymphosarcoma involves the lymph nodes and spleen. The predominant cell is the lymphocyte, which is actively mitotic. In appearance, it is slightly larger than the normal mature lymphocyte. Due to the increased numbers, the cells break through the follicles and begin to diffuse throughout the involved organs.

Diffuse lymphosarcoma is the classic form of the disease. Abnormal lymphocytes, showing a high degree of mitotic activity, predominate and may involve any organ in the body. The cells diffuse throughout the involved tissue and into the areolar tissue. This form of the disease is further identified by the type of lymphocyte present: lymphocytic lymphosarcoma in which the cells are normal-appearing mature lymphocytes, or lymphoblastic lymphosarcoma in which immature or blastic lymphocytes are present.

Reticulum cell sarcoma

Reticulum cell sarcoma, like lymphosarcoma, may involve any structure of the body. Normal tissue is replaced by increased numbers of reticular fibrils and reticulum cells. This condition is considered to be more highly malignant and invasive than the other malignant lymphomas. It is more locally aggressive and tends to metastasize more readily as well.

The signs and symptoms of the malignant lymphomas are produced as the result of the local invasion of the organs and structures in the body and the widespread dissemination of the disease. A painless and persistently enlarged lymph node mass is usually the earliest sign observed, although on occasion enlargement of the liver or spleen is the first indication that one of the malignant lymphomas may be present. Diagnosis can be confirmed only by biopsy and microscopic examination of lymph node tissue. As the disease progresses, constitutional symptoms become evident. These will vary depending on the body structures involved.

The modes of therapy for the malignant lymphomas include surgery, radiation therapy, and chemotherapy. Surgery is usually reserved for selected

Table 6-2. Treatment based on clinical staging*

Stage	Description	Therapy
I.	Local disease: one node or immediate adjacent nodes; no systemic manifestations as a rule	Local radiotherapy
II.	Regional disease: one group of nodes, adjacent groups of nodes, or nodes draining an area; may extend to include above or below the diaphragm	
	a. Regional disease without systemic symptoms	Radiotherapy
	b. Regional disease with systemic symptoms	Radiotherapy or chemotherapy
III.	Systemic disease: usually associated with systemic symptoms	Chemotherapy with radiotherapy to local areas

*From Nealon, T. F., Jr.: Management of the patient with cancer, Philadelphia, 1965, W. B. Saunders Co., p. 977.

patients with Stage I disease, in which the disease is localized in only one side of the neck, in one axilla, or in one groin area. In these instances, radical node dissection in the area is carried out. In some patients with bulky tumor masses in these areas, surgery may be employed to remove the tumor prior to radiation therapy or chemotherapy.

Radiation therapy may be utilized in treating any of the malignant lymphomas. Usually the high-voltage (200 to 250 kv.) or supervoltage (400 to 2,000 kv.) machines are used for irradiating the node-bearing areas. Aggressive therapy is deemed advisable for patients with early, localized lesions in an effort to eradicate the disease, and treatment should be carried out within a period of 2 to 3 weeks. Patients who are treated in this manner frequently develop erythema of the skin followed by desquamation. Due to the intensity of the therapy, they may also exhibit symptoms of radiation sickness—nausea, vomiting, anorexia, and a feeling of general malaise. Good nursing care is essential, and symptoms should be treated as they appear. Constant reassurance from the nurse can frequently minimize the fear, apprehension, and physical discomfort that the patient is experiencing.

Patients in whom the disease is no longer localized may also be treated with radiation therapy. Since the therapy cannot provide total eradication of the disease, a lower dosage is administered in an effort to provide long-term palliation and possibly prevention of recurrences.

Patients with widely disseminated and generalized disease may be treated by irradiation, chemotherapy, or a combination of both. Drugs most useful in the treatment of the malignant lymphomas are the polyfunctional alkylating agents, cyclophosphamide (Cytoxan) and more recently vinblastine (Velban). Vinblastine is administered intravenously at weekly intervals to the point of toxicity. The drug is highly active and may cause phlebitis and local tissue reaction at the site of injection. Nausea and vomiting may occur as early signs of toxicity. Delayed reactions include bone marrow depression, alopecia, and neuromuscular weakness. Neurologic symptoms such as mental depression, behavioral changes, and paresthesia may occur in from 5% to 20% of patients being treated with this drug.

Nursing care of the patient with a malignant lymphoma

Nursing care of patients who have one of the malignant lymphomas is essentially the same as that described for patients with leukemia. One important fact for the nurse to bear in mind when caring for the patient with leukemia or malignant lymphoma is that he will have his "ups and downs" and periods of remission or regression. It is important, too, for the nurse to keep in mind that the patient needs constant teaching with a view to discharge from the hospital and return to his family and community fully rehabilitated.

During 1965 many studies were conducted in relation to survival rate of patients with Hodgkin's disease. One follow-up study on 375 patients treated in the early or localized stage during the period between 1934 and 1959 showed the following: 57% were alive and free of disease 5 years after treatment was begun; 44% survived free of disease for a 10-year period; and nearly 40% had reached the 15-year mark. With this kind of evidence, the nurse has an even greater responsibility for rehabilitation of these patients who can still have many useful years ahead despite the diagnosis.

Bibliography

A cancer source book for nurses, New York, 1963, American Cancer Society, Inc.

Ackerman, L. V., and del Regato, J. A.: Cancer: diagnosis, treatment and prognosis, ed. 3, St. Louis, 1962, The C. V. Mosby Co.

Andrews, G. A., et al.: Studies of total body irradiation and attempted marrow transportation in acute leukemia, Acta Haemat., Basel **26:**129, 1961.

Ariel, I. M.: The use of radioactive isotopes in the treatment of lymphomas, Amer. J. Roentgen. **90:**311, 1963.

Arnold, Patricia: Total-body irradiation and marrow transportation, Amer. J. Nurs. **63:** 83, February, 1963.

Bluefarb, S. M.: Cutaneous manifestations of the malignant lymphomas, Springfield, Ill., 1959, Charles C Thomas, Publisher.

Brunner, L. S., Emerson, C. P., Ferguson, L. K., and Suddarth, D. S.: Textbook of medical-surgical nursing, Philadelphia, 1964, J. B. Lippincott Co.

Burchenal, J. H.: Symposium on cancer: current advances with clinical applications, Modern Med. **28:**145, 1960.

Burchenal, J. H., and Lyman, M. S.: Acute leukemias, Amer. J. Nurs. **63:**82, April, 1963.

Craver, L. F., and Miller, D. G.: Treatment and prognosis of Hodgkin's disease, CA **15:**246, 1965.

Cronkite, E. P., Moloney, W., and Bond, V. P.: Radiation leukemogenis. An analysis of the problem, Amer. J. Med. **28:**673, 1960.

Dameshek, W., and Gunz, F.: Leukemia, ed. 2, New York, 1964, Grune & Stratton, Inc.

Diamond, H. D.: The medical management of cancer, New York, 1958, Grune & Stratton, Inc.

Diamond, H. D., and Miller, D. G.: Chronic lymphocytic leukemia, Med. Clin. N. Amer. **45:**601, 1961.

Facts about leukemia, New York, 1963, American Cancer Society, Inc.

Geller, W.: Lymphoma and leukemia, GP **21:**125, May, 1960.

Golbey, R.: Chemotherapy of cancer, Amer. J. Nurs. **60:**521, 1960.

Gould, R. J., and Shaffer, B.: The surgical application of lymphography, Surg., Gynec. Obst. **114:**683, 1962.

Haut, A., Abbott, W. S., Wintrobe, M. M., and Cartwright, G. E.: Busulfan in the treatment of chronic myelocytic leukemia. The effect of long term intermittent therapy, Blood, vol. 17, no. 1, January, 1961.

Haynes, J. F., and Jannson, E. B.: Hodgkin's disease, Amer. J. Nurs. **58:**371, 1958.

Jackson, L., Wallace, L. S., Shaffer, B., Gould, R. J., Kramer, S., and Weiss, A. J.: The diagnostic value of lymphangiography, Ann. Intern. Med. **54:**870, 1961.

Krakoff, I. H.: Mechanisms of drug action in leukemia, Amer. J. Med. **28:**735, 1960.

Krakoff, I. H.: The management of chronic myeloproliferative disorders, Med. Clin. N. Amer. **50:**803, 1966.

Leukemia, New York, 1963, American Cancer Society, Inc.

McGrady, Pat: Leukemia: key to the cancer puzzle? Public Affairs Pamphlet No. 340, February, 1963.

Metropolitan Life Insurance Co.: Survivorship in Hodgkin's disease, Statistical Bulletin, vol. 46, December, 1965, pp. 8-10.

Miller, D. G., Budinger, J. M., and Karnofsky, D. A.: A clinical pathological study of resistance to infection in chronic leukemia, Cancer **15:**307, 1962.

Molander, D. W.: The malignant lymphomas, Am. J. Nurs. **63:**110, October, 1963.

Onidi, C.: The patient with a malignant lymphoma, Amer. J. Nurs. **63:**113, October, 1963.

Pack, G. T., and Ariel, I. M.: Treatment of cancer and allied diseases, vol. 9, Lymphomas and related diseases, ed. 2, New York, 1964, Hoeber Medical Division, Harper & Row, Publishers, Inc.

Price, G.: Leukemia nursing care, Amer. J. Nurs. **56:**604, 1956.

Reich, C.: The cellular elements of the blood, Clin. Sympos., vol. 14, no. 3, July-August-September, 1962, Ciba Corporation.

Rosenberg, S. A., Diamond, H. D., and Craver, L. F.: Lymphosarcoma. The effects of therapy and survival in 1,265 patients in a review of 30 years experience, Ann. Intern. Med. **53:**877, 1960.

Rubio, F., Jr.: Acute leukemia in patients past the age of 50, J. Amer. Geriat. Soc. **8:**644, 1960.

Schilling, R. F.: Principles for the management of patients with leukemia, Postgrad. Med. **26:**55, July, 1959.

Shafer, K. N., Sawyer, J. R., McClusky, A. M., and Beck, E. L.: Medical-surgical Nursing, ed. 3, St. Louis, 1964, The C. V. Mosby Co.

Smith, D. F., and Klopp, C. T.: The value of surgical removal of localized lymphomas, Surgery **49:**469, 1961.

Syverton, J. T., and Ross, J. D.: The virus theory of leukemia, Amer. J. Med. **28:**683, 1960.

The treatment of leukemia, Tuckahoe, N. Y., September, 1961, Burroughs Wellcome & Co.

Williams, H. M., Diamond, H. D., Craver, L. F., and Parsons, H.: Neurological complications of lymphomas and leukemias, Springfield, Ill., 1959, Charles C Thomas, Publisher.

Wilson, H. E.: Leukemia, Amer. J. Nurs. **56:**601, 1956.

Chapter 7

Management of the patient with a bone tumor

Primary malignant neoplasms of bone are uncommon and comprise only about 1% of all forms of cancer. Metastatic disease to bone, however, is relatively common, especially from a primary lesion of the breast, kidney, thyroid, or prostate. Other types of metastatic lesions of bone are also commonly found. Tumors in bone do present many difficult problems in terms of nursing care and, for this reason, must be discussed in considerable detail.

Prior to any discussion of these conditions, it is paramount that the nurse have a sound knowledge of the physiology of bone formation and its development.

PHYSIOLOGY OF BONE FORMATION

The formation of bone is a very complex process that begins in the very young embryo at about the eighth week of development. Cartilage and fibrous membranes are the tissues of origin for bone. There is a deposition of calcium salts primarily in the form of calcium phosphate laid down in these tissues within the intercellular substance.

When bone is formed from cartilaginous tissue, this is referred to as endochondral ossification. Most of the bones of the body are formed in this manner, namely, the bones of the thorax and limbs, the hyoid bone, and the greater portion of the bones of the skull. The flat bones of the face and cranial vault as well as a portion of the clavicle are formed from fibrous membrane, which is referred to as intramembranous ossification.

Bone cells lie in spaces in the matrix called lacunae, and the canaliculae are channels formed by fine projections of the cell body that grow out in the matrix. The lacunae and canaliculae connect with others and thereby form a continuous system of communicating cavities.

Bone tissue is formed in layers called lamellae. Depending on the arrangement of these layers, there will be the formation of cancellated bone or compact bone. The essential differences between the two types is that in cancellated or spongy bone the lamellae are arranged to form an interlacing latticework with large spaces, while in compact or hard bone they are arranged in layers to form solid masses.

When bone is being laid down, blood vessels penetrate the relatively avascular cartilage and enter the center of the shaft through an opening that later becomes the nutrient foramen. This blood supply then reaches the ends of the bone through smaller apertures known as epiphyseal canals. Once this occurs and blood comes in contact with the cartilage cells, there is a marked transition wherein the cartilage cell begins to disintegrate. This then leads to assimilation of calcium by the cartilage cell and deposition of the calcium into the surrounding tissues. Blood is supplied to long bones from three sources, namely, the nutrient artery, the periosteal arteries, and the epiphyseal arteries.

Periosteum is the fibrous membrane that envelops bone. It has a rich blood supply, consisting of small arteries and veins. These provide a continuous vascular network that completely ensheaths the bone.

Blood and lymph circulate through all parts of bone by means of the highly specialized Volkmann's canals and the haversian systems in bone. Volkmann's canals enter and leave the haversian systems. A haversian system is made up of a central canal containing both blood and lymph vessels around which there are concentric lamellae of bone deposited.

The exterior portion of all bones is compact bone while cancellous bone comprises the interior portion. Shafts of long bones are almost entirely compact bone. Within the shaft of long bones is the medullary cavity, which contains the bone marrow.

MALIGNANT NEOPLASM OF BONE

Any new growth arising in a bone or derived from cells that are components of skeletal tissue may be referred to as neoplasm of bone. This, then, may include tumors arising in bone itself, in cartilage, in bone marrow, or in the periosteum. Thus, tumors arising in primitive bone cells or osteoblasts, those arising in primitive cartilage cells or chondroblasts, those from primitive connective tissue or fibroblasts, as well as those arising in blood vessels of the bone and from bone marrow, all may be considered as neoplasms of bone. Bone metastasis is common from a variety of malignant lesions, especially from the breast, kidney, thyroid, lung, and prostate. Other malignant lesions are also known to give rise to bone metastasis, although with less frequency.

Primary malignant neoplasms of bone occur infrequently. In order of most common occurrence are osteogenic sarcoma, Ewing's sarcoma, plasma cell myeloma or multiple myeloma, reticulum cell sarcoma, and angiosarcoma. Of these, only the first three will be discussed in detail since they comprise the major bulk of malignant bone tumors.

When the physician is confronted with an individual in whom a primary

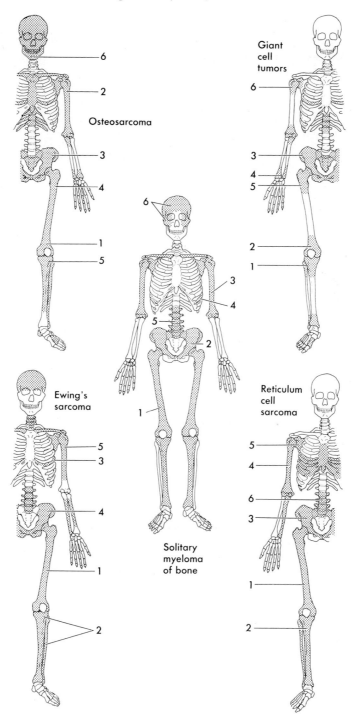

Osteosarcoma

Giant
cell
tumors

Ewing's
sarcoma

Solitary
myeloma
of bone

Reticulum
cell
sarcoma

Fig. 7-1. Schematic diagram of skeleton showing most frequent sites of bone cancer. Numbers, listed in numerical order, refer to the six most common sites for each tumor.

malignant neoplasm of bone is suspected, there are certain basic principles that he must be concerned with, namely:

1. For the patient who complains of persistent pain, swelling, or limitation of motion, accurate roentgenograms must be taken immediately.
2. A biopsy is actually the most accurate means of making a definite diagnosis.
3. An accurate pathological diagnosis must be made prior to any definite therapy to be undertaken, whether it be surgery or irradiation.
4. When utilizing roentgentherapy as the treatment of choice, it is imperative that the smallest dose that will be effective be employed.
5. When a diagnosis has been firmly established as being a malignant bone lesion, treat it without any delay as aggressively as may seem necessary to bring about a cure.

The age of the patient who is suspected of having a bone tumor is of utmost importance, especially since different types of tumors affect different age groups. Both osteogenic sarcoma and Ewing's sarcoma affect individuals in childhood and early adult life. Neither condition is seen after the age of 25 years. Giant cell tumor usually is found in individuals between 21 and 35 years of age, while plasma cell myeloma is rarely diagnosed before the age of 40 years and is most frequently diagnosed between 50 and 70 years of age.

Pain, swelling, and limitation of motion are the three major symptoms that indicate bone tumors and, for this reason, must be explored immediately. The pain is usually persistent and steadily increases in severity.

There are, literally, three forms of therapy available for any bone lesion, namely, surgery, irradiation, and chemotherapy. The primary form of treatment must be determined by the physician in terms of the symptoms presented by the patient, and the roentgenograms. Laboratory tests may also be of value in determining appropriate therapy.

METASTASIS TO BONE

Metastasis to bone is far more common than any primary malignant bone neoplasm. While both carcinomas and sarcomas do metastasize to bone, carcinomas metastasize more frequently than sarcomas. Metastasis may occur as a result of direct extension of an overlying soft tissue tumor, direct bloodstream invasion by cancer cell emboli, or by retrograde lymphatic infiltration. Prognosis in these cases is poor, and only palliative measures are possible. Chemotherapy and irradiation will frequently provide marked relief from symptoms.

MALIGNANT TUMORS OF BONE
Osteogenic sarcoma

Osteogenic sarcoma is a malignant tumor of bone that is seen mostly in adolescents. It invades the ends of long bones especially in the region of the knee (lower femur, upper tibia, and upper fibula), although any other bone may be involved. There is usually a triangular involvement beginning behind the epiphyseal line and involving the metaphysis. Mottling or increased density occurs in the cancellous portions of the bone, the cortex is then penetrated, the periosteum is raised, and a sunburst formation of new bone occurs.

On microscopic examination, osteogenic sarcoma exhibits a proliferation of preosseous connective tissue with many abnormal fibroblasts and osteoblasts. Malignant spindle cells of the fibroblastic series plus roentgenographic films showing more bone destruction than bone formation are fairly conclusive evidence that this is a highly aggressive tumor. These lesions are referred to as osteolytic forms of osteogenic sarcoma. Sclerosing forms of osteogenic sarcoma are characterized by new bone formation as a predominating feature.

The average duration of symptoms is approximately 9 months before medical advice and treatment are sought. When roentgen-ray examination is done for a suspected bone lesion, it is advisable for the physician to be alert to the possibility of a malignant neoplasm. If the suspicion is confirmed, the physician should obtain permission for an amputation prior to biopsy or frozen section since a positive report from either requires immediate intervention. It is also advisable to determine whether there is a palpable mass in the groin or axilla (depending on tumor site) since this is indicative of metastatic growth and possibly early demise as a result of pulmonary metastases. Cough, chest pain, and/or hemoptysis are generally signs of far-advanced disease with definite pulmonary metastasis.

Once the individual who has a suspected malignant neoplasm of bone has been hospitalized, the affected part should be kept at rest. This means that for the individual in whom the upper extremity is suspect, a sling or splint should be worn. If the lower extremity is involved, crutches should be provided, and with any trunk area involvement the patient should be kept on strict bed rest. These measures will, hopefully, prevent dissemination of the disease.

Treatment of osteogenic sarcoma must be individualized. There is no blanket blueprint that can be followed. In some instances, the lesion may be located in a site that renders the condition inoperable; the size of the tumor as well as its location and its rate of growth may cause the surgeon to adopt conservative rather than radical measures, and the refusal of the patient to permit amputation must influence the appropriate therapy to be undertaken. It must be recognized, however, that radical surgery is, at the present time, the most effective therapeutic measure available. This may mean amputation of a major portion of a limb, complete disarticulation of a limb, hemipelvectomy for a lower limb lesion, or, in the upper extremity, an interscapulothoracic amputation.

While it is a readily known fact that osteogenic sarcoma is a radioresistant tumor, use of telecobalt or million-volt irradiation can be of value in many instances without causing undue damage to the skin and soft tissues within the field of irradiation. Thus, for patients whose tumors are inoperable or for those who refuse any surgical procedure, there should be a concerted effort to control the disease by irradiation.

Prognosis is poor, with less than 10% surviving five years. Most succumb within two to three years as a result of pulmonary metastases.

At one time, fibrosarcoma and chondrosarcoma were included in the classification of osteogenic sarcoma. At the present time, the trend is to separate them, and to consider them as distinct entities. This has made a considerable change in the prognosis figure, since both of these conditions are far less malignant than osteogenic sarcoma.

Fibrosarcoma

Fibrosarcoma is now considered a primary bone tumor that is composed of fibroblastic elements and that fails to develop osteoid tissue either in its primary location or in any metastatic foci. This type neoplasm is uncommon and is rarely seen in children, although it may occur at any age. Surgical extirpation is the treatment of choice since this tumor is radioresistant and no chemotherapeutic agent has been shown to be effective in its control.

Chondrosarcoma

Since 1939, chondrosarcoma has been classified as a specific disease entity. Prior to that time, it was grouped with osteogenic sarcoma. This malignant neoplasm occurs in children and young adults, being seen most frequently in individuals between 10 and 25 years of age. Roentgen-ray examination shows this lesion as a circumscribed, multilobal area of increased density within which areas of dense calcification can be seen. At the margins of involvement, the periosteum is elevated and frequently shows reactive bone. The tumor is highly malignant, and pulmonary metastases occur early so that amputation rarely will produce a cure or even a 5-year survival. Microscopically, the tumor varies, although in the majority of cases there is cartilage and pre-cartilaginous connective tissue present in which areas of myxomatous or cystic degeneration can be observed. Here, again, early recognition of such a lesion may permit conservative treatment, but recurrence or late diagnosis requires a radical surgical procedure.

Ewing's sarcoma

Ewing's sarcoma can usually be differentiated from other types of primary malignant neoplasms of bone since it affects children and adolescents of the male sex more frequently than other individuals. It also invades the shaft of long bones rather than the ends of these same bones. This tumor tends to metastasize to other bones as well as to the lungs, and unlike other lesions it is highly radiosensitive. Unfortunately, this disease carries an exceedingly unfavorable prognosis.

While osteogenic sarcoma occurs more frequently than any other primary malignant neoplasm of bone, Ewing's sarcoma ranks second in this type of malignancy, with its peak incidence being between the ages of 10 and 15 years.

Since metastases occur early and frequently involve the skull, lungs, lymph nodes, and other viscera, it is logical that surgery may be far more traumatic than less conservative measures considering the prognosis. Since this lesion is highly radiosensitive, high-voltage radiation therapy is usually adequate to control the disease in this area where it has first arisen. Because of its inevitable early dissemination, however, it is often advisable to give some form of systemic therapy, such as nitrogen mustard, if there is the possibility of permanent cure. When metastatic lesions are evident, roentgentherapy can be only palliative, and dosage in lower concentration should be given that will relieve symptoms and cause regression without attempting complete sterilization of the metastatic lesions.

Multiple myeloma

Multiple myeloma, a disease of unknown etiology, involves the plasma cells of the bone marrow. While some authorities consider this to be a primary tumor of bone, others contend that it is a disease of the blood-forming organs, specifically, the bone marrow. There is multiple involvement of the skeletal system with the flat bones, vertebrae, pelvis, ribs, and skull being invaded by the plasma cell. Other organs are frequently the site of invasion, as well as the liver, spleen, lymph nodes, gonads, lungs, adrenal glands, kidneys, skin and subcutaneous tissue, and the gastrointestinal tract.

This condition, like other lesions of the skeletal system, is uncommon. It occurs more frequently in men than in women and is seen most commonly after the fifth decade of life. The prognosis is poor, except where a solitary tumor exists (plasmacytoma). This solitary lesion may occur in the nasal cavity, paranasal sinuses, tonsil, tongue, nasopharynx, or thyroid. The lesions of multiple myeloma may remain localized for many years before widespread dissemination occurs.

As a result of multiple involvement of the skeletal system, patients with multiple myeloma experience severe bone pain, pathologic fractures, and muscle spasm. Anemia, hyperproteinemia, and renal dysfunction with excretion of Bence Jones protein in the urine are significant findings as well that lead to the diagnosis of this disease.

Invasion of bone is usually multiple and medullary and causes distention of the cortex and periosteum, resulting in severe pain. With the continued proliferation of these plasma cells, there is weakening of the shafts of long bones and of the bodies of vertebrae, ribs, or clavicle, leading to collapse and spontaneous fracture. On roentgen-ray examination, the picture is usually one of multiple round, punched-out osteogenic lesions that show little or no evidence of bony repair about the periphery of the lesions. On occasion, the predominant picture may be one of a generalized osteoporosis.

As more and more displacement of normal marrow components occurs, anemia and thrombocytopenia develop, and at times a pancytopenia may be observed. This leads to increased susceptibility to infection, particularly upper respiratory or urinary tract infections that may be complicated by septicemia. Epistaxis, bleeding from the gums, and gastrointestinal hemorrhages are common.

Many biochemical alterations are brought about by this disease characterized almost always by a great rise in the globulin fraction leading to hyper-proteinemia. The serum calcium level is frequently elevated as a result of the bone destruction taking place, thereby resulting in hypercalcemia. This can be a major problem since nausea and vomiting occur, leading to loss of fluid and electrolytes and constipation. Neurological symptoms including apathy, weakness, and drowsiness may be observed. Severe hypercalcemia can lead to various cardiac aberrations, vascular collapse, and death.

Treatment for multiple myeloma is palliative, and the goal in both medical and nursing care is the prolongation of life with a minimum of disability and discomfort. Surgery, ionizing radiation, and chemotherapy may be employed but none have proved too satisfactory.

Surgery is extremely limited, except in selected cases, with a single tumor (plasmacytoma) such as may be found in the tonsil, submaxillary gland, or thyroid. In some instances, there has been a favorable response to surgery.

Radiation therapy is at times effective in treating solitary lesions either alone or in combination with surgery. Perhaps it has its greatest value in relieving bone pain. On occasion, steroids may be given in combination with irradiation for further reduction of discomfort from bone pain.

Chemotherapy has limited usefulness in the treatment of multiple myeloma. To date, phenylalanine mustard (Alkeran), cyclophosphamide (Cytoxan), and urethane are the only drugs that may provide temporary control of symptoms. The steroids and ACTH have demonstrated ability to modify the biochemical alterations and, at times, have been a lifesaving measure in this disease. It is unfortunate, however, that such therapy merely increases susceptibility to infection, to which the patient is already prone.

In order to minimize complications, it is essential to keep the patient as active as possible since inactivity encourages increased rate of bone demineralization and muscle wasting and predisposes to hypostatic infections.

Miscellaneous forms of primary neoplasms

Other forms of primary malignant neoplasms of bone that occur infrequently include giant cell tumor, primary reticulum cell sarcoma of bone (a rare and rather controversial lesion), and angiosarcoma of bone. The reader desiring more detailed information on these lesions is referred to highly specialized cancer textbooks listed in the bibliography.

Nursing care of the patient with a bone tumor

The patient with a bone tumor is faced with many serious problems. Since the majority of these lesions occur in children and young adults, many decisions must be made by their parents, including the need to give permission for amputation of a limb to save a life. This is usually necessary if the diagnosis is osteogenic sarcoma, fibrosarcoma, or chondrosarcoma.

To most individuals the thought of losing a limb is almost unbearable, and emotional reactions of fear and distress are to be expected. The nurse must realize that this is a major adjustment for the patient to make. A comprehensive plan of care for the immediate preoperative and postoperative period should be developed. It must be sufficiently flexible so that with modification it can be continued throughout the convalescent and rehabilitation period.

Once the patient has been informed that amputation is necessary, the nurse can help him to accept the procedure. A calm manner of approach, a sincere interest in him as an individual, and reinforcement of what he has been told by the doctor will help to allay much fear and apprehension. Watching him closely and listening carefully to what he says may often provide clues that other members of the health team will be required to follow up.

Usually the doctor will explain the operation to the patient and tell him what to expect when he comes out of anesthesia. On occasion, he will have someone who has undergone the same procedure and has made a full recovery visit the patient. This is frequently reassuring. Children, however, may not be told about the surgery until the morning of the day of operation.

On the morning of surgery, an intravenous infusion is usually started before the patient goes to the operating room as a means of maintaining adequate fluid and electrolyte balance. Blood is usually available and may be started during the surgery, if signs of shock or hemorrhage occur.

Following the surgery, the patient is usually returned to the recovery room. Vital signs should be checked immediately, and the stump must be watched for any evidence of hemorrhage. A heavy tourniquet is kept at the bedside at all times following amputation, and the nurse should apply it at the first sign of bleeding until the physician arrives. For the first 12 to 24 hours, the stump is usually elevated on a rubber-covered pillow to decrease edema and lessen bleeding or serous oozing.

In the case of a lower extremity amputation, when the patient is allowed out of bed, the nurse should teach him how to get in and out of a chair and how to balance on one leg without support. She also shares responsibility with the physical therapist in assisting the patient to walk with crutches. She may be the person to measure the patient for crutches. One of several methods may be used for this measurement: (1) take the height of the patient and subtract 16 inches; (2) measure from 2 inches below the axilla to the base of the heel; or (3) have the patient lie flat in bed with arms at his sides and then measure from the axilla to a point 6 inches out from the side of the heel. It must be remembered that even with careful measurement some alteration may be necessary when the crutches are used.

Whether a prosthesis is to be worn or not, the patient should be taught how to care for his stump as soon as it is completely healed. The stump should be washed daily and massaged gently. It should be inspected carefully for any signs of redness, skin irritation, or abrasion. Usually to shape the stump in preparing for a prosthesis, a firm bandage is applied and may be kept in place day and night. Usually the patient can be taught to apply this for himself, but in some cases the nurse can instruct a family member to do it for him. The bandage should be removed, the stump washed, powdered, and exposed to the air for a short period of time and then rebandaged at least twice a day. Stump socks will be needed when the prosthesis is worn. These must be washed daily and, for this reason, the patient should have several pairs on hand at all times. He should be instructed that if they begin to wear out, they should not be mended since this may be a source of stump irritation. The nurse should advise him that he will probably wear out one sock a month when he begins to use his prosthesis.

For some patients, simple amputation will be inadequate to control the disease, and more radical surgery will be necessary. This may entail hip (or shoulder) disarticulation or hemipelvectomy or interscapulothoracic amputation. Needless to say, many more serious problems present themselves for the nurse and the patient when such radical surgery becomes necessary.

As well as having the multiple problems of the amputee, the patient who requires a hip disarticulation frequently develops urinary retention. At the first indication of retention, a Foley catheter should be inserted and left in place until voluntary voiding is possible. Because the wound is close to the anus, antibiotics are prescribed to minimize chance of wound infection. These patients will, in all probability, have more difficulty in learning to use crutches as well as prosthetic devices and will need much encouragement from the nurse. She must set realistic goals for the patient to prevent severe frustration and depression if the goals that have been set are too extensive for him to attain. The patient's family will also have many fears, and the nurse can help them to accept the need for mutilating surgery. She is in the position to answer their numerous questions, but she must be certain of what both patient and family have been told by the doctor. Her reinforcement of what he has told them frequently adds to their comfort. This means that there must be open channels of communication with the entire health team. The nurse is the logical member of the team to see that this occurs since she is with the patient more of the time than the doctor, physical therapist, social worker, or others.

When the tumor involves the upper femur, pelvic bones, or both, the surgical procedure required is hemipelvectomy. This entails unilateral removal of the patient's lower extremity, buttock, and innominate bone. If the lesion is located in the upper extremity the surgical procedure requires removal of the entire upper extremity, the scapula, part of the clavicle, and all the muscular attachments to the shoulder girdle. This is referred to as interscapulothoracic amputation.

The patient who must undergo hemipelvectomy (hind quarter amputation) requires special nursing care since this is about the most radical procedure that can be performed. A Foley catheter is required for several days postoperatively because these patients have a loss of bladder tone. In order to prevent abdominal and gastric distention, a Levin tube is inserted prior to surgery and is usually connected to a Gomco machine for at least 48 hours postoperatively, after which time the patient can usually tolerate a soft diet.

Blood transfusions of whole blood, or in some instances of plasma, may be necessary for several days postoperatively. Antibiotic therapy is indicated to minimize wound infection or, for that matter, any type of infection that might complicate surgery. Since there is profuse drainage from the wound for several days, drains should be left in place, again, to minimize danger of infection.

In most instances, the patient is allowed out of bed in a chair on the second

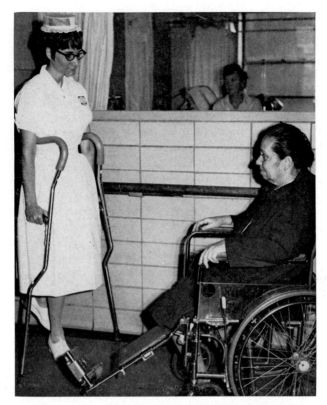

Fig. 7-2. Nurse demonstrates use of crutches. (Courtesy James Ewing Hospital, New York, N. Y.)

or third postoperative day, and soon thereafter he is encouraged to begin walking on crutches. Frequently, it is the nurse who provides the encouragement for early ambulation, and her attitude will be of considerable importance in helping the patient accept what seems to him a cruel injustice. Preoperatively, the nurse must tell the patient what he can expect, the plans for his immediate postoperative care, and long-range goals that may involve his prognosis, his future job possibilities, and his total rehabilitation. This may also involve the family, and, here again, honest, straightforward answers to questions, a calm manner of approach, and realistic goal-setting will ensure a satisfactory mental outlook for recovery and rehabilitation. It is also important, preoperatively, that the nurse help the patient to adjust to this radical surgery with psychological preparation and instructions in crutch walking and proper body mechanics, as well as insight into the difficulties he will encounter postoperatively. She must be aware of all community resources available to him, in order to help him cope with the numerous problems to be faced postoperatively. On occasion, such teaching preoperatively would only increase fear and apprehension; the nurse must take this into consideration before such teaching is undertaken preoperatively.

The patient and his family as well as the nurse must recognize that progress is slow and requires persistence from all involved. The nurse, cognizant of the multiple problems these patients present and having the background knowledge needed to cope with these problems, will enjoy a gratifying experience as well as a challenging one.

Multiple myeloma. The patient with multiple myeloma presents many nursing care problems due to the complexity of the disease and its many symptoms. While it is important to keep the patient as active as possible and to keep him ambulating to prevent bone demineralization, muscle wasting, and hypostatic infections, the nurse must recognize that such activity may cause increased pain, muscle spasm, and pathologic fracture. The nurse must avoid any jarring or bumping of the bed, since the patient experiences an exaggerated sensitivity to any movement. She must prewarn the patient if she is planning to touch him or move him in any way because he needs time to move more slowly in an attempt to minimize muscle spasm, bone pain, and pathological fracture.

Patients with multiple myeloma are prone to develop pathological fractures readily due to lytic lesions, and, for this reason, the nurse has the responsibility of maintaining good body alignment, especially for the patient who is bedridden. The patient should be offered the opportunity to turn on his own if he is not too weak to do so; if he is too weak, the nurse should obtain additional help. The nurse should keep in mind that when help is needed the change in position must be made gradually with extremities supported.

These patients frequently may require braces to prevent excess strain and to keep them ambulatory as long as possible. The nurse must be certain that such devices fit properly to ensure maximum protection and comfort.

Here, again, the nurse who is a good listener can evaluate the patient's needs in terms of how much he can ambulate, the appropriate position that is most helpful for him in the bed, and how much activity will be most beneficial for him. When the patient is totally bedridden, the nurse must recognize that his position should be changed at frequent intervals to prevent bedsores and muscle contractures.

In order to reveal new areas of fractures, periodic roentgen-ray examination of weight-bearing bones should be done. This will enable the physician and the nurse to obtain the appropriate prosthetic devices needed.

Because of pain and debilitation, the patient may become reluctant to move. The nurse must realize that he may not be able to reach items normally reached without difficulty and that this may cause him to become easily frustrated. Since the patient is so uncomfortable, he is in the position to determine his particular needs, and the nurse should go along with his suggestions.

Ambulation is of utmost importance to keep the patient in the best possible physical condition. This requires that ambulation be increased progressively with pain tolerance as the major consideration. If the patient is bedridden, elevation of the head of the bed must be attained gradually until a sitting position is possible. This should be followed by dangling before the upright position is attempted.

The nurse must be alert to any signs of infection since these patients have an inadequate defense against such conditions. Any indication of potential infection warrants close scrutiny. It is also necessary to protect the patient from extreme fatigue and from others who may have minor infections. At the first indication of infection, the patient should be turned frequently, and, here, the nurse can be of assistance in supporting his extremities while he is turning. Deep-breathing exercises should be instituted to avoid possible respiratory infection, since these patients are prone to pneumonia. Antibiotic therapy is frequently employed as a precautionary measure when infections are suspected. Forcing fluids may be helpful in preventing urinary tract infections. It must be remembered, however, that milk or any other foods high in calcium should be restricted because of the possible onset of hypercalcemia. This may entail obtaining assistance from the dietitian in order to plan for a diet that will be acceptable to the patient and in accord with the required dietary regime. The dietitian can also help the patient accept his dietary restrictions and can provide his family with the information concerning his dietary limitations in preparation for discharge.

The nurse is in a unique position to help the patient and his family to accept his illness and to function at a maximum level within his limitations. By encouraging the patient to do as much as he can for himself, the nurse can help the patient to assume an active role in his own care and can lessen his fear of being a burden on others. She must exercise considerable patience since these tasks, no matter how minor they are, will take much longer than before his illness.

As the disease progresses, the patient will need help to accept increasing limitations in what he can or cannot do for himself. The nurse can help him accept modified and unfamiliar activities and learn how he can rechannel his efforts and interests in order to maintain some degree of independence.

Since bone tumors occur relatively infrequently, the nurse rarely has had previous experience. She will need to understand the pathology involved and what occurs to the patient as a result. With a clear knowledge of the nursing problems and an understanding of the physical and emotional impact of a bone tumor on the patient, the nurse will find caring for him an interesting and challenging test of her nursing abilities. Her own ingenuity and utilization of all available resources will contribute to the welfare of the patient and to her own sense of satisfaction.

Bibliography

A cancer source book for nurses, New York, 1963, American Cancer Society, Inc.

Ackerman, L. V., and del Regato, J. A.: Cancer: diagnosis, treatment, and prognosis, ed. 3, St. Louis, 1962, The C. V. Mosby Co.

Ariel, I. M., and Hark, F. W.: Disarticulation of an innominate bone (hemipelvectomy) for primary and metastatic cancer, Ann. Surg. **130:**76, 1949.

Barnes, G. H.: Skin health and stump hygiene, Artif. Limbs **3:**4, Spring, 1956.

Brunner, L. S., Emerson, C. P., Jr., Ferguson, L. K., and Suddarth, D. S.: Textbook of medical-surgical nursing, Philadelphia, 1964, J. B. Lippincott Co.

Brunnstrom, S., and Kerr, D.: Leg amputee: pre-prosthetic training (rehabilitation), Series No. 3, West Orange, N. J., 1951, The Kessler Institute for Rehabilitation.

Cancer manual for public health nurses: Washington, D. C., 1963, U. S. Department of Health, Education and Welfare, Public Health Division of Chronic Diseases, Cancer Control Branch.

Chondrosarcoma, Cancer Bull. **11**:93, 1959.

Coley, B. L.: Neoplasms of bone, ed. 2, New York, 1960, Paul B. Hoeber, Inc., Medical Book Department of Harper & Row, Publishers.

Covalt, D. A.: Rehabilitation of the amputee, South M. J. **46**:57, 1953.

Dembo, T., Levitor, G., and Wright, B.: Adjustment to misfortune—a problem of social-psychologic rehabilitation, Artif. Limbs **3**:4, Autumn, 1956.

Field, J. B., editor: Cancer: diagnosis and treatment, Boston, 1959, Little, Brown & Co.

Jaffe, H. L.: Tumors and tumorous conditions of the bones and joints, Philadelphia, 1958, Lea & Febiger.

Knocke, L.: Crutch walking, Amer. J. Nurs. **61**:70, October, 1961.

Levy, S. W.: The skin problems of the lower extremity amputee, Artif. Limbs **3**:20, Spring, 1956.

Lichenstein, L.: Bone tumors, ed. 3, St. Louis, 1965, The C. V. Mosby Co.

McLean, F. C., and Urist, M. R.: Bone, ed. 2, Chicago, 1961, University of Chicago Press.

M. D. Anderson Hospital and Tumor Institute: Tumors of bone and soft tissues, Chicago, 1965, Year Book Medical Publishers, Inc.

Pack, G. T., McNeer, G., and Coley, B. L.: Interscapulothoracic amputation for malignant tumors of the upper extremity. A report of thirty-one consecutive cases, Surg. Gynec. Obstet. **74**:161, 1942.

Rusk, H. A.: Rehabilitation medicine, St. Louis, 1958, The C. V. Mosby Co.

Shafer, K. N., Sawyer, J. R., McCluskey, A. M., and Beck, E. L.: Medical-surgical nursing, ed. 3, St. Louis, 1964, The C. V. Mosby Co.

Step into action, U.S.P.H.S., Pub. No. 980, Superintendent of Documents, Washington, D. C.

Young, E. L., and Barnes, W. A.: Hemipelvectomy, Amer. J. Nurs. **58**:361, 1958.

Chapter 8

Management of the patient with a tumor of the brain or spinal cord

Before any consideration can be given to a discussion of tumors of the brain or spinal cord and the nursing problems inherent in the care of the patient, it is essential to present, for review purposes, some of the major highlights of the anatomy of the nervous system.

PHYSIOLOGY OF THE CENTRAL NERVOUS SYSTEM

It is a well-known fact that the nervous system consists of a central portion composed of the brain and spinal cord and a peripheral portion composed of the cranial nerves, the spinal nerves, and the autonomic nervous system. The brain (encephalon) is divided into three major parts: (1) the prosencephalon or forebrain and (2) the mesencephalon or midbrain—together these comprise the cerebrum; and (3) the rhombencephalon, which includes the brain stem and associated structures. To be more explicit, the rhombencephalon includes the cerebellum, the pons, and the medulla oblongata. The spinal cord, which emerges from the skull through the foramen magnum, is continuous with the brain. The brain is encased in the bones of the cranial cavity while the spinal cord descends in the vertebral column in which it is enclosed. Covering the brain and spinal cord are the dura mater, arachnoid, and pia mater, the meninges.

The brain appears to be a large oval mass divided into right and left hemispheres by the longitudinal fissure. The two hemispheres are connected by the corpus callosum. Both hemispheres have marked convolutions (gyri) that are separated by fissures called sulci. Lying under the occipital lobes of the cerebrum is the cerebellum. This structure is divided into a middle portion, the vermis, and two lateral hemispheres. It is connected to the pons by three bands of fibers called peduncles. These three bands of fibers are referred to as: (1)

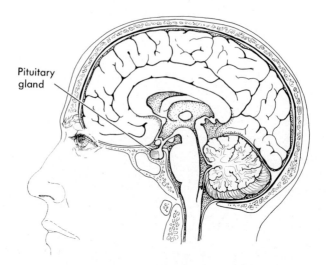

Fig. 8-1. Cross section of the brain showing the stem and cord.

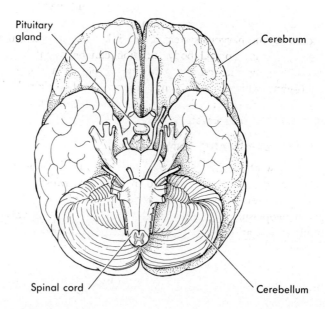

Fig. 8-2. Undersurface of the brain.

the superior cerebellar peduncle, which connects the cerebellum with the mid-brain; (2) the middle cerebellar peduncle, which unites the cerebellar hemi-spheres after passing through the pons and across the midline; and (3) the inferior cerebellar peduncle, which contains fibers of the dorsal spinocerebellar tracts of the cord, and connects with the medulla.

The roots of the twelve cranial nerves emerge from the undersurface of the brain. From this view, the hypophysis (pituitary gland) and the optic chiasma can also be identified, as can the two rounded ridges behind the pons and on the inferior aspect of the medulla, the pyramids that are composed of highly important nerve pathways.

Anatomically, the cerebral hemispheres are divided into special areas including the lobes and the olfactory structures. These include the frontal, parietal, occipital, and temporal lobes. Each cerebral hemisphere has a hollow space called the lateral ventricle. These lateral ventricles communicate with the third ventricle in the midbrain by means of the interventricular foramen (Monro). This third ventricle lies in the midline of the brain just below the corpus callosum. The fourth ventricle, which is found in the medulla, is connected to the third ventricle by means of the aqueduct of Sylvius. Cerebrospinal fluid, believed to originate in the choroid plexuses of the pia mater, circulates through the ventricles, passes through the foramen of Magendie and foramens of Luschka into the subarachnoid space of the brain and spinal cord as well as the central canal of the spinal cord where it is also reabsorbed by arachnoid villi and enters the venous bloodstream, thus causing a circulation of the fluid through and over the brain and spinal cord.

The twelve pairs of cranial nerves, thirty-one pairs of spinal nerves, and the autonomic nervous system (sympathetic and parasympathetic divisions) comprise the peripheral nervous system.

In essence, the nervous system is the link between external and internal environments so that normal body function can be maintained. Nerve stimulation travels along the sensory pathways through various connections to the effector organs, which bring about a response to the original stimulation. Thus, continuous adjustments are being made as a result of the coordinating mechanism provided by the nervous system.

TUMORS OF THE BRAIN AND SPINAL CORD

In a review of the literature, there are far more tumors affecting the brain and spinal cord than can be covered in this book. Most authorities have classified these into seven or eight categories, many of which may or may not be malignant neoplasms. Those malignant lesions most commonly observed will be discussed; information regarding the less common lesions can be found in reference books if the reader wishes more information about them. Most common tumors include the gliomas (glioblastoma, astrocytoma, oligodendroglioma, and medulloblastoma) and nerve cell tumors (neuroblastoma and the retinoblastomas).

In order to make an accurate diagnosis of a brain tumor or a lesion within the spinal cord, it is essential that a detailed neurological history and a meticulous physical examination be carried out keeping in mind the chronological order of development of the symptoms.

For the most part, from the history, the patient will indicate changes such as: (1) focal seizures affecting one extremity or the face; (2) subtle changes in relation to visual, auditory, olfactory, or gustatory phenomena; or (3) even flushing, perspiring, epigastric pain, or nausea. Headache may be the only complaint that is offered. This may have existed for many months, especially in the individual who is harboring an intracranial tumor. Loss of sensation may be a major complaint of an individual with a spinal lesion.

Once a tumor is suspected, roentgenographic examination of the skull and/or spinal cord should be done immediately. Pending the results of this examination, such diagnostic procedures as pneumoencephalography, ventriculography, encephalography, myelography, and angiography may be considered or even scheduled.

If a spinal cord tumor is suspected, the patient will frequently reveal a history of progressive back pain or neck pain associated with weakness of muscle groups and loss of acute perception of light touch and pain stimuli. Frequently, a rapidly expanding lesion of the cord will cause paralysis of an extremity or bowel or bladder dysfunction.

Tumors of the brain rarely, if ever, metastasize through the bloodstream or lymphatics. They may, in some instances, produce implants far remote from the primary tumor within the cerebral axis or even attached to the meninges.

Gliomas usually invade adjacent brain tissue as a result of infiltration from the primary site. Malignant meningiomas frequently invade the skull and extend into the scalp.

The gliomas constitute nearly half of all intracranial tumors. The major types of gliomas encountered include the astrocytomas, glioblastoma multiforme, medulloblastomas, and oligodendrogliomas.

Astrocytomas occur at any age and may arise in various sites within the central nervous system. In childhood and adolescence, they are likely to involve the cerebellum, brain stem, and hypothalamic region, while in adults cerebral hemispheres are involved. These tumors appear as firm cysts of variable size. They are usually filled with a yellow-colored fluid. Microscopically, fine and coarse neuroglial fibers occupy the matrix. They form a crisscross arrangement between the cells from which they are derived. The cell bodies vary considerably in size and shape.

Glioblastoma multiforme occurs in adult life most often between the ages of 45 and 55 years. The tumor characteristically involves the white matter of the brain, the frontal lobe (or lobes) and/or the temporal lobe being most frequently affected. In some instances the corpus callosum is involved and serves as a link between tumors in both hemispheres. The lesion appears as a rather circumscribed mass that is more or less spherical in shape. The cut surfaces have a mottled appearance produced by an opaque creamy-yellow necrosis. Variable amounts of hemorrhage also can be observed, adding to the mottled effect.

Medulloblastomas comprise approximately 7% to 8% of all intracranial tumors of neuroepithelial origin. They occur most frequently in children during the first decade of life, with a second peak of incidence occurring in young adults between 20 and 24 years of age. Males are affected more frequently than females. These lesions are soft and somewhat friable. They are usually moderately demarcated from the cerebellar tissue. Their cut surfaces are gray-white or pink. It is not uncommon, especially in the larger lesions, to observe central areas of necrosis.

Oligodendrogliomas occur most frequently in adults. They arise most commonly in the cerebral hemispheres and, on rare occasions, in the cerebellum or within the spinal cord. These tumors have a gray-pink appearance. They are usually well-defined lesions and tend to be solid masses. Many of the lesions have heavy deposits of calcium around the periphery.

Neuroblastomas and retinoblastomas are the common nerve cell tumors. Since these are tumors that occur only in children, discussion of them will be found in Chapter 9 on tumors of childhood.

Whatever the type or location of the glioma, it is essential that a diagnosis be confirmed. Surgical verification and microscopic diagnosis are of paramount importance even in instances in which surgical extirpation is impossible. When a lesion can be excised, the surgery should provide as wide an excision as possible that is consistent with the anatomical location of the tumor. Following surgery, deep x-ray therapy offers the best means of controlling whatever may remain of the original tumor.

Nursing care of the patient with a brain or spinal cord tumor

When a patient is admitted to the hospital with a diagnosis of intracranial or spinal cord tumor, the implications for nursing care may be extremely variable. Much of the special preoperative care will depend upon the actual condition of the patient. Some patients may be fully ambulatory and capable of maintaining activities of daily living without assistance while others may not be able to provide even minimal self-care. For the comatose patient, the nurse will be called upon to utilize every nursing skill at her command in providing care.

Patients with supratentorial lesions are likely to have seizures of one kind or another. For these patients, the nurse should make certain that bed rails are available and in place as a precautionary measure. The patient should be provided with a small, firm pillow since there is a possibility of smothering during a seizure if he is face down in the pillow. A padded tongue blade should be kept at the patient's bedside table at all times, readily available to prevent the patient from biting his tongue during a seizure.

In many instances patients have been receiving anticonvulsant drug therapy for a period of time. Upon admission to the hospital, quite often these drugs must be withdrawn for the purpose of preoperative diagnostic studies. These patients should be kept in bed as much as possible—the nurse should keep in mind that they are likely to have seizures more frequently and are therefore more prone to injury.

If the patient has an increased intracranial pressure, accurate recording of intake and output is essential. Furthermore, fluid intake should be restricted since excess fluid will lead to an increased hydration of the brain, precipitating herniation into the tentorial notch or foramen magnum, and death could ensue.

It should be remembered that minimal sedation is necessary for the patient with a brain tumor since fluctuation in the level of consciousness is one of the most useful indicators of impending danger. When the intracranial pressure is within normal limits, the patient may be given barbiturates, chloral hydrate, or even paraldehyde. Since headache is a prominent symptom, aspirin can be given safely. If this is not adequate to relieve the headache, codeine in conjunction with the aspirin will usually suffice. It is essential to avoid drugs that will affect the respiratory system. Morphine sulfate is contraindicated for this reason, as well as for the fact that it has a miotic effect, which would mask a danger signal wherein there is progressive dilatation of one pupil indicative of increasing intracranial pressure.

When constipation presents a problem, magnesium sulfate is one of the safest drugs to use since it will not only serve as a cathartic but will also help decrease intracranial pressure at the same time.

The comatose patient must be watched closely for bladder distention. The patient should be catheterized as often as necessary to prevent overdistention. He should be catheterized just prior to surgery even though there is no evidence of distention, since the surgery may be prolonged and parenteral fluids will be administered during the procedure. An adequate supply of blood should be available for immediate use during the operative procedure.

Prior to surgery, the preoperative care will be similar to that for any major surgical procedure. The patient who has been ambulatory will need additional reassurance and psychological support to reduce anxiety and apprehension.

Oftentimes, the nurse can learn a great deal from the patient by letting him express his fears and raise questions. She can frequently clarify or further reinforce the information he has received from his doctor. This may be all that is necessary, but, again, the nurse has to know what the patient has been told. She can frequently help the patient's family in a similar fashion at this stressful period.

The night before surgery, the hair may be removed with clippers. The head should not be shaved until the morning of operation, and in many instances, this will be done in the operating room. Tiny nicks in the skin, always produced by the shaving process, increase the chances of infection from bacterial growth.

Following surgery, the patient's head should be kept elevated for about 6 hours or until consciousness returns, to minimize the possibility of intracranial hemorrhage. Likewise, if surgery has been performed with the patient in a sitting position, he should be kept in a sitting position with a backrest for the same period of time. In this instance, the nurse will be expected to suction the patient's mouth and nose whenever necessary to prevent aspiration. It is essential that a clear airway be maintained as this is an important factor in maintaining the intracranial pressure within normal levels postoperatively as well as during the surgical procedure.

The patient should be turned at least every hour until he is capable of moving by himself. His head will need to be turned at least every half hour to prevent the development of pressure areas of the scalp.

Vital signs must be checked every 15 minutes until stable. If the systolic pressure falls below 100 mm., the head should be kept level until the blood pressure rises again, when the head should be elevated once more. If the blood pressure continues to fall even with the head flat, pillows should be used to elevate the legs, and blood transfusions are initiated.

The nurse should record the general condition of the patient, his level of consciousness, and his motor status as indicated by hand clasp and toe movement at least hourly.

In most instances, the patient will return from the operating room with a slow intravenous drip of 5% glucose in distilled water. Fluids by mouth are withheld for the first 36 hours postoperatively to prevent retching or vomiting, which can produce an increase in intracranial pressure. After this time lapse, fluids may be given orally as tolerated. Oxygen may be administered by mask or tent to prevent further injury of nerve cells in the immediate postoperative period due to anoxia. Postoperative pain can be alleviated by injection of codeine once the patient is sufficiently conscious to be disturbed by headache. When the danger of vomiting has passed, the patient can usually tolerate codeine and aspirin by mouth. Antibiotics are administered as a prophylactic measure to minimize the possibility of infection in most cases.

By the second postoperative day, the patient can usually have food as tolerated, progressing from liquids to a soft diet and then to a regular diet.

Ambulation is determined by the degree of comfort of the patient. By the second postoperative day, the bed can usually be raised to a full sitting position. If the patient does not complain of discomfort, he should be allowed to sit on the side of the bed, dangle his feet, and progressively ambulate. This is accomplished around the fifth postoperative day.

In many instances, the patient with a spinal cord lesion will undergo laminectomy. Following such a procedure, the nursing care will vary according to whether the surgery has been performed by a neurosurgeon, an orthopedist, a general surgeon, or a cancer specialist. The type of nursing care will depend on whether the surgeon believes in early ambulation or conservative therapy.

In some instances, the patient may be allowed to have the head of the bed raised the first day postoperatively and progress to full sitting, dangling, out of bed in a chair, and finally walking position. Other surgeons believe in keeping the patient flat in bed with a small, firm pillow under the head for 7 days before progressive ambulation is initiated. Another factor that must be considered by the nurse is the region of the spinal cord involvement—cervical, thoracic, lumbar, etc., since each area presents specific nursing care problems. For example, the patient who has a lumbar lesion will present problems relating to the use of a bedpan not only for urinating but also for defecation. Usually the "fracture" bedpan should be offered since raising the patient high enough for the regular bedpan can be a very painful procedure for him. Turning him on his side and placing the bedpan in position will probably help considerably.

The patient who has undergone laminectomy should be turned frequently during the first 48 hours postoperatively. This is often best accomplished by use of a drawsheet under the patient. It should be rolled tightly up to him with at least one nurse on each side of the bed to assist with turning. The patient should not be expected to turn by himself at this time. Following this period, the nurse should teach the patient the principles involved in "logrolling" so that he can begin to help himself in turning. It may be necessary, at this time, to provide side rails for the patient's use in turning. They will also serve as a protective device against possible rolling out of bed.

Lesions occurring in the cervical or thoracic region are also treated surgically by laminectomy. These patients should not be allowed to use their arms for any reason during the first 48 hours postoperatively. This means, then, that they must be given complete nursing care including being fed by the nurse, an aide, or a volunteer. They should not be allowed even a small firm pillow under the head since this can cause trauma to the surgical area.

Regardless of the region of cord involvement, these patients will experience a considerable amount of pain postoperatively, and medication should be given judiciously. The nurse will have to evaluate the status of the patient, but she must realize that pain does exist for at least 4 to 5 days following surgery and, in some cases, even longer.

Patients who have had a lesion in the lumbar or lumbosacral region must be watched closely for bowel and bladder function. Frequently they will need to be catheterized or will require cathartics to be able to void or to have a bowel movement. This may be due to nerve damage or to the fact that they experience so much discomfort on having to use a bedpan that they ignore the physical impulse.

Unless specific dietary orders are written by the physician, food can be given as tolerated by the patient and need not be liquid to soft to regular. The nurse must evaluate the type of food to be offered from how the patient has reacted and what he says he would like to eat. She must remember, however, that if a regular diet is provided, the patient will need assistance to cut his meat or to dig out his baked potato. She should not expect that he will be able to do this for himself, especially when he is flat in bed.

Once the patient is allowed to be out of bed in a chair, the nurse should check on his condition at least every 15 minutes. As a matter of fact, he should probably be returned to bed after this period of time on his first experience at sitting up, especially if he has been flat in bed for 1 week or 10 days. This period can be extended progressively, but the nurse must make certain that the patient has a bell cord close at hand to ring if he feels he needs anything. If the nurse recognizes that each patient will react differently following surgery, she can anticipate his individual needs and help him recuperate and become rehabilitated as quickly as possible.

TUMORS METASTATIC TO THE NERVOUS SYSTEM

Tumors metastatic to the central nervous system comprise the majority of tumors of the nervous system. Once a primary tumor metastasizes to the brain, or on very rare occasion, to the spinal cord, the situation is an almost hopeless one since these lesions are most often fatal. Many primary lesions produce metastases to the central nervous system and, more specifically, to the brain.

Such metastatic lesions spread via the bloodstream since there are no lymphatics within the central nervous system. These lesions will vary considerably in their gross characteristics. Many are spherical in shape, some are solid and firm, and still others show signs of degenerative change. Presenting symptoms will be determined by the location of the metastatic lesion.

Treatment for metastatic lesions is quite different from treatment for a primary lesion of the central nervous system. Since this type lesion represents widespread dissemination of disease, surgery is rarely indicated. For the most part, these patients are treated with radiation therapy and/or chemotherapy. There is no possible chance that surgical intervention would bring about a long-term survival or cure.

Whether radiation therapy or chemotherapy is employed will, in most instances, depend on where the primary lesion occurred and whether or not it is responsive to irradiation, or chemotherapy, or both.

Nursing care, therefore, will be dependent upon the type of therapy the patient is receiving. Since nursing responsibilities for patients undergoing radiation therapy or chemotherapy will be essentially the same as those discussed previously, it is suggested that the nurse refer to them for her specific responsibilities (Chapter 5).

The nurse is in a unique position to provide reassurance to her patient since she is with him more than anyone else. She should recognize that despite the presence of metastatic disease, the patient may still have a considerable period of time in which he can be relatively comfortable. For this reason, the nurse has a responsibility for teaching, guiding, and clarifying for the patient in view of rehabilitation to his maximum level of health.

He should be helped to accept as much responsibility for self-care as his condition permits. Frequently this will mean teaching him a different approach to carrying out activities of daily living from the manner to which he has been accustomed. This may be time-consuming, but the nurse should recognize its importance for the welfare of the patient.

The nursing care plan should be evaluated daily in order that the goals set for the patient are realistic, since he can easily become frustrated if he cannot see progress for his efforts. It should be emphasized again that open channels of communication must be maintained for the patient to derive optimal benefit from his therapy.

To reiterate, the aspects of nursing care that must be followed most obviously include:

1. Ensuring adequate food intake in order to maintain proper nutrition.
2. Ascertaining that the patient develops regular habits with regard to elimination.
3. Making certain that he keeps up a good personal appearance, especially in respect to personal hygiene.
4. Ascertaining that he gets appropriate rest, whether this means administration of sedative, ataractic drugs, or appropriate type of baths.
5. Providing for physical, occupational, and recreational therapy in so far as his condition permits.

6. Maintaining accurate and detailed records pertaining to the patient's behavior, attitudes, cooperation, etc.

7. Treating him as an individual, respecting his rights as an adult and not expecting that he can be dictated to, corrected, just because he is ill.

If the nurse will plan for the psychological as well as the physical care of the patient who has either a brain or a spinal cord tumor, the effective execution of such a plan will provide optimum welfare for the patient as well as tremendous satisfaction to the nurse who cares for him.

Bibliography

A cancer source book for nurses, New York, 1963, American Cancer Society, Inc.

Beeson, P. B., and McDermott, W., editors: Cecil-Loeb textbook of medicine, ed. 11, Philadelphia, 1963, W. B. Saunders Co.

Brain, L., and Norris, S., editors: The remote effects of cancer on the nervous system, vol. 1, New York, 1965, Grune & Stratton, Inc.

Chusid, J., and McDonald, J.: Correlative neuroanatomy and functional neurology, Los Altos, Calif., 1964, Lange Medical Publications.

Covalt, D. A., et al.: Early management of patients with spinal cord injury, J.A.M.A. **151**:89, 1953.

Davis, L., editor: Christopher's textbook of surgery, ed. 7, Philadelphia, 1960, W. B. Saunders Co.

de Gutierrez-Mahoney, C. G., and Carini, E.: Neurological and neurosurgical nursing, ed. 3, St. Louis, 1960, The C. V. Mosby Co.

Feiring, E. H.: Recent advances in neurosurgery, New York J. Med. **59**:1569, 1959.

Field, J. B., editor: Cancer: diagnosis and treatment, Boston, 1959, Little, Brown & Co.

Gilbertson, E. L., and Good, C. A.: Roentgenographic signs of tumors of the brain, Amer. J. Roentgen. **76**:226, 1956.

Hart, B. L., and Rohweder, A. W.: Support in nursing, Amer. J. Nurs. **59**:1398, 1959.

Hodges, L. R., and Taufic, M.: Tumors of the brain and rehabilitation after craniotomy, Amer. J. Nurs. **58**:58, 1958.

Jordan, V., et al.: Halo body cast and spinal fusion, Amer. J. Nurs. **63**:77, August, 1963.

Jourad, S. M.: How well do you know your patients? Amer. J. Nurs. **59**:1568, 1959.

Klingon, G. H.: Neurologic problems in cancer, Med. Clin. N. Amer. **45**:585, 1961.

Knowles, L. N.: How can we assure patients? Amer. J. Nurs. **59**:1568, 1959.

Larson, C. B., and Gould, M.: Calderwood's orthopedic nursing, ed. 5, St. Louis, 1961, The C. V. Mosby Co.

MacKenzie, M., and Baldwin, M.: Cerebral seizures, Amer. J. Nurs. **57**:312, 1957.

Manter, J. T., and Gatz, A.: Essentials of neuroanatomy and neurophysiology, Philadelphia, 1961, F. A. Davis Co.

Martin, M. A.: Nursing care in cervical cord injury, Amer. J. Nurs. **63**:60, March, 1963.

Mullan, S.: Essentials of neurosurgery, New York, 1961, Springer Publishing Co., Inc.

Pack, G. T., and Ariel, I. M., editors: Treatment of cancer and allied diseases; vol. 2, The nervous system, ed. 2, New York, 1959, Paul B. Hoeber, Inc., Medical Book Department of Harper & Row, Publishers.

Peyton, W. T.: Tumors of the brain in the elderly, Geriatrics **14**:697, 1959.

Pool, J. L., Ransohoff, J., and Correll, J. W.: Treatment of malignant brain tumors, primary and metastatic, New York J. Med. **57**:3983, 1957.

Potanos, J., Pool, J. L., and Gleason, A. M.: Cerebral edema, Amer. J. Nurs. **61**:92, March, 1961.

Russell, D. S., and Rubenstein, L. J.: Pathology of tumors of the nervous system, ed. 2, Baltimore, 1963, The Williams & Wilkins Co.

Willis, R. A.: Pathology of tumors, ed. 3, London, 1962, Butterworth & Co.

Chapter 9

Tumors of childhood

Within the past twenty years, the major causes of death during infancy and childhood in the United States have changed considerably. This is due, in large measure, to the dramatic improvements in the control of infectious diseases plus the decrease in infant mortality. Recognition of cancer and its allied diseases as a major child health problem has resulted from the increasing number of deaths reported from these diseases in the juvenile age group.

Cancers and benign tumors are now among the foremost causes of death in children between the ages of 5 and 14 years, exceeded only by accidental deaths, and are the third greatest cause of death in children from 1 to 4 years of age as well.

Childhood tumors differ as a group from those seen in adults. Malignant neoplasms of infants and children arise from tissues of mesenchymal origin while those observed in the adult most frequently arise from epithelial tissue.

The more common types of malignant lesions observed in childhood are the leukemias and lymphomas, intracranial tumors including the eye and its orbit, tumors of the bones and cartilaginous tissues, and tumors derived from the adrenal medulla and from the kidney. While childhood tumors include a great variety, each of which is uncommon, together they form a fairly large proportion of the whole. Although cancers of all types can occur in childhood and no organ or site can be considered immune, lesions common in the adult are observed only in rare instances in children. For example, carcinoma of the skin is so rare as to be a medical curiosity, primary carcinoma of the lung is almost unknown, and malignant melanoma is extremely unusual. It has also been observed that certain types of tumors predominate in various age groups, while other types prevail only in later life.

LEUKEMIA

Leukemia accounts for the greatest number of malignant neoplasms in children. It occurs most frequently as acute leukemia in the juvenile age groups, particularly of the lymphocytic or lymphoblastic type. Fortunately, this type is most responsive to the forms of therapy available today, and re-

103

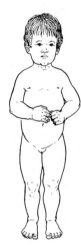

Common types of cancer in children

Ages 0-5

Wilms' tumor
Glioma of retina
Medulloblastoma of brain
Neuroblastoma
Acute leukemia
Somatic sarcoma

Fig. 9-1.

Common types of cancer in children

Ages 6-10

Hodgkin's disease
Leukemia (often acute)
Cerebellar tumors
Kidney tumors

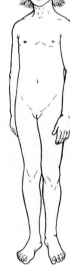

Fig. 9-2.

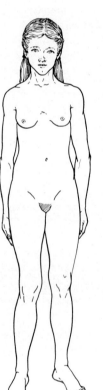

Common types of cancer in children

Ages 11-20

Brain tumors
Hodgkin's disease
Lymphosarcoma
Leukemia
Ewing's sarcoma of bone
Osteogenic sarcoma of bone

Fig. 9-3.

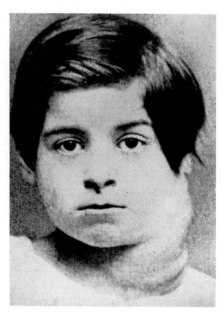

Fig. 9-4. Dr. Damon's patient, John S., 8 years of age in 1863. This probably was the first photograph of a child with leukemia to be published. (Courtesy Dr. Harold Dargeon, Memorial Center, New York, N. Y.)

missions that may last from several weeks to many months can frequently be expected.

The clinical picture is quite similar regardless of the cell type involved. Fever, prostration, weakness, occasional headache, ulceration of the mucous membranes, purpura, hemorrhage, weight loss, and fatigue present a syndrome similar to that seen in the presence of overwhelming sepsis. Many of these symptoms represent the hypermetabolic demands of the rapidly dividing cells. Lymphadenopathy and splenomegaly are common occurrences and are manifested by complaints of abdominal fullness, gastrointestinal distress, and enlarged lymph nodes. The liver may be somewhat enlarged as well.

The disease has a rapid onset and rarely responds to aggressive therapy for any long period of time. Until recently it has always been fatal. There are, however, over 50 children in the United States who are living and well over 5 years after onset of leukemia. One of them is living over 12 years since onset of the disease.

MANAGEMENT OF THE CHILD WITH ACUTE LEUKEMIA

In many instances, after a child is suspected of having acute leukemia, the pediatrician will refer him to a special cancer hospital clinic for more accurate diagnosis and treatment. When such a tentative diagnosis is made by the pediatrician, the parents will undoubtedly become extremely fearful and apprehensive. This fear and apprehension are frequently communicated nonverbally to the child.

Clinic visit

As a result of referral from the pediatrician, both the child and his parents may be extremely nervous and tense. Showing an interest in the patient and the parents, listening to them and attempting to answer their questions, explaining clinic procedures and routines, and clarifying details that may not be fully understood (in accordance with the explanations provided by the physician) may be of considerable help. Being available to provide emotional support as needed and to enlist assistance from other services to help in the solution of problems for the patient and his parents is a major nursing responsibility. All too frequently, long waiting periods occur. These in many instances increase anxiety and apprehension in the parents and lead to an increased fatigue in the child. Every effort should be made to avoid such long waiting periods but, when unavoidable, diversional therapy should be employed for both the child and his parents. If the child is acutely ill, provision of an area where he may rest quietly will be of value to him and will provide considerable relief to his parents as well. If hospitalization is indicated, this often causes an emotionally traumatic experience for both the child and his parents.

Establishment of a good rapport with both the patient and his parents is of paramount importance on the first clinic visit since this will often be a predominating factor in terms of whether follow-up visits will be continued or not. The nurse must be supportive and give reassurance to both the patient and the parents if further advice and follow-up will be accepted.

Hospitalization

Once it has been established that hospitalization is essential for the child, both parents and child will experience feelings of insecurity—the child on being left alone in a strange environment, and the parents on leaving their youngster probably for the first time. Having some of the child's personal belongings at his bedside, such as a doll, a baby blanket, or a toy dog, will often help in overcoming the strangeness of the environment to some degree. Introduction of both the child and his parents to roommates as well as to other personnel on the ward and to the physical organization of the floor may greatly add to increased feelings of security for all concerned.

As soon as the child has been admitted, he will feel more secure and his parents will be more willing to accept his admission if they can be enlisted to help. Frequently, the parents can assist in helping the child change into hospital clothing, take his temperature, collect a urine specimen, and help with other activities including providing much-needed nourishment. This will, frequently, help the parents to realize that the nurse is not trying "to take over" for them. The nurse should make certain that the child is not left alone when his parents must leave. She must also make every attempt not to become the "mother figure" for the child, thereby competing for the child's affections over those he has for his parents. The "separation anxiety" may be overcome if the child is not left alone when his parents leave.

In the presence of nausea and vomiting, administration of oral medications may be difficult, and intravenous feedings may be just as much of a problem; when intravenous fluids are prescribed, the nurse must observe the rate of flow closely, prevent infiltration into the tissues, and record intake and output accurately. Preparation for this or any other treatment or procedure with appropriate explanations is essential. These explanations must be at the appropriate level so that the child is well aware of what is being done for him. The child may become even more discouraged when repeated blood tests and sternal and/or iliac crest marrows must be repeated, especially when hematomas or multiple discoloration are seen from such tests. In some cases, the child may not feel that any progress is being made in relation to his illness, and in many instances this may be true.

Bleeding from the mouth and gums is a common complication and may be the first indication of the illness. Even the slightest trauma produces bruising. Special oral and skin care is essential but may present a problem due to the fact that the lips tend to crack and bleed easily. Mouthwashes or medicated solutions may be prescribed to loosen the crusts or exudate that accumulate. Soft cotton applicators should be used for this purpose. Toothbrushes should be avoided.

Overwhelming infection is another complication frequently observed. Every effort should be made to prevent this from occurring, and meticulous ob-

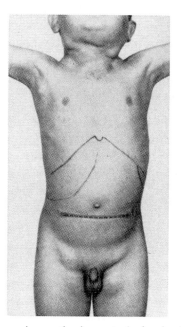

Fig. 9-5. Patient showing adenopathy in acute leukemia. Cervical, supraclavicular, axillary, inguinal, and femoral adenopathies, as well as splenohepatomegaly, are conspicuous. Owing to earlier diagnosis and the response to present-day chemotherapy, these findings are becoming less common except in advanced cases. (Courtesy Dr. Harold Dargeon, Memorial Center, New York, N. Y.)

servance of good technique must be employed to prevent cross-infection. Antibiotic therapy will be essential to counteract infection, and here again care must be taken if the antibiotic is given by injection. Sites for injections must be rotated to prevent bruising and bleeding.

Fatigue is a symptom commonly present. This may be due to the decreased red blood cell and hemoglobin level or to toxic effects of chemotherapy. Frequent rest periods should be provided. Transfusions of whole blood or packed red blood cells may be ordered. This entails close observation of the child for transfusion reactions.

The nurse must be alert to signs and symptoms of toxicity from medications the child is receiving since these are frequently administered to the point of toxicity to produce a remission. Adequate nutrition may be difficult at this time, and the nurse should make every effort to see that a well-balanced diet is taken. Small, frequent meals, attractively served and in a pleasant environment, may be helpful. Catering to the child's likes whenever possible will also ensure adequate food intake.

Inherent in the nursing care plan is preparation and teaching with a view toward discharge. Throughout the hospital stay the nurse should be alert to opportunities for teaching and should make every effort to secure parental participation in the various aspects of the child's care. She should recognize that one or more remissions and relapses may occur before the terminal stage. Emotional support will be essential for the parents at these various stages.

The nurse can reinforce what the physician has told the parents with regard to necessary care once the child is to be discharged. Explanations regarding adherence to medical instructions should be given, and the nurse should provide an opportunity for the parents to raise questions if there is any doubt in their minds. On occasion, referral to a public health nursing agency may be beneficial in assisting the parents when the child is discharged.

TUMORS OF BONE

Malignant tumors of bone are seldom seen before the fourth year of life. These tumors show a predilection for the ages between 5 and 25 years with a peak incidence in early adolescence. The types most commonly encountered in childhood and early adolescence are osteogenic sarcoma, chondrosarcoma, Ewing's sarcoma, and reticulum cell sarcoma.

The behavior of these tumors is consistent, the usual symptom being pain, sometimes coincident with trauma. Swelling and tenderness sometimes occur over the involved bone. However, the initial complaint is pain, and this may persist for weeks and even months before a palpable tumor is noted. (See Chapter 7 for pathology, treatment, and nursing care.)

INTRACRANIAL TUMORS

Tumors of the central nervous system comprise an important group of neoplasms in children. The astrocytomas and medulloblastomas are the more common types observed. Gliomas of the brainstem occur infrequently.

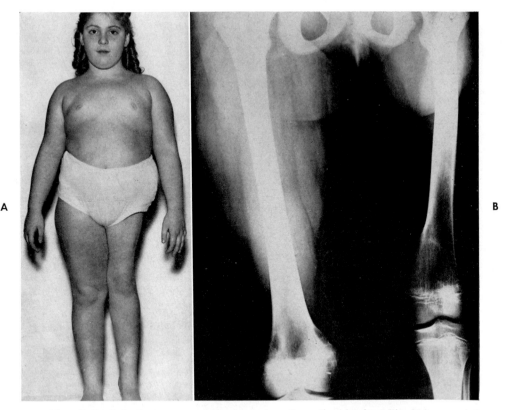

Fig. 9-6. Ewing's sarcoma of the femur in a 7-month-old infant. The lesion presents an unusual appearance with marked osteoporosis and considerable periosteal reaction over the entire shaft. Angulation is probably due to spontaneous fracture. **A,** The patient about 8½ years later. Following initial therapy the lesion regressed, and the patient has had no evidence of disease since. Atrophy and shortness of the affected leg are very apparent. **B,** Roentgenogram taken when the patient was 11 years of age shows shortness of the affected femur but no angulation or other evidence of disease. (Courtesy Dr. Harold Dargeon, Memorial Center, New York, N. Y.)

The symptoms produced depend on the site affected and on the degree of intracranial hypertension produced. This is influenced by the fact that in the infant and child the easily expandable head may permit a tumor to develop to a considerable size before signs or symptoms become evident.

Vomiting and headache are the most common early manifestations of these tumors. Staggering gait, diplopia, enlargement of the head, increasing loss of vision, and convulsions are other symptoms that may result from intracranial neoplasms. (See Chapter 8 for pathology, treatment, and nursing care.)

RETINOBLASTOMA

Retinoblastoma is a malignant primary tumor of neuroepithelial origin. It arises from the granular layer of the retina, occurs predominantly in infants and young children, and may be noted at birth. It is seldom observed after the fifth year.

The tumor may arise unilaterally or bilaterally with one third to one half of the patients having bilateral lesions. These are believed to represent independent growths in the two eyes and not extensions from a single primary growth. There may be an interval lapse of several months before the second eye becomes affected.

The tumor is gray-white or pink-white in color, and it may be moderately firm, although there may be necrotic, hemorrhagic, or calcified areas present. In many instances, the cells are small with scanty cytoplasm and darkly stained nuclei. On occasion, necrosis appears to destroy the tumor completely.

As the disease progresses, the tumor may break through the globe to invade the orbital structures and the sinuses. Once this occurs, the tumor grows rapidly and produces widespread metastases to the bones and viscera.

If the disease is unilateral, prompt enucleation of the eye must be accomplished. When the disease is bilateral, the therapy of choice is removal of the orbital contents of the more seriously affected eye and irradiation of the other one. This has provided encouraging results in some instances; however, the eventuality of loss of vision even following irradiation must be considered. The advantage offered by irradiation is the possibility of saving the vision in the remaining eye, although this aim is not always attained.

It is generally agreed that patients who have recovered from retinoblastoma should be made aware of the possible occurrence of the disease in their offspring.

NEUROBLASTOMA

The neuroblastoma is one of the most common of the malignant tumors seen in infants and children. It may arise from any part of the sympathetic nervous system. The greatest number originate in the adrenal medulla, although the celiac plexus and thoracic sympathetics are also relatively frequent primary sites.

The primary lesion may be small and present no symptoms. As a matter of fact, symptoms in the beginning are so few as to render an early diagnosis difficult. Frequently, a fairly large proportion of these neoplasms will be noticed first through metastases. Failure to gain weight, symptoms of anemia, and fever may cause the physician to search for the underlying cause. When there are metastases to bone, these may appear as a mass growing in some area such as the skull, or they may cause pain and disability as in metastases to the femur or pelvis. Because of the frequency of osseous metastases, some authorities recommend a complete skeletal survey if the diagnosis of neuroblastoma is suspected. In addition, examination of bone marrow aspiration may reveal the characteristic pseudorosettes of the neuroblastoma even in the absence of roentgenographically demonstrable osseous metastases.

In some infants, the first indication of neuroblastoma will be from massive infiltration of the liver. Occasionally, a mass appearing in the back will be the first sign that such a lesion is present. The most common presenting complaint, however, is presence of an abdominal mass.

The tumor mass is usually extremely vascular and friable. When the pseudo-capsule is invaded, there is a rapid extension along the tissue planes, nerve trunks, and lymphatics.

The treatment for neuroblastoma consists of surgical removal of the primary tumor followed by irradiation. Even when the lesion is not totally resectable, it is believed that as much as is consistent with the safety of the patient should be removed.

Although this disease is frequently widespread when diagnosed, radiation therapy is indicated. Preoperatively, irradiation may be of value in shrinking the tumor mass and decreasing its vascularity. This is extremely important, especially if it is recognized prior to surgery that only a partial resection can be carried out. Some authorities, however, are in accord that decrease in the size of the tumor by surgery will make the remaining lesion more radioresponsive.

Neuroblastoma is believed to hold a unique place among all human malignancies in that it can, at times, change from a malignant neuroblastoma to a benign ganglioneuroma by maturation of its cells. In some cases, the neuroblastoma seems to regress entirely. For this reason, treatment is stressed for it is felt that if the tumor growth is held in check long enough, the lesion may reverse its course.

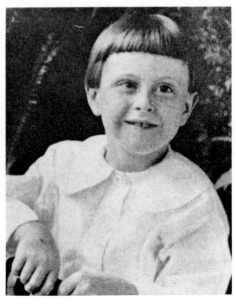

Fig. 9-7. Boy with neuroblastoma reported by Coley and by Cushing and Wolbach. This patient is living and well over 56 years later. (Courtesy Dr. Harold Dargeon, Memorial Center, New York, N. Y.)

WILMS' TUMOR

This renal tumor constitutes about 25% of all malignant tumors in children and is composed of embryonic tissues. It occurs most frequently between the ages of 4 months and 8 years, with the average age being 5 years. It affects males and females equally.

Most often, the presenting symptom is that of an asymptomatic abdominal mass frequently discovered accidentally by the parent. It may be on either side of the abdomen or flank, and on occasion it may be bilateral.

An intravenous or retrograde pyelogram is an important aid to diagnosis of this tumor since it usually reveals a dislocation of the kidney pelvis either upward or downward depending on the location of the tumor within the kidney. This, along with the history and clinical manifestations, serves to establish a tentative diagnosis prior to surgery. Biopsy is contraindicated since this is a highly malignant tumor.

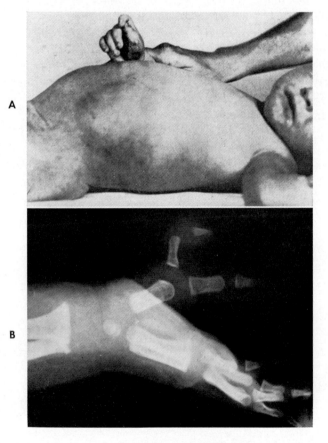

Fig. 9-8. A 2-year-old boy with Wilms' tumor of the left kidney. **A,** The left abdominal mass is outlined. A supernumerary thumb was removed earlier; the scar is visible. **B,** Preoperative roentgenogram showing extra thumb. (Courtesy Dr. Harold Dargeon, Memorial Center, New York, N. Y.)

The tumor is generally well encapsulated. It is bluish in color, usually smooth in appearance, and may have a knobbed or lobulated surface. When cut, the substance is gray-white or yellow and appears soft and at times vascular. In some, gelatinous and edematous areas are interspersed between fibrotic sections.

Wilms' tumor may spread by direct infiltration to involve the omentum and neighboring organs in the peritoneal cavity. It can also metastasize by means of venous extension or even through lymphatic channels to any or all organs of the body. It metastasizes early to the lungs. In some cases, the tumor grows into the renal vein and ultimately reaches the inferior vena cava.

Wilms' tumors may grow rapidly, but the size alone bears no direct relationship to prognosis. If there is no evidence of metastasis, with proper treatment the prognosis varies inversely with age—the younger the patient, the better the chance of cure.

The best results in the treatment of Wilms' tumor have been obtained by a combination of surgery and irradiation. Once the diagnosis has been made, a nephrectomy should be performed through a transabdominal incision. In this way, the renal pedicle can be ligated early prior to manipulation of the tumor. This will prevent tumor cells from becoming dislodged and disseminated into the bloodstream. As soon as possible thereafter radiation therapy should be initiated.

SOFT TISSUE SARCOMAS

Tumors of the supporting structures of the body are not uncommon. These may be found in fat, muscle, or connective tissue as well as in other structures. They may appear at any age and are often observed at, or shortly after, birth. They may present as benign tumors that undergo malignant change early in life.

One of the most frequent of childhood lesions is the rhabdomyosarcoma. It may occur in the genitourinary tract, the diaphragm, or the head or neck region. This tumor spreads by direct extension as well as by way of the lymphatics. Other sarcomas of the soft tissues are fibrosarcoma, liposarcoma, malignant neurilemomas, and synoviomas.

One of the most common benign lesions in white children is the hemangioma. It is extremely rare in the Negro race. When it is cutaneous in location, it is readily diagnosed; however, hemangiomas may occur subcutaneously, viscerally, or in bone. Death may result from hemorrhage, pressure, or serious interference with function in the area involved before external signs are evident.

Sarcoma of soft tissues should be treated by wide local excision. Rarely is radical surgery indicated, nor should amputation be considered necessary. These soft tissue tumors vary in their sensitivity to irradiation with the majority of them being radioresistant. In general, the majority respond poorly to chemotherapy as well.

•   •   •

Nursing care of the child with a malignant disorder

To hear the statement, "Your child has cancer," can be one of the most traumatizing experiences for a parent. This frequently creates an immediate picture of death following a long, lingering, and painful illness. It frequently means revision of long-term goals for the child and planning on an almost day-to-day or week-to-week basis. It is imperative that once such a diagnosis is confirmed, the parents be given an accurate diagnosis, an explanation of the appropriate therapy, the probable length of the illness, the course to be expected, and the probable expense involved.

When a child is stricken with cancer, the nurse has a major responsibility for providing emotional support and physical care for him, and she must also consider the parents and provide them with emotional support as well. Frequently they will require more attention in this respect than the patient.

Specific nursing care is related to the site of involvement, the type of treatment required, and the degree of progress that is made by the patient. Any therapy, surgical, irradiation, or purely palliative medical treatment will challenge all resources the nurse has at her command. General, rather routine nursing measures must also be employed to maintain optimum health and conserve powers of resistance for the child. Expert nursing care is required regardless of the prognosis, and the nurse must establish good interpersonal relations with both the child and his parents if she hopes to function effectively.

Whenever feasible, the child should not be placed in a single room since contact with other children makes the adjustment to hospitalization more tolerable. Care must be taken, however, to ascertain that none of the children are harboring, or have, upper respiratory infections since the child with a malignant neoplasm is particularly prone to such infections.

The child with a malignant neoplasm frequently is malnourished since digestive disturbances such as anorexia, nausea and vomiting, and diarrhea or constipation often occur. This means careful planning with the dietitian to see that likes and dislikes are taken into consideration. Small, frequent feedings should be offered that are especially high in calories and proteins, and further supplemented with minerals and vitamins. This will help to prevent or correct any deficiencies that may develop. The nurse should provide for a few moments of rest before the tray is served. She should schedule treatments so that none are administered immediately before or after the meal is served.

Unless contraindicated, water or other fluids should be offered periodically between meals to help prevent dehydration and to assist in the removal of any toxic substances that might be present. For the child who cannot tolerate nourishment by mouth, gavage feedings or parenteral fluids should be provided.

For the acutely ill child, the nurse must be alert to the need for frequent change of position and frequent bathing and/or sponging to prevent infection, loss of body tone, and the development of pressure areas on the skin. Both urinary elimination and defecation must be watched closely to prevent bladder distention or dehydration and fecal impaction or diarrhea; each of these conditions may interfere with proper nutrition and rest.

It is most important that the child get adequate rest and sleep in order to conserve much-needed strength. This will entail planning for periodic rest periods throughout the day and preparing the child for bed early in the evening. Medications for pain should be offered when needed, and sedatives should be given as necessary to induce required sleep. The ingenious nurse can frequently eliminate the use of large doses of medication by employing appropriate nursing measures that will eliminate the need for large doses of pain medications and sedatives. Good body alignment in bed will promote proper rest and sleep and will also aid in prevention of posture deformities.

Frequently, the physical condition of the child can change in a matter of minutes or even seconds. Every possible type of equipment that might be needed should be close at hand for this reason. Oxygen equipment and medications, as well as mouth gags, airways, and side rails, should be available for emergency use.

The nurse must recognize that the child will have periods of remission as well as regression, and her nursing care plan must take this into consideration. Once the child can begin to feel secure in the hospital situation, he can begin to function independently as far as his physical condition will permit. After he has overcome his fears of hospitalization and can feel free to talk, the nurse should encourage him to verbalize his fears and to release inner tensions. Whenever he is physically able, diversional and occupational therapy should be provided, and if the child is of school age, tutors or other substitutes should be encouraged to keep him alert and reassured.

The nurse should be aware of the fact that the child is entitled to and should be given an honest and simple answer to his questions. An outright falsehood should never be offered to the child because if he accidentally learns the truth, his confidence in the doctor and/or the nurse, or even in his parents, may be seriously impaired, causing increased difficulty in his future care.

When the child's condition becomes terminal, he should not be apprised of the situation. Younger children are more readily handled at this stage because they are not fully aware of what "death" really means. The older child or the teen-ager, on the other hand, must be handled with special care, and the hope of continued life must never be completely shut off from him. The situation must be handled in accord with the philosophy of the hospital and that of the doctors who have responsibility for the patient.

In many instances, the nurse must be capable of helping the parents to accept the form of therapy (radical surgery, irradiation, or chemotherapy), and she will, of necessity, have to accept the prevailing philosophy of the institution in which she works. Verbalizing approval is not adequate since her words will provide little or no reassurance to the parents or to the patient.

Probably one of the most challenging situations the nurse will encounter is caring for the child in terminal stages of his disease. This will be discussed in greater detail in the chapter on advanced disease.

In caring for the child who has a malignant neoplasm, the nurse must utilize every skill at her command. Not only does she have to provide emotional support and physical care for the patient, but she also needs to provide emotional support to the parents and, hopefully, avoid their becoming overly dependent on her and the other nursing personnel. Caring for the child with cancer can provide one of the most challenging experiences the nurse will ever encounter.

Bibliography

Ariel, I. M., and Pack, G. T., editors: Cancer and allied diseases of infancy and childhood, Boston, 1960, Little, Brown & Co.

Ariel, I. M., and Pack, G. T.: Cancer of infancy and childhood, New York J. Med. **60**:404, 1960.

Bill, A., et al.: Common malignant tumors of infancy and childhood, Pediat. Clin. N. Amer. **6**:1197, 1959.

Bozeman, M. F., Orbach, C. E., and Sutherland, A. M.: Psychological impact of cancer and its treatment. III. The adaptation of mothers to the threatened loss of their children through leukemia, Cancer **8**:1, 1955.

Blakemore, W. S., and Ravdin, I. S.: Current perspectives in cancer therapy, New York, 1966, Hoeber Medical Division, Harper & Row, Publishers, chap. 20, pp. 167-180.

Collins, V. P.: The treatment of Wilms' tumor, Cancer **11**:89, 1959.

Dargeon, H. W.: Cancer alerts, New York State J. Med. **58**:402, 1958.

Dargeon, H. W.: Lymphosarcoma in childhood, Amer. J. Roentgen. **85**:729, 1961.

Dargeon, H. W.: Childhood cancer; a growing health problem, Ca **12**:51, 1962.

Dargeon, H. W.: Leukemia in children: some current considerations, Ca **12**:87, 1962.

Dargeon, H. W.: Juvenile cancer: considerations on the etiology, Ca **12**:139, 1962.

Dargeon, H. W.: Neuroblastoma: the unpredictable tumor, Ca **12**:188, 1962.

Dargeon, H. W., and Tan, C.: Thoracic tumors of childhood, Arch. Surg. **78**:660, 1959.

Dytz, W., and Stout, A. P.: Kaposis sarcoma in infants and children, Cancer **13**:684, 1960.

Editorial: Advances in the control of cancer in infants and children, J. Pediat. **54**:406, 1959.

Friedman, S., Karon, M., and Goldsmith, G.: Childhood leukemia: a pamphlet for parents, U. S. Department of Health, Education, and Welfare, Public Health Service, 1963.

Gross, R. E.: The surgery of infancy and childhood, Philadelphia, 1958, W. B. Saunders Co.

Gutowski, F.: Nursing the leukemic child with central nervous system involvement, Amer. J. Nurs. **63**:87, April, 1963.

Kieswetter, W. B., and Mason, E. J.: Malignant tumors in childhood, J.A.M.A. **172**:1117, 1960.

Kinzel, R. C., Mills, S. D., Childs, D. S., Jr., and De Weerd, J. H.: Wilms' tumor: a review of 47 cases, J.A.M.A. **174**:1925, 1960.

Lyman, M. S., and Burchenal, J. H.: Acute leukemia, Amer. J. Nurs. **63**:63, April, 1963.

Management of children with cancer, Cancer Bull. **13**:50, 1961.

Martin, L. W., and MacCollum, D. W.: Hemangiomas in infants and children, Amer. J. Surg. **101**:571, 1961.

Murphy, M. L.: Leukemia and lymphoma in children, Pediat. Clin. N. Amer. **6**:611, 1959.

Ng, E., and Low-Beer, B. V. A.: The treatment of Wilms' tumor, J. Pediat. **48**:763, 1956.

Pack, G., and Ariel, I.: Tumors of the soft somatic tissue, New York, 1958, Paul B. Hoeber, Inc., Medical Book Department of Harper & Row, Publishers.

Petrakis, N. L.: Malignant disease in children, J. Chron. Dis. **12**:368, 1960.

Radler, H. B.: All about an operation, New York, 1956, The Society of Memorial Center.

Radler, H. B.: Inside the hospital, New York, 1955, The 100 League.

Riker, W., and Bigler, J.: Unpredictability of tumors of childhood, Pediatrics **24:**666, 1959.

Rosenberg, S. A., Diamond, H. D., Dargeon, H. W., and Craver, L. F.: Lymphosarcoma in childhood, New Eng. J. Med. **259:**505, 1958.

Southwick, H. W., Slaughter, D. P., and Majarakis, J. D.: Malignant disease of the head and neck in childhood, Arch. Surg. **78:**678, 1959.

Stowens, D.: Pediatric pathology, Baltimore, 1966, The Williams & Wilkins Co.

Williams, H. M., Diamond, H. D., and Craver, L. F.: Pathogenesis and management of neurological complications in patients with malignant lymphomas and leukemias, Cancer **11:**76, 1958.

Willis, R. A.: The pathology of the tumors of children, Springfield, 1962, Charles C Thomas, Publisher.

Chapter 10

Management of the patient with an endocrine disorder

Coordination of the many biological processes of the body depends on the integrating influences of the central nervous system and the endocrine system. The hypophysis (pituitary body) plays a unique role as a link between these two integrating systems. This link is established in the embryo when the neural and somatic ectoderms merge as the hypophysis. It is carried in postnatal life by a system of vascular channels that connect the hypothalamus to the adenohypophysis and by neural pathways that link the hypothalamus to the neurohypophysis. By these connections, the central nervous system and that part of the endocrine system controlled by the pituitary join to exert their regulatory control over many body processes involved in growth, differentiation, reproduction, maintenance of homeostasis and the metabolic state.

THE HYPOPHYSIS

The hypophysis is an organ of multiple functions, many of which are well defined while others are only suspected. It exercises its effect essentially through the production of various hormonal fractions that, either directly or indirectly, affect the other endocrine glands.

The fully developed hypophysis varies in weight from 0.4 to 1.1 grams and is about the size of a pea. It occupies the hypophyseal fossa of the sella turcica of the sphenoid bone.

It consists of the adenohypophysis and the neurohypophysis, each of which has major divisions and subdivisions.

The anterior lobe is responsible for integrating activities of the entire system. Present evidence indicates that there are at least six hormones secreted by this portion of the gland. The somatic (growth) hormone acts directly upon the growth of body tissues by regulating cell division. After growth has been completed, the hormone presumably plays a role in maintaining and replenishing the protein of the tissues. It also has important effects upon carbohydrate metabolism.

Table 10-1. The hypophysis*

Gland	Major divisions	Subdivisions	
Adenohypophysis	Lobus glandularis	1. Pars distalis	Anterior lobe
		2. Pars tuberalis	
		3. Pars intermedia	
	Lobus nervosus (neural lobe)	1. Process infundibularis	Posterior lobe
Neurohypophysis	Infundibulum (neural stalk)	1. Pediculus infundibularis	(stem)
		2. Bulbus infundibularis	(bulb)
		3. Labrum infundibularis	(rim)

*International Commission on Anatomical Nomenclature.

Thyrotropic hormone (TSH) stimulates the enzymatic breakdown of stored thyroglobulin, thereby forcing the liberation of thyroxin from the thyroid gland. It stimulates the activity of the thyroid and causes hypertrophy and hyperplasia of the gland with loss of colloid. The blood level of thyroxin determines the amount of thyrotropic hormone produced at any given time.

The adrenocorticotropic hormone, or corticotropin (ACTH), controls secretion of adrenal cortex secretions. It stimulates production of hydrocortisone, aldosterone, and other steroid hormones. The rate of ACTH production is, however, regulated by the concentration of these hormones in the blood. Physiological actions of the adrenal hormones affect electrolyte metabolism, carbohydrate and protein metabolism, renal function, and resistance to disease.

Three gonadotropic hormones, the follicle-stimulating hormone (FSH), the luteinizing hormone (LH), and the lactogenic hormone, are also produced by the anterior lobe.

The follicle-stimulating hormone is essential for growth of the graafian follicles in the female, and for the spermatogenesis and enlargement of the seminiferous tubules of the testes in the male.

The luteinizing hormone stimulates the interstitial tissue of the ovary and testes. It causes formation of the corpus luteum provided that maturing follicles are present. It acts upon the ovary only when it has been primed by FSH.

Lactogenic hormone prepares the breasts for lactation during pregnancy and stimulates milk production after delivery. It acts in conjunction with estrogen and progesterone.

The anterior pituitary gland, then, acts as a control center and is, in turn, subject to regulation through the nervous system and by the concentration of the circulating hormones elaborated by the target glands. It is capable of responding, then, to alterations in the physiologic and biochemical conditions of the body.

The secretory principles of the posterior lobe are not fully established; however, several hormones have been established as arising from this lobe.

Antidiuretic hormone (ADH) controls water reabsorption in the kidney tubules and prevents or inhibits the onset of diabetes insipidus. Oxytocin causes uterine muscle to contract and may (in some cases) be a galactogogue. Intermedin, the melanocyte-stimulating hormone, stimulates pigment production in the skin. The vasopressor principle, vasopressin, increases blood pressure by arteriolar and capillary constriction.

THE THYROID GLAND

The thyroid gland, located in the lower anterior midline of the neck, consists of two lateral lobes with a connecting median isthmus. The isthmus passes in front of the trachea while the lateral lobes extend from the thyroid cartilage to the sixth tracheal ring. The gland is enclosed in a capsule of fibrous connective tissue and is firmly fixed to the cricoid and thyroid cartilages by means of pretracheal fascia. The gland weighs about 20 grams and is relatively richly supplied with lymphatics. The blood supply is derived from the external carotids and the subclavian vessels.

Microscopically, the gland consists of closely packed small sacs or acini filled with colloid. The follicles vary in size and tend to be spherical in shape.

The thyroid has a major function of producing thyroxin, the hormone that accelerates metabolism and is also essential for growth and development. Iodine or iodine ion is absorbed from the gastrointestinal tract; some is excreted in the urine, and some is selectively removed by thyroid cells. The iodine plus tyrosine forms thyroxin, which then combines with a globulin to form thyroglobulin. This substance is stored in the thyroid follicles until needed.

Essentially all diseases of the thyroid gland are associated with structural abnormalities. Any abnormal enlargement of the gland, regardless of the cause, is referred to as goiter. Some of these do undergo malignant change, although an accurate percentage is not available.

Carcinoma of the thyroid occurs more frequently in females than in males, the ratio being 3:1. It is seen between the ages of 40 and 70 years, with the median age being about 50. It is also observed in childhood and in young adults.

Carcinoma of the thyroid has been classified according to the degree of malignancy produced: (1) low-grade malignancy, the adenomas that invade the blood vessels; (2) moderately malignant, the papillary adenocarcinomas; and (3) highly malignant, such as the small cell and giant cell carcinomas.

Signs and symptoms vary. Usually, an enlargement or swelling in the neck is the first indication of any tumor being present. This is oftentimes noticed by the patient himself or by a relative or friend. Occasionally it is found at the time of a routine physical examination. As the tumor enlarges, symptoms arise as the result of pressure, that is, hoarseness due to pressure on the larynx, dysphagia due to pressure on the esophagus, and so forth.

In some cases, the presenting symptom is an enlarged cervical node. This is usually indicative of metastatic disease. These tumors have a predilection for metastasizing to the bones. Here, again, this may be the initial manifestation of the disease, especially when there has been a fracture of the humerus, a rib, or the femur. The other most common site for metastases is the lung, although this usually is a late manifestation. Despite metastatic disease, however, long survivals are common.

Treatment for carcinoma of the thyroid is surgical excision. Depending on whether the lesion is a solitary nodule or multiple nodules, well localized or diffuse, lobectomy or total thyroidectomy may be performed. If the lesion is a papillary carcinoma, some surgeons advocate lobectomy combined with prophylactic neck dissection on the same side.

The most common complications observed (during or after surgery) include hemorrhage, paralysis of the laryngeal nerve, hypoparathyroidism, and respiratory difficulty.

In some patients with postoperative local recurrence, treatment by irradiation may be extremely valuable since many malignant tumors have proved to be remarkably radiosensitive.

Nursing care of the patient with a thyroid carcinoma

The preoperative nursing care of the patient with carcinoma of the thyroid will not differ essentially from that required for any patient having thyroid surgery. He will need adequate explanations prior to any diagnostic tests so that he will know what to expect.

Common diagnostic procedures such as the basal metabolism determination, various blood chemistries, and tests employing radioactive iodine may be employed. A lateral roentgenogram of the soft tissues of the neck may prove of value in demonstrating calcification within the tumor or compression of the trachea.

When the patient is to have a basal metabolism test, he should be given detailed explanations of what to expect during the test as well as the necessary preparation beforehand. The nurse should explain the importance of a good night's sleep before the test is done and the need for being as quiet as possible the day of the test. The patient should be instructed not to carry out any activities that morning since this will alter the results of the test as well. By informing the patient that he will lie on a comfortable bed during the test, that his nostrils will be closed with a clamp, and that he will breathe through his mouth from a tube that supplies oxygen, she can allay his apprehension when the nose clamp is applied. This can be a terrifying experience for the patient since he may feel that he cannot breathe, which, in itself, may make the results of the test inaccurate.

Several tests may be carried out utilizing radioactive iodine. If such tests are ordered, the nurse should observe the patient closely for signs of apprehension. Explanation will minimize his fears of ingesting a "radioactive" substance.

Prior to surgery, the patient should be informed that he may be a little hoarse and may have some difficulty in swallowing when he awakens after the operation due to irritation produced by the endotracheal catheter. He should be told that this will be temporary and that it will subside after the edema disappears.

If the patient is to go to the recovery room following the operation, he should be informed that he will not awake in his own room but that he will be in a place where he will receive expert attention until he is fully conscious. In most instances he is placed in a Fowler's or semi-Fowler's position with the head, neck, and shoulders well supported. He must be observed closely, assisted in coughing and expectorating mucus. If the secretions are thick, the nurse may have to suction him frequently to ensure an open airway.

As soon as he has reacted from anesthesia he should be asked to speak in order to determine the possibility of injury to the recurrent laryngeal nerve. Every half hour or so, he should be encouraged to speak as another check for such injury. Steam inhalations (benzoin or cold steam) will keep the air moist and help soothe the irritated mucous membranes of the respiratory passages, thereby making breathing less difficult. Usually, on return to his room, the patient will have an intravenous infusion running. Once the nausea subsides (and some patients do not experience this at all), fluids should be offered orally. A soft diet can frequently be tolerated even the first or second postoperative day.

The nurse should constantly be alert to the possibility of hemorrhage and should check the dressings at frequent intervals. Not only should the dressing itself be checked, but the nurse should slip her hand gently under the patient's neck and shoulders since blood may drain back to this area. Any evidence of swelling, increased tightness of the dressing, hoarseness, or increasing respiratory distress should be watched for since these may be signs of hemorrhage into the tissues. The physician should be notified immediately if any of these signs are observed.

The alert, observant nurse can greatly enhance a rapid and uncomplicated recovery for the patient who has undergone surgery for carcinoma of the thyroid.

THE ADRENAL GLANDS

The adrenal glands are crescent-shaped glands located on the upper poles of the kidneys. They weigh 3 to 5 grams each. The glands are enclosed in a tough connective tissue capsule and are embedded in adipose tissue. The capsule penetrates into the deeper portions of the gland and is contiguous with the septa that divide the organ into its characteristic zonal layers.

Each gland consists of an outer section, the cortex, which is firm and distinctly yellowish in color due to the presence of lipid-filled cells, and an inner portion, the medulla, which is softer, less firm, and has a dark red-brown cast. The cortex is divided into three layers or zones as a result of the penetration of trabeculae from the capsule. These include: (1) the zona glomerulosa, which is the outermost zone, the thinnest layer, and the cells are grouped rather loosely together in ill-defined clusters; (2) the zona fasciculata, the widest layer, and the cells, particularly rich in fats, are arranged in strands that extend parallel to one another from the glomerular to the reticular layers; (3) the innermost layer is the zona reticularis, and the cells in this area are arranged in an irregular network and contain lipid droplets as well as considerable pigment.

The glands have an unusually rich blood supply as well as lymphatic supply. They are innervated chiefly by branches of the splanchnic nerves.

The adrenocortical hormones include: (1) the glucocorticoids, cortisone, and hydrocortisone; (2) the mineralocorticoids, desoxycorticosterone and aldosterone; (3) the sex hormones, androgens and estrogens. Epinephrine (Adrenalin) is secreted by the adrenal medulla, and a second hormone, norepinephrine (arterenol) is also formed in this area of the gland. All of these substances have important functions within the body.

Malignant neoplasms of the adrenal gland are not observed very frequently and consist primarily of the neuroblastomas of infancy and childhood. (See Chapter IX.)

THE MAMMARY GLAND

Although the breast is not actually considered an endocrine gland, it is being presented here since it is affected by many secretions of hormonal origin.

To describe a "normal" breast adequately is somewhat difficult since the gland is never at rest. Factors in the environment that may produce emotional stress, allergies, or any reactions that may affect the endocrine glands may in turn affect the functioning of the breast.

The mammary gland is considered to be an accessory organ of the reproductive system and has as its major function the secretion of milk for

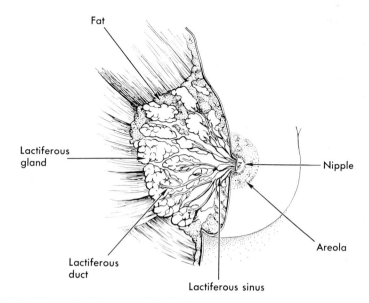

Fig. 10-1. Schematic diagram of the breast.

nourishment of the infant. The gland is structurally and embryologically related to the glands of the integument.

Mammary glandular tissue, adipose tissue, and connective tissue are all contained within the breast with the connective tissue filling in between and around the glandular tissue. Dense fibrous bands (Cooper's ligaments) extend from the dermis into the gland to perform a suspensory function. Two primary structures, the acini (alveoli) and the ducts, make up the glandular system of the breast. The acini serve as the secretory organs while the ducts act as the channels through which the secretion passes to the orifices of the nipple. The ductal system is a complex one due to the variation in size. As a result, ducts are referred to as interlobar, intralobar, interlobular, and intralobular. The acini are lined by layers of cuboidal epithelium. The epithelium lies upon a single layer of unstriated muscle fibers that is continuous around the ducts and acini. These unstriated muscle fibers have been described as myoepithelial cells and possess the faculty of proliferation, either alone or in conjunction with the epithelium.

The subepithelial connective tissue lies immediately outside the layer of unstriated muscle fibers and consists of delicate connective tissue with a fine fibrillar matrix in which a few cells (some bipolar and others stellate) are scattered. The next layer, elastica, surrounds the ducts and terminates abruptly where the acini begin. Encircling the outside of all ducts is a loose fibrous connective tissue that should be distinguished from the supporting fibrous connective tissue of the breast.

The amount of subcutaneous fat in the breast may vary considerably, and, in some instances, may be essentially absent. The subcutaneous fat is intersected by the ligamenta suspensoria. These ligaments arise from the superficial fascia enclosing the breast and, after branching, are inserted into the dermis. The gland is abundantly supplied with blood vessels and lymphatics.

The nipple projects from the surface of the breast as a conical or cylindrical structure at about the level of the fourth intercostal space just below the center of the breast. It is covered by a layer of epidermis continuous with the openings of fifteen to twenty lactiferous ducts that end on its surface.

Extreme structural variations are observed in the breast according to its functional state. Glandular tissue is sparse in the breast of the nonpregnant but sexually mature female, and the tubules have a ductlike appearance; furthermore, there is proportionately more adipose and connective tissue present. Changes occur, however, in the course of pregnancy. Tubules enlarge to become buds, which, in turn, enlarge to form acini, while the stromal tissue decreases proportionately in preparation for lactation. When lactation ceases, the stromal tissue again increases. Following menopause, the fibrous involutional type of gland is seen.

The ovarian hormones, estrogen and progesterone, have been established as the primary agents responsible for growth of the mammary glands. It is generally recognized that estrogen causes duct growth, while progesterone is concerned with development of the lobule-alveolar system. Evidence has also been presented that adrenal and hypophyseal hormones play a synergistic role in the development of the mammary glands.

Estrogen is primarily responsible for enlargement of the breasts occurring at puberty and with successive menstrual cycles. Estrogen has the ability to produce extensive growth of the duct system of the breast. It has also been suggested to have an accessory and direct action on the stromal tissue, producing hyperemia and increased vascular permeability, thereby allowing other hormones and metabolites greater access to the mammary tissue.

Pituitary hormones are necessary for growth of the mammary glands as is evidenced by the inability of estrogen and progesterone to produce mammary development in hypophysectomized animals. At the present time, prolactin is the only pituitary hormone known to have specific mammogenic activity, acting directly on the mammary gland. In addition to this, growth hormone has a nonspecific action on mammary tissue, as it has on all tissues of the body.

The human mammary glands are subject to many diseases. From a practical standpoint, carcinoma is the most important lesion. Below the age of 20 years it is considered as a medical curiosity. From 20 to 30 years of age, the disease is rare, and from 30 to 50, there is a steady increase in the incidence of the disease before it begins to level off. A second peak is observed after the age of 65, after which there is a steady incline until the end of the life-span.

According to the American Cancer Society, carcinoma of the breast is the leading type of cancer in females, accounting for approximately 25% of all cancers in women. The disease is almost exclusively found in women, with less than 0.5% occurring in males.

While the exact cause of human breast cancer is unknown, there are various factors that have been suggested as possible etiological origins. Familial inheritance has been well established by a series of statistical studies of the heredity of patients with the disease from Norway, Holland, Denmark, and England.

There is considerable evidence that mammary function has a definite relationship to the development of breast cancer. Studies have substantiated the fact that unmarried women have more breast cancer than married women and that the incidence of the disease diminishes sharply as the number of children increases.

All breast carcinomas are adenocarcinomas that may be classified as noninvasive and invasive. They are derived from the mammary epithelium. The noninvasive type is the intraductal tumor, which consists of large masses of tumor cells confined to the ducts. It is not uncommon to observe necrosis of the central portion of the tumor. Scirrhous, medullary, and diffuse anaplastic tumors make up the invasive types seen. Other specific types of breast tumors seen occasionally are the papillary carcinoma and Paget's carcinoma of the breast. The papillary carcinoma is the least malignant form and the most easily cured of all forms of mammary carcinoma. Paget's carcinoma is a multicentric intraductal form of carcinoma involving the large ducts beneath the nipple and extending along them to the skin surface. The so-called Paget cells grow within the nipple epithelium and produce erosion of the nipple surface.

Inflammatory carcinoma of the breast is a very virulent type, and invariably its prognosis is grave. The clinical features are striking—the entire breast is enlarged, indurated, edematous, abnormally warm and red. The inflammation is due largely to capillary congestion and invasion of the subdermal lymphatics.

Carcinoma of the breast usually arises as a single focus in one breast with almost half of these tumors occurring in the upper, outer quadrant and another one fourth of them originating in the central portion. Tumors in the upper, outer quadrant tend to metastasize first to the axillary lymph nodes while those from the central portion metastasize to the internal mammary chain of lymph nodes. From the axillary and/or internal mammary chain, secondary drainage extends into the nodes at the base of the neck, and other metastasis may spread through the bloodstream. While the regional nodes

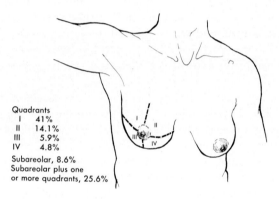

Quadrants
  I   41%
  II   14.1%
  III   5.9%
  IV   4.8%
Subareolar, 8.6%
Subareolar plus one
or more quadrants, 25.6%

Fig. 10-2

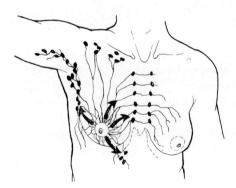

Fig. 10-3

Fig. 10-2. Incidence of breast cancer according to quadrants.
Fig. 10-3. Mode of dissemination of breast cancer.

are the commonest site of spread initially, distant metastases to bones, skin, lungs, contralateral nodes, liver, and brain do occur.

There are numerous views concerning the choice of treatment for carcinoma of the breast. These views vary from radiation therapy alone for primary breast cancer to a combination of radiation therapy and radical mastectomy, or a third possibility of simple mastectomy followed by radiation therapy. More recently, two other surgical procedures have been introduced for carcinoma of the breast. These procedures are referred to as the extended radical mastectomy with chest wall resection and the superradical mastectomy in which the sternum is split and the lymph nodes are dissected from the mediastinum.

Radiation therapy may be used as a primary form of therapy, or it may be used preoperatively or postoperatively, or in total combination. In some cases it may be saved for treatment of local recurrence and/or distant metastases.

Nursing care of the mastectomy patient

A patient who has carcinoma of the breast and who must undergo radical mastectomy can be extremely terrified. The mere connotation of the word "cancer" can create inner turmoil. The fact that a breast must be removed to many women means loss of their femininity. Culturally, too, the loss of a breast often means disgrace. Fear of mutilation and fear of death further increase anxiety and apprehension.

The nurse should realize that anxiety, with its multiple manifestations, is an entirely normal reaction at this time. In fact, if the patient appears overly cheerful, the nurse should be concerned since this may be an indication that the patient has not accepted the diagnosis, which may lead to numerous difficult situations following surgery. The patient needs the greatest understanding in the preoperative period, and the nurse must observe closely in order to be able to reassure the patient and help her to express her fears. Sometimes, when the physician knows definitely that a radical mastectomy will be performed, a short visit from an individual who has made a satisfactory adjustment to her mastectomy may help the patient to accept the surgery more readily.

The patient may be in the hospital only one or two days prior to surgery, so that the nurse must be alert to her response to various treatments and diagnostic procedures. Common preoperative procedures include the following: (1) a roentgenogram of the chest to ascertain that there is no metastasis; (2) an electrocardiogram to determine any evidence of heart disease; (3) blood typing and cross-matching so that blood will be available at the time of surgery; and (4) complete blood count that may indicate evidence of anemia or infection. Other blood chemistries may be ordered depending on the physical status of the patient at the time of admission.

The patient is informed by the surgeon that there is a possibility of radical surgery if it is indicated because of the trauma that might result when the patient recovers from anesthesia and becomes aware of the extensiveness of the wound. In radical mastectomy, the entire breast, the pectoral muscles, all

Table 10-2. Clinical staging system,* cancer of the breast†

T (local tumor)	N (regional lymph nodes)	M (distant metastasis)
T_1 Tumor of 2 cm. or less in its greatest dimension Skin not involved, or involved locally with Paget's disease	N_0 No clinically palpable axillary lymph node(s) (no metastasis suspected)	M_0 No distant metastasis M_1 Clinical and radiographic evidence of metastases except those to homolateral axillary or infraclavicular lymph nodes
T_2 Tumor over 2 cm.; or with skin attachment (dimpling); or nipple retraction (subareolar tumors) No pectoral muscle or chest wall attachment	N_1 Clinically palpable axillary lymph nodes that are not fixed (metastasis suspected) N_2 Clinically palpable homolateral axillary or infraclavicular lymph node(s) that are fixed to one another or to other structures (metastasis suspected)	
T_3 Tumor of any size with any of the following: skin infiltration, ulceration, peau d'orange, skin edema, pectoral muscle or chest wall attachment		

Clinical stage classification

Stage I	Stage II
No clinically palpable axillary lymph node(s) (no metastases suspected) (N_0) Tumor of 2 cm. or less in its greatest dimension (T_1) Skin not involved (T_1) or involved locally with Paget's disease (T_1) No distant metastasis (M_0) $T_1N_0M_0$ or Tumor over 2 cm. (T_2); or Skin attachment (dimpling) (T_2); or Nipple retraction (subareolar tumors) (T_2) No pectoral muscle or chest wall attachment (T_2) No distant metastasis (M_0) $T_2N_0M_0$	Clinically palpable axillary lymph node(s) that are not fixed (metastasis suspected) (N_1) Tumor of 2 cm. or less in its greatest dimension, as in Stage I (T_1) Skin not involved, as in Stage I (T_1), or Paget's disease, as in Stage I (T_1) No distant metastasis (M_0) $T_1N_1M_0$ or Tumor over 2 cm. as in Stage I (T_2); or Skin attached (dimpling); or Nipple retraction (subareolar tumors), as in Stage I (T_2); or No pectoral muscle or chest wall attachment, as in Stage I(T_2) No distant metastasis (M_0) $T_2N_1M_0$

*American system developed by The Joint Committee on Cancer Staging and End Results Reporting.

†Courtesy American Cancer Society, Inc.; reprinted from Ca **12:**195, 1962.

Table 10-2. Clinical staging system, cancer of the breast—cont'd

Clinical stage classification		

Stage III

No clinically palpable lymph node(s) (no metastasis suspected) (N_0)

Tumor of any size with any of the following associated findings: skin infiltration, ulceration, peau d'orange, skin edema, pectoral muscle or chest wall attachment (T_3)

No distant metastasis (M_0) $T_3N_0M_0$ or

Clinically palpable axillary lymph node(s) that are not fixed (metastasis suspected) (N_1)

Tumor of any size with any of the following associated findings: skin infiltration, ulceration, peau d'orange, skin edema, pectoral muscle or chest wall attachment (T_3)

No distant metastasis (M_0) $T_3N_1M_0$ or

Clinically palpable homolateral axillary or infraclavicular lymph node(s) fixed to one another or to other structures (metastasis suspected) (N_2)

No distant metastasis (M_0) $T_3N_2M_0$ or

Any combination of N_2 with M_0 $T_1N_2M_0$ or
                                            $T_2N_2M_0$

Stage IV

Any stage, with distant metastases (M_1)

Summary of stage groupings

Stage I $T_1N_0M_0$ or $T_2N_0M_0$

Stage II $T_1N_1M_0$, $T_2N_1M_0$ (includes all N_1M_0 except for T_3)

Stage III $T_3N_0M_0$, $T_3N_1M_0$, $T_3N_2M_0$, $T_1N_2M_0$, $T_2N_2M_0$ and includes any combination of either T_3 or N_2 with M_0

Stage IV Any clinical stage of disease with distant metastasis (M_1)

fat, fascia, and adjacent tissues along with the axillary lymph nodes are removed en bloc. Drains may be inserted to help remove the serous fluid that collects under the skin, thereby delaying healing and predisposing to infection. In some hospitals a Hemovac is used for this purpose, which enables the patient to be up and about with greater ease and eliminates the need for constantly reinforcing dressings.

When the patient returns from the recovery room she is usually placed in a semi-Fowler's position with the affected arm elevated and supported on a pillow. This helps to prevent, or at least lessen, lymphedema that commonly occurs postoperatively due to interference with the circulatory and lymphatic systems.

The patient should be encouraged to cough deeply and to take deep breaths at frequent intervals. This is of paramount importance since the dressing tends to constrict the chest, and the patient may develop congestion in the lungs due to inadequate expansion of the lung tissue. Coughing deeply and taking deep breaths may cause considerable pain—the nurse can assist the patient by supporting the chest on both sides.

Pain may be quite severe for the first few days postoperatively, and narcotics should be given as necessary unless contraindicated by respiratory complications or specific orders by the physician.

The patient is usually allowed out of bed the day after surgery. She will

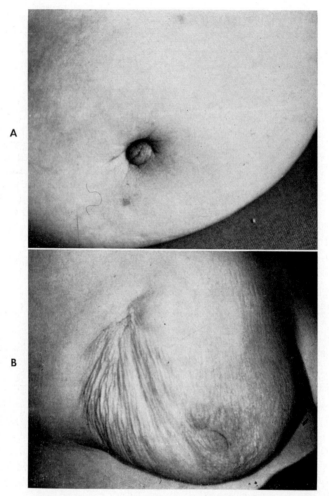

Fig. 10-4. A, Nipple retraction. **B,** Dimpling. (Courtesy Dr. Arthur Holleb, Memorial Center, New York, N. Y.)

need help for the first few days since use of muscles to sit up in bed and stand up will cause pulling and pain in the operative site. Supporting the affected arm will lessen the tension and thereby lessen the discomfort produced by motion.

A major objective of nursing care after mastectomy is to restore normal function to the affected arm. The patient should be encouraged to flex and extend her fingers once she has returned from the recovery room. Another exercise that can be initiated at the same time is to have the patient move the forearm by turning the palm first up and then down. The nurse must reassure the patient that this will not cause any injury at the operative site and that it will enhance a speedy return of normal arm function.

The surgeon will indicate when formal exercise pattern can be started.

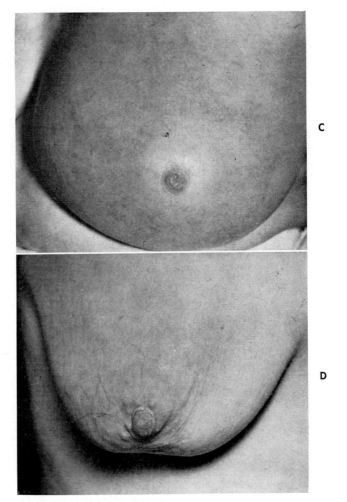

Fig. 10-4, cont'd. C, Edema of breast due to carcinoma. **D,** Paget's disease of breast. (Courtesy Dr. Arthur Holleb, Memorial Center, New York, N. Y.)

This usually depends on the extensiveness of the surgery and whether skin grafting was required. The exercises, therefore, may be initiated as early as the third postoperative day, or they may not be permitted until the seventh postoperative day. The nurse should explain to the patient that these exercises are essential to prevent shortening of muscles, contracture of joints, and loss of muscle tone, all of which reduce normal function of the affected arm.

In some centers, where a number of patients with mastectomy are hospitalized at the same time, these may be done in group exercise classes where patients may all be in different stages of recovery at the same time. This often encourages individual patient progress and is helpful in raising morale for all concerned.

A number of basic exercises are used that will serve to restore arm and

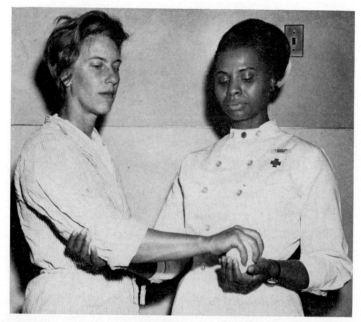

Fig. 10-5. Nurse teaches patient to flex and extend fingers and hand using rolled Curlex. (Courtesy James Ewing Hospital, New York, N. Y.)

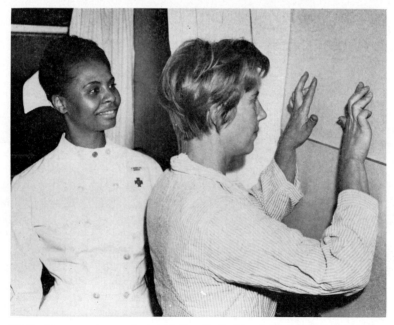

Fig. 10-6. Nurse assists patient with "wall climbing." (Courtesy James Ewing Hospital, New York, N. Y.)

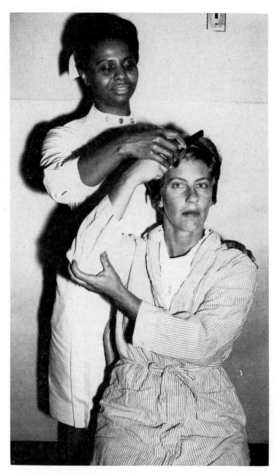

Fig. 10-7. Nurse assists patient to comb her hair. Comb is held in the hand on the operative side. (Courtesy James Ewing Hospital, New York, N. Y.)

shoulder function. A small handbook entitled "Help yourself to recovery" is available for use by nurses in teaching patients and for distribution to patients on approval from their surgeon. This can be obtained from the local chapter of the American Cancer Society, Inc. Another handbook is also available from Memorial Center for a nominal cost of twenty-five cents. This is "A handbook for your recovery"; it adds a more personal touch, since it was written by a patient who had had a similar operation. Routine exercises can become tiresome and prove boring many times. For this reason, when the patient is ready for discharge, substitute exercises can be offered whereby the patient can sweep the floor, wash dishes, and so forth. In this way she is obtaining the same benefits from exercise but feels that she is accomplishing something in her home as well.

Following radical surgery, many patients are reluctant to look at the wound. Every effort should be made to have the patient see it while she is

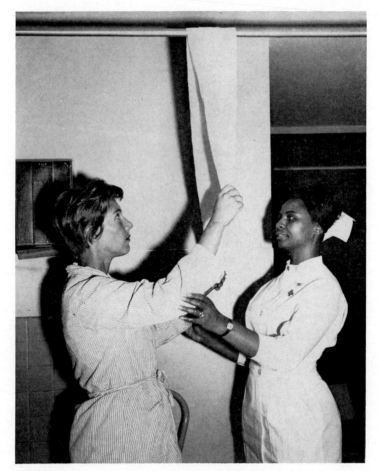

Fig. 10-8. Nurse assists patient with arm exercises. Curlex used as a lever. (Courtesy James Ewing Hospital, New York, N. Y.)

still in the hospital. She will need to be informed that the redness, swelling, and irregularity will gradually disappear. She also needs to be instructed that any signs of increasing redness, infection, or tenderness should be reported at once to her surgeon. She needs to know that in time the scar will be less prominent, the surrounding tissues will become softer, and the tissues will become more normal in color.

As soon as the wound has healed, the patient will be able to bathe the area. A soft washcloth should be used gently and the area patted dry, since vigorous rubbing may cause injury to the newly healed tissues. Cocoa butter or cold cream, gently applied to the wound area (after healing), will prevent dryness and scaling and will promote a more rapid return to near normal appearance of the skin. These, as well as cornstarch or plain talcum powder, will also lessen itching.

Once the prospect for discharge from the hospital is a reality, the physi-

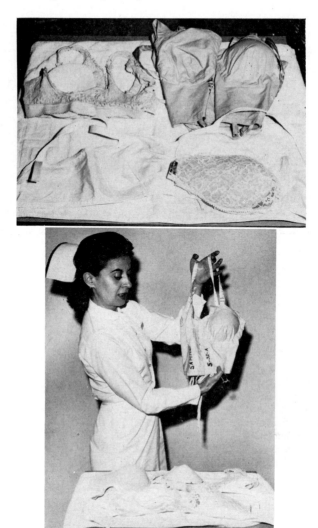

Fig. 10-9. Sample types of available prosthesis. (Courtesy Memorial Center, New York, N. Y.)

cian will tell the patient how much activity she can undertake and how much rest she will need. He will usually have a similar type discussion with the patient's husband (if she is married) or with other members of the family. The nurse should follow up on these explanations and help the patient and her husband or family to continue living as they did prior to the surgery—as normal as is compatible with the patient's condition.

Even though physically the patient is well enough to be discharged, she is seldom able to obtain a prosthesis at this time, since the wound is still too new to permit its use. The nurse can use cotton and provide appropriate padding, which can either be sewed into the patient's brassiere so that her deformity is not obvious or, with a small piece of cotton material and snaps, cotton wadding can be inserted to fill in for the breast that has been lost.

Whenever possible, the patient should be advised about the availability of a prosthesis before she leaves the hospital, even though its use may not be possible for several weeks to several months later. She needs to know the various types that can be obtained such as one made of foam rubber, another filled with fluid, and still a third filled with air. She should be instructed to try each type before purchasing any, since each individual differs in terms of suitability.

The patient who has undergone radical mastectomy for carcinoma of the breast can present a challenging and rewarding experience to the nurse who is interested, alert, and creative. Psychological skills, technical skills, and rehabilitative measures will all be essential in order to afford an uncomplicated rehabilitation and return to optimum health for the patient and her family.

Bibliography

A cancer source book for nurses, New York, 1963, American Cancer Society, Inc.

Ackerman, L. V., and del Regato, J. A.: Cancer: diagnosis, treatment and prognosis, ed. 3, St. Louis, 1962, The C. V. Mosby Co.

Alexander, S. E.: Nursing care of a patient after breast surgery, Amer. J. Nurs. 57:1571, 1957.

Alrich, E. M.: Blank, R. H., and Allen, M. S.: Carcinoma of the thyroid, Ann. Surg. 153:762, 1961.

American Cancer Society, Inc.: Help yourself to recovery, New York, 1957, American Cancer Society, Inc.

Bard, M.: The use of dependence for predicting psychogenic invalidism following radical mastectomy, J. Nerv. Ment. Dis. 122:152, 1955.

Bard, M.: Emotional control in mastectomy nursing, RN 21:76, 1958.

Bard, M., and Sutherland, A.: Psychological impact of cancer and its treatment. IV. Adaptation to radical mastectomy, Cancer 8:656, 1955.

Blakemore, W. S., and Ravdin, I. S., editors: Carcinoma of the breast, chap. 22, Current perspectives in cancer therapy, New York, 1966, Harper & Row, Publishers.

Britton, R. C., and Nelson, P. A.: Causes and treatment of postmastectomy lymphedema of the arm, J.A.M.A. 180:95, 1962.

Brunner, L. S., Emerson, C. P., Jr., Ferguson, L. K., and Suddarth, D. S.: Textbook of medical-surgical nursing, Philadelphia, 1964, J. B. Lippincott Co.

Cancer manual for public health nurses, Washington, 1963, U. S. Department of Health, Education, and Welfare, Public Health Service.

Cassidy, C., and Vander Laan, W.: Laboratory aids to diagnosis in thyroid disease, New Eng. J. Med. 258:828, April 24, 1958.

Copeland, M. M.: Precancerous lesions of the breast, how to treat them, Postgrad. Med. 27:332, 1960.

Cutler, M.: Tumors of the breast, Philadelphia, 1962, J. B. Lippincott Co.

Egan, R. L.: Cancer diagnosis with mammography, Radiology 75:894, 1960.

Egan, R. L.: Mammography, Springfield, 1964, Charles C Thomas, Publisher.

Egan, R. L.: Mammography, Amer. J. Nurs. 66:108, January, 1966.

Field, J. B., editor: Cancer: diagnosis and treatment, Boston, 1959, Little, Brown & Co.

Frazell, E. L., and Foote, F. W.: Papillary cancer of the thyroid: a review of twenty five years of experience, Cancer 11:895, 1958.

Garland, L. W.: The management of cancer of the breast, Surg. Clin. N. Amer. 42: 853, 1962.

Grollman, A.: Clinical endocrinology and its physiology, Philadelphia, 1964, J. B. Lippincott Co.

Haagensen, C. D., and Cooley, E.: Radical mastectomy for mammary carcinoma, Ann. Surg. **157:**166, 1963.

Hayles, A. B., Kennedy, R. L., Beahrs, O. H., and Woolner, L. B.: Management of the child with thyroidal carcinoma, J.A.M.A. **173:**21, 1960.

Higginbotham, S.: Arm exercises after mastectomy, Amer. J. Nurs. **57:**1573, 1957.

Hilkemeyer, R.: Nursing care of cancer patients in hospital and home, Cancer **8:**122, 1958.

Ingleby, H., and Gershon, C. J.: Comparative anatomy, pathology, and roentgenology of the breast, Philadelphia, 1960, University of Pennsylvania Press.

Kendall, B. E., Arthur, J. E., and Patey, D. H.: Lymphangiography in carcinoma of the breast, Cancer **16:**1233, 1963.

Kraft, R. O., and Black, G. E.: An approach to the problems of mammary carcinoma, Surg. Clin. N. Amer. **41:**1219, 1961.

Lanes, P.: Primary aldosteronism, Amer. J. Nurs. **61:**46, August, 1961.

Lewison, E. F.: The psychologic aspects of breast cancer, GP **13:**99, 1956.

McClintock, J. C.: Early treatment of cancer of the thyroid gland, Postgrad. Med. **27:**416, 1960.

Neylan, M. P.: Anxiety, Amer. J. Nurs. **62:**110, May, 1962.

Pollack, R. S.: The surgical treatment of carcinomas of the breast, Surg. Clin. N. Amer. **42:**839, 1962.

Pollack, R. S.: Treatment of breast tumors, Philadelphia, 1958, Lea & Febiger.

Quinn, J. C.: The impact of mastectomy, Amer. J. Nurs. **63:**88, November, 1963.

Radler, H. B.: A handbook for your recovery, New York, 1955, The Society of Memorial Center.

Robbins, G. F., Berg, J. W., Bross, I., de Padua, C., and Sarmiento, A. P.: The significance of early treatment of breast cancer, Cancer **12:**688, 1959.

Shafer, K. N., Sawyer, J. R., McCluskey, A. M., and Beck, E. L.: Medical-surgical nursing, ed. 3, St. Louis, 1964, The C. V. Mosby Co.

Segaloff, A., editor: Breast cancer, St. Louis, 1958, The C. V. Mosby Co.

Smith, G. W.: When a breast must be removed, Amer. J. Nurs. **50:** 335, 1950.

Sutherland, A. M.: Psychological factors in surgical convalescence, Ann. N. Y. Acad. Sci. **73:**491, 1958.

Taylor, G.: Radical mastectomy, Amer. J. Nurs. **63:**396, 1963.

Urban, J. A.: Treatment of early cancer of the breast, Postgrad. Med. **27:**389, 1960.

Warner, M.: Advice for your post-mastectomy patient about her prosthesis, RN **26:**67-68, April, 1963.

Wilkins, L.: The diagnosis and treatment of endocrine disorders in childhood and adolescence, Springfield, 1957, Charles C Thomas, Publisher.

Zintel, H. A., and Nay, H. R.: Postoperative complications of radical mastectomy, Surg. Clin. N. Amer. **44:**313, 1964.

Chapter 11

Management of the patient with a gastrointestinal disorder

The gastrointestinal tract has numerus functions among which are the ingestion, digestion, absorption, and utilization of foodstuffs. Alimentation is a highly complex process that involves not only the organs of the gastrointestinal tract but also the accessory organs including the salivary glands, liver, gallbladder, and pancreas.

The major functions of the gastrointestinal tract are primarily motor functions, i.e., propulsion of food along the tract, mixing movements, and tonic contractions so that the organs will not become distended. Each portion of the tract differs in the degree to which it carries out these motor functions due to the anatomical differences in each segment.

Anatomically, the gastrointestinal tract can be described as a tube or canal divided into segments varying in size and structure according to their function. It extends from the oropharynx of the mouth to the anal canal, which passes through the pelvic floor to the anus and is surrounded by internal sphincters. It is lined with mucous membrane throughout and is supported by a layer of fibrous connective tissue, beneath which is a thin layer of muscularis mucosa. Outside this is an inner circular and an outer longitudinal layer of muscle. Either a fibrous or a serous coat covers the muscle layers.

Food enters the mouth where it is mixed with enzymes and masticated. Deglutition carries or propels food through the esophagus into the stomach. The stomach is described as a collapsible, saclike dilatation of the alimentary canal that serves as a temporary receptacle for food while it undergoes further digestion. It is located directly beneath the diaphragm in the epigastric, umbilical, and left hypochondriac regions. It has a cardiac or esophageal orifice and a pyloric orifice both of which are guarded by sphincters. The blood supply is derived from the branches of the celiac plexus. The vessels run along the greater and lesser curvatures and anastomose freely. Venous blood is returned into the portal vein.

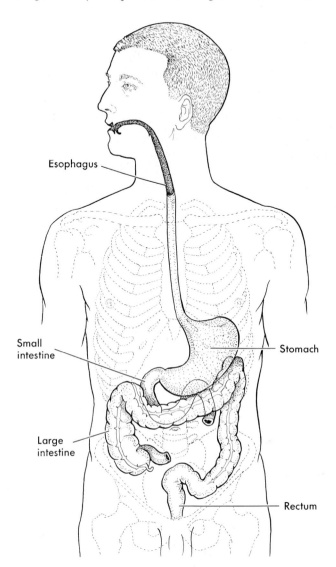

Fig. 11-1. Schematic diagram of gastrointestinal tract.

Three types of glands are found in the gastric mucosa. The cardiac glands, chiefly mucus, are located close to the cardiac orifice. The fundic glands contain chief cells or central cells. These cells secrete pepsinogen. Parietal cells are also found in the fundus and secrete hydrochloric acid. The pyloric glands represent the third type gland of the stomach. Both pepsinogen and hydrochloric acid are essential for the digestive process.

The small intestine is divided into three segments, namely, the duodenum, the jejunum, and the ileum. The duodenum is a somewhat C-shaped tube. The concave portion surrounds the head of the pancreas. It is divided into superior, descending, transverse, and ascending segments. It terminates at the duodenojejunal flexure. The superior segment is in contact with the liver and the neck of the gallbladder and forms the lower border of the epiploic region. The liver and transverse colon lie anteriorly, while the head of the pancreas, the common bile duct, and the portal vein lie posterior to this segment.

The right kidney and the renal vessels are anterior to the descending segment of the duodenum while the transverse colon lies behind it. Medially, it is in contact with the head of the pancreas, and posteriorly the common bile duct descends between the pancreas and the duodenum and enters the descending portion with the pancreatic duct at the ampulla of Vater. The vena cava lies behind the transverse portion. Behind the ascending portion are the aorta and the left renal vessels. Both the transverse and the ascending segments are covered with peritoneum. The jejunum and the ileum comprise the mesenteric portion of the small intestine with the ileum being the larger of the two segments. Peyer's patches characterize the ileum.

In the mucosa of the small intestine are the villi, between the bases of which are the crypts of Lieberkühn and Brunner's glands. Much of the absorption of foodstuffs takes place in the villi.

Beginning at the ileocecal valve and extending to the anus is the large intestine, which surrounds the small intestine. It is divided into numerous segments: the cecum, the vermiform appendix, the ascending colon, the transverse colon, the descending colon, the sigmoid colon, the rectum, and the anal canal. This portion of the gastrointestinal tract is mainly concerned with the absorption of water and the formation of waste products that will be excreted by the process of defecation.

PHYSIOLOGY AND GENERAL FUNCTIONS OF THE GASTROINTESTINAL TRACT

The major functions of the gastrointestinal tract, as was stated previously, are motor functions, that is, propulsion of food along the tract, mixing movements, and tonic contractions, so that the organs will not become distended. Once food enters the mouth, a series of motions are initiated and the process of digestion is begun. Solid foods are masticated and broken down into pieces that can be swallowed with ease. At the same time saliva is mixed with the food, making it a soft mass. The process of swallowing, or deglutition, forces the food mass into the esophagus where peristaltic action carries it through to the stomach. Peristalsis is the progressive movement along a hollow viscus that consists of a coordinated contraction and relaxation of the ring of muscle fibers in the organ, that is, muscle fibers above the food mass contract while those below relax, thus propelling the food along through the tract.

When the food mass enters the stomach the smooth muscle fibers stretch, allowing the stomach wall to relax. Peristaltic action begins in the body of the stomach, and the waves or contractions serve to mix the food with gastric juice. Protein digestion begins at this point. The mixing motion causes churning of the food mass, which breaks down in finer particles. From time to time, small amounts of the stomach contents pass into the duodenum. Anywhere from 1 to 6 hours is required for the complete passage of the gastric contents into the duodenum. Three distinct types of movements occur in the small intestine, and these are responsible for the mixing of the contents with the intestinal juices, bringing the contents into closer contact with the absorbing surface, and moving it through to the large intestine. These motions are usually referred to as segmentation, peristalsis, and pendular movement. Haustral churning takes place in the large intestine and is responsible for the passage of the contents through the ascending, transverse, and descending colon to the sigmoid, where it remains until defecation occurs.

The gastrointestinal tract is supplied with an extensive nervous system, commonly referred to as the myenteric plexus, which extends from the esophagus to the anus. This plexus includes afferent nerve fibers, ganglionic cells, and efferent nerve fibers. It is assumed that the afferent nerve fibers pick up the sensations from the mucosa of the tract as well as from the serosa. These, in turn, pass across the ganglionic cells to the efferent nerve fibers, which go to all of the smooth muscle fibers and, in all probability, to most of the glands of the tract.

The myenteric plexus is probably responsible for both excitation and inhibition of these various structures, as well as for the control of the special motor functions of propulsion and mixing movements.

The gastrointestinal tract is innervated by both parasympathetic and sympathetic nerve fibers. It is believed, however, that nerve fibers from both systems probably synapse with ganglion cells in the myenteric plexus and that the myenteric plexus is responsible for excitation or inhibition of the tract. Stimulation of the parasympathetic nerve fibers will, in general, produce an increase in muscle tone, an increase in motility, and a relaxation of the sphincter muscles. The opposite occurs when the sympathetic nerve fibers are stimulated.

Needless to say, any one or all of the organs may be affected by cancer. When a malignant neoplasm affects any organ, the major concern relates to fluid and electrolyte balance since fistulas, drainage tubes, and so forth produce gross alterations.

SIGNS AND SYMPTOMS OF DYSFUNCTION OF THE GASTROINTESTINAL TRACT

It is most unfortunate that the symptoms of gastrointestinal disorders do not forewarn the possible presence of a malignant neoplasm. They are, for the most part, symptoms that may be present in any mild gastrointestinal disorder, and for this reason early diagnosis of a malignant neoplasm is a rare occurrence.

Anorexia may be present; on the other hand, the individual may have a good appetite or a desire for certain foods. Either condition may be affected by a change in emotional state, chemical or vascular variations, or impulses that are transmitted to the midbrain from the viscera by way of the vagus, pelvic and/or splanchnic nerves, or other organs.

Nausea is a second symptom often suggestive of an early malignant neoplasm. This can be defined as a revulsion for food. It is frequently associated with imbalances in the autonomic nervous system such as salivation, sweating, and tachycardia.

Vomiting is the sudden, forceful ejection of the contents of the stomach through the mouth. It is, in many instances, preceded by a sensation of nausea. The vomiting center in the medulla is activated directly by afferent impulses that arise within the gastrointestinal tract.

Constipation occurs when materials in the colon move too slowly through the large intestine. As a result, an excess amount of water is absorbed, causing the materials to become hard and dry, and evacuation becomes difficult. When the material is moved too rapidly through the colon, there is little opportunity for water absorption. This results in frequent, loose stools, or diarrhea.

Hematemesis, or the vomiting of blood, may cause the individual to seek advice from the physician, but not always. Here, again, this symptom does not necessarily suggest a diagnosis of malignant neoplasm. It may just as readily be a symptom of gastric ulcer, esophageal varices, or even disturbance of the clotting mechanism. Chronic gastritis with resultant erosion of the blood vessels may also be the cause of hematemesis. Thus, a diagnosis of malignant neoplasm of the stomach may not be considered.

Melena may be another symptom. This is defined as the passage of black, tarry stools or stools in which blood is present, but not in gross amounts. This, again, is not conclusive evidence that a malignant neoplasm is present, and all too often the individual is not really aware of the symptom. In all too many instances, awareness of blood in the stool suggests to the individual that he has hemorrhoids.

MALIGNANT DISORDERS OF THE GASTROINTESTINAL TRACT AND THEIR MANAGEMENT

Malignant neoplasms can occur in any area of the gastrointestinal tract, although they are relatively uncommon in the small intestine.

Numerous tests and procedures are available for the physician's use in confirming a diagnosis of malignant neoplasm. These include the following: gastrointestinal series (G.I. series); barium enema; endoscopy-esophagoscopy, gastroscopy, sigmoidoscopy, proctoscopy, proctosigmoidoscopy, or anoscopy; gastric analysis; insulin tolerance test; Papanicolaou balloon studies; gastric decompression; intestinal decompression; stool examinations; and biopsy. Any of these may confirm a diagnosis of malignant neoplasm.

Esophagus

Carcinoma of the esophagus causes obstruction of this organ, thereby making the swallowing of food more difficult as the tumor increases in size. This lesion most frequently develops in the middle or lower third of the esophagus. Dysphagia of a mild or intermittent nature may be the initial symptom of an early lesion. As time elapses, the individual may find it more and more difficult to swallow solid foods. Regurgitation and gradual weight loss are danger signals of this malignant neoplasm. As a member of a community, the nurse has a major responsibility to recommend an individual with any of these symptoms to see his physician immediately.

Unfortunately, even when first symptoms appear, the disease is already beyond early stages. In some instances, the disease has not extended to a stage of inoperability. In such cases, an esophagectomy is performed. The tumor is excised along with a margin of normal tissue, and the surrounding lymph nodes are dissected at the same time. When the lower third of the esophagus is involved, part of the stomach may be removed as well, due to its close proximity. This, then, is referred to as an esophagogastrectomy. If the lesion is too far advanced and the patient cannot tolerate major surgery, a gastrostomy may be the procedure of choice.

Preoperatively, the patient with a malignant neoplasm of the esophagus is in a poor state of nutrition. Attempts are made to replace nutritional deficiencies and to reestablish normal fluid and electrolyte balances. For this reason, it is imperative that the nurse maintain an accurate account of intake and output. If fluids can be taken orally, they should be high in caloric value and should be forced.

Skin care is of utmost importance to prevent the development of decubiti. Bony prominences must be protected, position must be changed at hourly intervals, and frequent backrubs with massage are required to avoid this complication.

Frequent mouth care is required to eliminate odor, foul breath, and a "bad taste." Mouthwashes should be offered prior to meal times and should be alternated so that they do not become identified with the foul taste in the mouth.

Since surgery for carcinoma of the esophagus frequently requires thoracic surgery, the patient should be taught principles relative to the need for coughing and turning postoperatively. He should also be aware of the fact that fluids by mouth will be restricted, a nasogastric tube will be necessary, and intravenous fluids will be required.

Following surgery, the first concern is maintenance of a patent airway. The nasal catheter is usually inserted to extend as far as the esophagogastric anastomosis or through it. This is always attached to continuous suction and after 3 to 5 days is removed. Following this, fluids are started by mouth and are increased daily. Soft foods are introduced gradually, and following discharge a regular diet is offered as tolerated. Depending on the patient's ability to tolerate a soft diet or a regular diet, the nurse is responsible for teaching both the patient and his family regarding his nutritional needs. She may, in some instances, need to consult with the dietitian regarding his nutritional needs. Both the nurse and the dietitian can reinforce his daily food intake following discharge. It may also be necessary to have both a social worker and a visiting nurse participate in his care when he goes home, and it will be the responsibility of the nurse to make the necessary arrangements.

Once again, emotional, psychological, and spiritual support must be offered since this type of surgery is extremely anxiety-producing along with being a most uncomfortable procedure.

Stomach

When a diagnosis of carcinoma of the stomach is made, the average lay person immediately associates this with impending death. Unfortunately many medical men also have the impression that such a diagnosis signifies a "hopeless" condition. The incidence of carcinoma of the stomach is particularly high in such countries as Japan, Iceland, Costa Rica, Chile, and Hawaii. The great consumption of smoked fish and smoked meats is believed to be a contributory factor. Other predisposing factors include: polyps; benign tumors, especially adenomas; atrophic gastritis; and chronic gastric ulcer, particularly within one half inch or so of the greater curvature, or in the pyloric segment, or in the posterior wall away from the curvatures.

Although no segment of the stomach is immune to carcinoma, these growths most commonly occur in the pyloric segment or in the region of the lesser curvature. They usually infiltrate rapidly and spread to regional lymph nodes as well as to the liver.

Carcinoma of the stomach has eight principal routes by which it spreads. These are the following: (1) in the stomach wall; (2) in the duodenal and esophageal walls; (3) to neighboring or distant lymph nodes via the lymphatic vessels; (4) to adjacent organs or to the abdominal parietes; (5) to distant organs via the bloodstream; (6) by the peritoneal cavity; (7) by transplantation; and (8) by transluminal implantation.

Clinical features of carcinoma of the stomach will vary according to the site of the lesion, the type of growth, and its size. Although many symptoms may be present, there are no pathognomonic signs of early gastric cancer. Nu-

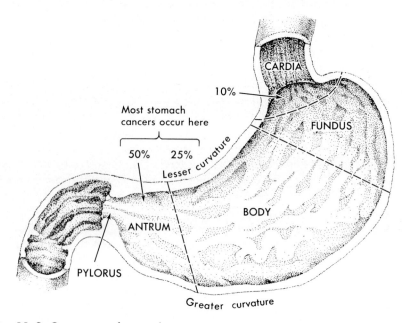

Fig. 11-2. Occurrence of stomach cancer.

merous symptoms, including epigastric pain or discomfort, dysphagia, nausea and vomiting, anorexia, and weight loss, are described by the patient, all of which may not necessarily alert the physician to look for a malignant lesion.

When gastric carcinoma is suspected, there are a number of diagnostic procedures that may be used to ascertain an accurate diagnosis. Of utmost importance is an accurate, complete, and detailed history accompanied by complete physical examination, including a rectal examination and numerous blood chemistries. Gastric analysis accompanied by cytologic study of gastric washings will also aid in diagnosis. A gastrointestinal series will be of value in pointing up any filling defects, altered pyloric function, diminished or absent peristalsis from involved areas of the wall of the stomach, etc. A complete blood count will verify or disprove any evidence of anemia. If, however, after these procedures have been carried out the diagnosis is still uncertain, an exploratory laparotomy is indicated. When surgery is contemplated, the patient must be evaluated with regard to his age, general physical status, general nutritional status, state of hydration, and amount of blood loss.

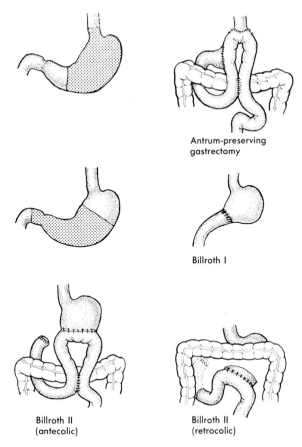

Fig. 11-3. Types of gastrectomy.

Once the diagnosis of gastric cancer has been made and the patient's status has been evaluated, surgery can be performed. If there is sufficient evidence that the lesion can be removed completely (and the patient's physical condition warrants it), radical surgery is the procedure of choice. Usually the patient will be admitted to the hospital about 3 days before such surgery is contemplated for further blood work, electrocardiogram, and roentgenographic examination. Preoperatively, the patient should receive a light, well-balanced, nutritious, nonresidue diet. In addition, vitamins B and C are given routinely. If the patient shows signs of dehydration or of fluid and electrolyte imbalance, these conditions must be corrected prior to surgery. Intravenous solutions of 5% glucose in saline can be given to combat dehydration. This will also stimulate both renal and hepatic function. Blood transfusions may be indicated prior to surgery especially if the hemoglobin or the hematocrit is lowered. Even when blood transfusion is not required prior to surgery, blood is usually started shortly before the patient is taken to the operating room and may be continued over the first 24 hours following the surgery. Gastric lavage is usually carried out once or twice daily following hospitalization and then 1 or 2 hours before the operation.

When total gastrectomy is the procedure of choice, this will probably involve a block dissection of the entire stomach, the first portion of the duodenum, the greater omentum, the upper leaf of the transverse mesocolon, the gastrosplenic omentum, the spleen, the tail and body of the pancreas (in many cases), the lesser omentum into the porta hepatis and as far to the right as where the hepatic artery gives off its feeding branches to the liver, the soft tissues around the cardia, and a cuff of the distal portion of the esophagus. All regional lymph nodes are excised and the vagus nerves must be isolated and severed.

Following surgery, the patient is usually maintained on intravenous feedings the first 3 or 4 days. Small sips of water can be given in the majority of

Table 11-1. Indications for total gastrectomy*

1. Carcinomatous leather-bottle stomach and diffuse gastric cancer
2. Large infiltrating gastric sarcomas of lymphoid origin, especially when they involve the proximal half of the stomach
3. Diffuse adenomatous polyposis of the stomach
4. Cancers involving the proximal half of the stomach, which include those situated at or near the cardia and those arising high up on the lesser curvature
5. Large or multiple leiomyosarcomas of the stomach, especially when the proximal half of the stomach is the seat of the lesion
6. Gastric ulcers situated at or about the cardia which are unsuitable for resection by Pauchet's method (rare)
7. Recurrent anastomotic ulcer following sub-total gastrectomy combined with vagotomy (rare)
8. Recurrent peptic ulcer associated with the Zollinger-Ellison syndrome

*From Maingot, R.: Abdominal operations, New York, 1961, Appleton-Century-Crofts, p. 355.

cases on the third postoperative day, and if well tolerated a liquid diet is started on the fourth day following surgery, at which time the nasogastric tube can be removed. Most patients can then gradually progress to a semisoft or soft diet and then to full diet as tolerated.

No surgical procedure is entirely without complications, and total gastrectomy may be accompanied by a variety of such complications and sequelae. These are listed in Table 11-2.

Nursing care for these patients begins at the time of admission to the hospital. The nurse assumes responsibility for assisting the physician in overcoming nutritional disturbances as well as fluid and electrolyte imbalances. Accurate measurement of intake and output will be an essential procedure. Since respiratory complications may occur in the immediate postoperative period, the nurse can minimize the chances of pneumonia or atelectasis by teaching the patient preoperatively the technique of deep breathing and use of coughing exercises that will aid in improving muscle function. By offering the patient oral mouthwashes at frequent intervals, she can promote elimination of oral sepsis. Rigid adherence to giving medications as ordered may correct avitaminosis and other disorders such as anemia. She can prepare the patient prior to gastric lavage so that he understands why such a procedure is necessary and can, therefore, be more cooperative when it is performed. This will be helpful for the physician and less disagreeable for the patient at the same time.

Postoperatively, the nurse has major responsibilities in terms of accurate observation for adverse reactions to blood transfusions, measurement of intake

Table 11-2. Complications and sequelae of total gastrectomy*

I. Immediate
   A. Chest complications: atelectasis, pneumonia, bronchopneumonia, cardiac failure, embolism
   B. Peritonitis and subphrenic abscess
   C. External fistula due to breaking down of anastomosis
   D. Wound infections and disruption of abdominal wounds
   E. Steatorrhea
   F. Acute small gut obstruction
   G. Avitaminosis, especially deficiencies in vitamin B
   H. Phlebothrombosis and thrombophlebitis
II. Late
   A. The "dumping syndrome"
   B. Hematological complications
   C. Dysphagia; stenosis of the esophagoenteric stoma
   D. Symptoms caused by nutritional, metabolic, and functional derangements, e.g., hypoproteinemia, steatorrhea, loss of weight, anorexia
   E. Intestinal obstruction
   F. Incisional hernia
   G. Recurrence of growth

---

*From Maingot, R.: Abdominal operations, New York, 1961, Appleton-Century-Crofts, p. 356.

and output, administration of medications that will usually include morphine sulfate for pain, ferrous sulfate for secondary anemia, vitamin B 12, antibiotics, and so forth. The patient will need supportive care in turning, deep breathing, and coughing, and the nurse can be of great value in assisting him at these times. In most cases, the patient can be discharged about 2 weeks after surgery. The nurse will need to make long-range plans so that the patient understands thoroughly what he can and cannot do, what he can or cannot eat, and how to care for himself adequately when he goes home. The importance of the follow-up visits to his surgeon should be stressed.

Many patients will develop symptoms that specifically point to the "dumping syndrome." Such conditions may occur early following surgery once the patient has returned to a regular diet of three meals daily. In other instances, patients may develop symptoms referred to as the late syndrome, once a normal dietary regimen has been adopted. Either group of symptoms may last for as short a period of time as 1 year—or they might never disappear.

In some instances, the patient will undergo surgery for a total gastrectomy

Table 11-3. Dumping syndrome*

I. Early syndrome: usually the onset is fairly sudden and occurs a few minutes after the meal is finished; any or all of the following symptoms may be present:

  A. Nausea and weakness with a feeling of distention in the epigastrium.

  B. A general and unpleasant sensation of warmth all over the body, which may be accompanied by a cold sweat standing out on the forehead and face.

  C. The patient is conscious of the action of his heart and may say that it "seems to fill the whole chest"; there is also a general sense of fatigue and sometimes extreme exhaustion so that he is compelled to lie back and shut his eyes; in addition, there may be dizziness and pallor.

  D. Eructation of wind, borborygmi, and sometimes explosive diarrhea.

  E. The average attack lasts about 45 minutes and is accompanied by a rise in pulse rate and blood pressure, but there is no significant change in the blood sugar level, which steadily rises throughout.

II. Late syndrome: usually these symptoms occur during the second or third hour after a meal and coincide with a precipitate fall in blood sugar.

  A. Gradual onset of a fine tremor of the hands and legs, which is associated with profuse sweating and a sense of anxiety.

  B. Tremors may be accompanied by vertigo, exhaustion, and lassitude.

  C. In some instances, there is a distinct sensation of hunger and emptiness.

  D. Palpitation, throbbing in the head, a feeling of faintness, and occasional loss of consciousness may occur.

  E. Glycosuria and postprandial diuresis are common.

  F. Marked fall in blood pressure during attack.

  G. Late syndrome is much less serious than the early variety, and often patients will not complain about the syndrome unless they are specifically questioned on the matter.

---

*Adapted from Maingot, R.: Abdominal operations, New York, 1961, Appleton-Century-Crofts, pp. 399-403.

through the transthoracic approach. These patients will return to the floor and be placed in an oxygen tent. Water seal drainage is usually instituted if an intercostal or abdominal drainage tube has been inserted. In order to avoid repetition, care of the patient in an oxygen tent with water seal drainage will be discussed in detail in Chapter 13 in the section on carcinoma of the lung.

The patient can usually be removed from the oxygen tent within 12 to 14 hours. If cyanosis occurs, this may be indicative that the patient has excessive bronchial secretions, bronchial obstruction, hemothorax, or pneumothorax. Such complications may be prevented or minimized if the patient has been taught deep breathing exercises and how to cough properly. Coughing should be encouraged shortly after pain medication has been administered. Changes of posture will also aid in the expulsion of bronchial secretions, while inhalation of compound tincture of benzoin in steam or cold steam may help to render the mucus less tenacious. Early ambulation should be encouraged since many complications may be avoided if the patient becomes active. It cannot be overemphasized that physical, physiological, psychological, and spiritual support are essential for a smooth recovery for the patient and a less apprehensive period for his family.

Small intestine

Malignant lesions develop less frequently in the small intestine than in any other part of the alimentary tract—when present they are found most often at the upper end of the jejunum or the lower end of the ileum. Unfortunately, there are no early symptoms—the symptoms are usually those of intestinal obstruction, intestinal bleeding, a palpable mass in the abdomen, or perforation. Adenocarcinoma, malignant lymphoma, and sarcoma are the types of malignant neoplasms most commonly encountered. Except for certain lymphosarcomas, treatment of neoplasms of the small intestine is surgery. Prognosis is poor since these tumors tend to metastasize relatively early before the primary tumor has attained a considerable size. Also, due to the abundance and extreme functional activity of the lymphatics in this region, a considerable portion of the bowel wall is involved before symptoms appear, thereby making early diagnosis almost impossible.

Patients with malignant neoplasms of the small intestine are generally admitted to the hospital in a debilitated state, or in a state of acute or chronic intestinal obstruction. Preoperatively, it usually is necessary to give blood transfusions since anemia is inevitably present. Fluid and electrolyte imbalances are corrected by intravenous therapy with glucose and saline, and any other electrolytes as indicated from laboratory findings. Decompression of the proximal intestine is carried out by insertion of either a Miller-Abbott or a Cantor tube connected to continuous suction. The patient is usually acutely ill and will require painstaking nursing care.

Since the patient is acutely ill, he will usually be placed on complete bed rest. Frequently, there will have been considerable weight loss, and for this reason care must be taken to ascertain that bony prominences are protected to prevent formation of decubiti.

Ileostomy. Inasmuch as malignant lesions occur in the jejunum or in the lower end of the ileum, an ileostomy will be the procedure of choice in most instances, with wide excision of the lesion so that normal tissue is viewed in the pathological specimen. Since the contents of the ileum are semiliquid, special bags have been developed to collect the drainage. On occasion, a visit and talk from a patient who has adjusted well to this procedure is helpful. It can often allay fear and apprehension for the patient.

The patient is usually placed on a low-residue diet for 3 to 5 days prior to surgery and will receive only clear fluids for the 24 hours before the operation takes place. Sulfonamides or intestinal antibiotics are usually prescribed to lower the bacterial count and to prevent infection of the suture line postoperatively. With the insertion of a nasogastric or intestinal tube, accurate recording of intake and output is essential in order to maintain a normal fluid and electrolyte balance. The nurse must also be aware of symptoms that indicate any fluid or electrolyte imbalance so that it can be corrected immediately.

Abnormal losses of fluids and electrolytes from the intestinal tract can occur as a result of vomiting, diarrhea, and/or use of a nasogastric or Miller-Abbott tube. This may lead rapidly to severe imbalances, since in severely ill

Table 11-4. Physiological effects of splenectomy*

 I. Changes in the blood:
   A. Red blood cells: Following splenectomy there is a transient erythrocytosis, the red cells tend to be thinner, and some of them contain nuclear remnants described as Cabot or Howell-Jolly bodies.
   B. Platelets: The number of platelets is increased temporarily—thrombocytosis.
   C. White blood cells: There is an increase in the total number of white cells, this being almost entirely due to an increase in the number of polymorphonuclear leukocytes. The white blood count slowly returns to normal, there may be a slight eosinophilia, and with this there is often an increase in the number of mast cells.
 II. Enlargement of the lymph nodes: There is a slight general enlargement of all the lymph nodes in the body, due to compensatory increased hematopoietic activity.
III. Changes in the bone marrow: The yellow marrow in the long bones is gradually replaced by red marrow, this change usually being complete within 6 months. After about one year the bone marrow returns to its former state.
 IV. Changes in the reticuloendothelial system: As the spleen contains a large collection of lymphoid tissue and a considerable amount of reticuloendothelial elements, the specialized cells of the remaining portion of this system undergo marked proliferation.
  V. Hypertrophy of accessory spleens.
 VI. An increase of iron in the liver and copper in the tissues.
VII. Diminished resistance to infection (especially under 12 years of age).
VIII. Diminished metabolic activity of the liver.
 IX. Splenosis.

---

*Adapted from Maingot, R.: Abdominal operations, New York, 1961, Appleton-Century-Crofts, p. 445.

patients the amount of fluid lost may approach 15 to 20 liters, and suction as well as indwelling tubes can account for considerable fluid loss.

Many disturbances can result from large amounts of intestinal fluid losses. These losses may result in:

1. Changes in osmolarity of blood serum caused by the difference in concentration of sodium (Na^+) in the intestinal fluids as compared with blood. This can result from the loss of gastric juice and fluids through a Miller-Abbott tube where a greater proportion of water is lost in comparison to the amount of sodium ion. This results in an elevation of sodium concentration with a loss of water.

2. Where diarrhea is a presenting problem, bile and pancreatic fluids make up a large part of the excretion; thus there is a lower concentration of sodium ion with no change in the osmolarity. However, there is considerable alteration in electrolyte balance since, with a nasogastric or Miller-Abbott tube, the amount of chloride ion loss is much greater than that of sodium ion. This can lead to alkalosis. Diarrhea, on the other hand, results in acidosis. Fluids must be replaced along with the electrolytes that have been lost.

When an ileostomy has been performed, an ileostomy bag must be placed over the stoma so that fecal drainage will not pour out over the abdomen and into the incision. This will promote healing and prevent complications. For the first few days, the drainage may be extremely minimal; however, when peristalsis returns and the patient begins to eat, drainage may be profuse. Usually within six weeks following surgery, the edema disappears and the stoma will be at its normal size, at which time a permanent ileostomy bag can be applied. This permanent bag will usually last from 1 to 2 years and is made of a form of plastic material or rubber.

The patient should be taught how to change the bag, how to care for it, and proper care of the skin around the stoma. A belt is usually worn to hold the bag securely in place. The elastic band at the bottom of the bag can be removed and the fecal material allowed to flow into the toilet. The bag can then be washed by using a small Asepto syringe filled with soapy lukewarm water followed by rinsing with clear warm water. Every 2 or 3 days the bag should be changed. At this time, the skin area should be washed and dried thoroughly before replacing the bag. The bag that has been removed should be washed thoroughly in soapy water and allowed to soak in a weak solution of vinegar or chlorine household bleach. This will not only eliminate odors but will also increase the life of the bag.

The patient who has had an ileostomy may have considerable difficulty in adjusting and will, therefore, need a great deal of encouragement, emotional support, and instruction. In some instances, it is advisable that a referral be made to the visiting nurse service for follow-up care in his home after discharge. She can then reinforce teaching of care, proper diet, etc. A member of the family may be taught how to care for the patient, especially if he seems reluctant or hesitant. Here, again, the visiting nurse can provide the necessary support so that appropriate care is maintained.

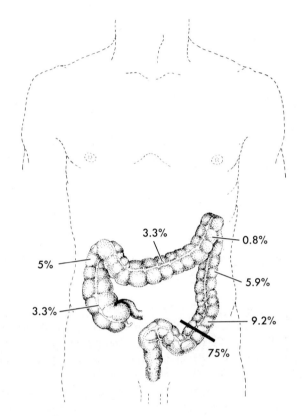

Fig. 11-4. Locations of cancer of colon and rectum.

Large intestine

It is estimated that cancer of the colon and rectum will strike 73,000 Americans this year, more than any other type of cancer except skin.* Although the etiology of these lesions is still not known, much progress has been made with regard to treatment and earlier diagnosis. It is a well-known fact that there are numerous lesions that, if not removed, can be considered as premalignant lesions. Among these are isolated polyps, pseudopolyps, familial polyposis, adenomas, papillomas, leiomyomas, argentaffinomas, and so forth. For this reason, it is deemed essential that at the time of an annual physical examination, every person over 40 years of age have a proctoscopic examination as part of the routine physical.

In the early stages of the disease, the symptoms are extremely vague or, in many instances absent. The chief presenting symptoms do, however, fall into one of three areas: mainly, abdominal pain, alteration or change in bowel function, or rectal bleeding.

Cancer of the colon has a tendency to grow slowly and to remain localized

---

*1967 Cancer facts and figures, New York, 1966, American Cancer Society, Inc., p. 22.

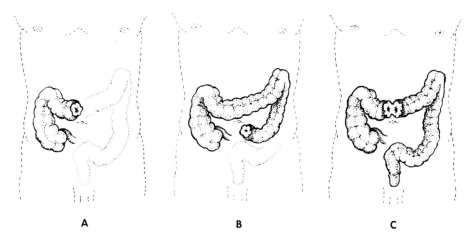

Fig. 11-5. Types of colostomies. **A** and **B,** Permanent colostomies following abdominoperineal resection. **C,** Transverse colostomy, may or may not be permanent.

for a considerable period of time. Extension of the lesion may occur by: direct spread in the bowel wall; direct infiltration of adjacent tissues or spread by continuity; invasion of the lymphatic vessels and glands; bloodstream invasion resulting in metastasis to distant sites; transperitoneal implantation; and/or intraluminal transplantation of cancer cells.

Diagnostic measures must be undertaken in a specific sequence if a malignant lesion is suspected and if surgical treatment is to be effective. A careful history with a meticulous physical examination that includes a digital rectal examination may well be diagnostic in approximately 50% of cases; proctoscopy and sigmoidoscopy are extremely important as diagnostic tools. If the diagnosis still remains inconclusive, other x-ray procedures may prove of value, especially a flat plate of the abdomen, a barium enema, a double contrast enema (barium enema followed by insertion of air to distend the bowel), and laboratory examination of blood and stools. If diagnosis is still uncertain, a laparotomy is indicated.

Preoperatively, general measures to correct the systemic effects of the lesion and to improve the patient's health status are employed. This may involve blood transfusions, replacement of fluids and electrolytes, a high-protein, low-residue diet, supplementary vitamins, antibiotics, colonic irrigations, and introduction of a Miller-Abbott tube. In most instances, prior to surgery, the insertion of a Foley catheter is advisable since these patients experience considerable problems with voiding postoperatively. Obviously, the patient's emotional status must be evaluated as well as his cardiovascular and renal status prior to any form of surgical intervention. When a permanent colostomy is anticipated (or even considered), the patient should be made aware of this. Sufficient time should be allowed to answer his questions, allay his fears, and assist him to accept the procedure that will in no way interfere with his normal social or economic life.

These same principles apply as well to carcinoma of the rectum. The operative procedures may vary, however, depending on the extent of involvement. In some instances, a dry colostomy may be the procedure of choice; a wet colostomy may need to be the procedure finally decided upon depending on the extent of involvement, while a partial pelvic exenteration may be the procedure required (Chapter 12).

When an individual is faced with rectal or colon surgery, his previous experiences with such problems will vividly color his reaction to it. He may react in any number of ways to such a situation, in terms of his training as a child with regard to bowel elimination, his attitudes toward the diagnosis of cancer, his reaction to body image, his role in the family or community, or his reaction to life itself. For these reasons, it is essential that the nurse develop a good rapport with the patient and provide the necessary understanding and

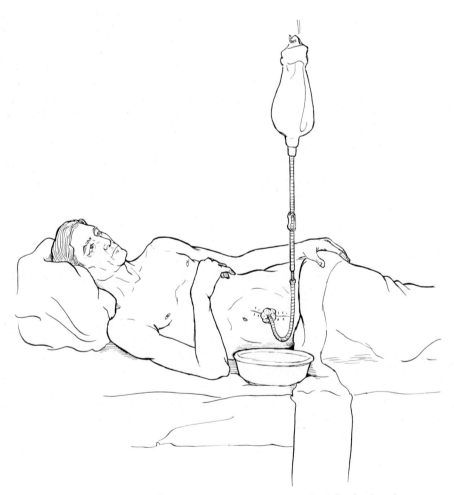

Fig. 11-6. A-C, Colostomy irrigation. **A,** Alternative method for bed patient.

emotional support that will prove invaluable through the various phases of his illness and hospitalization.

To help in meeting the need for understanding and emotional support, the nurse must be understanding and nonjudgmental so that the patient will feel free to verbalize his feelings, fears, and questions and not have them cut off abruptly by a noncommittal response. In order to do this, the nurse must be aware of her own needs and understand her own feelings so that she can feel comfortable in discussing the patient's problems with him. Merely verbalizing assent can lead to the patient's inacceptance for the operative procedure required and a loss of faith in his surgeon as well as in himself.

The patient usually needs assistance in accepting the varied diagnostic procedures that take place prior to therapy. Reinforcement and clarification of such procedures can allay fear, make the patient accept them, and make him cooperate in their being performed.

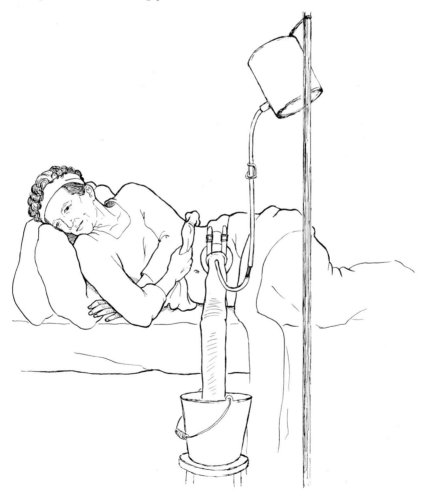

Fig. 11-6, cont'd. B, Another alternative method for bed patient.

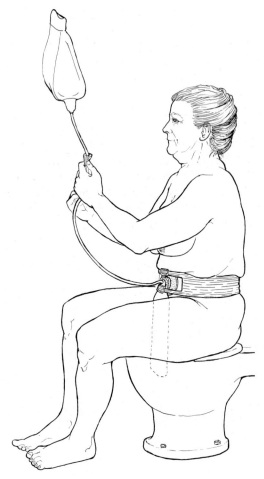

Fig. 11-6, cont'd. C, Ambulatory patient irrigates colostomy in bathroom.

Colostomy. Following surgery, the nurse is required to help the patient who has had a permanent colostomy adjust to living with it. All of the nursing measures in the immediate postoperative period must be adhered to (maintenance of adequate respiratory exchange, turning from side to side to prevent accumulation of fluid in the lungs, frequent checking of vital signs, constant observance of dressings for excessive bleeding, etc.). Early ambulation is essential to prevent complications including pneumonia, urinary tract infection, and thrombophlebitis. Medication for pain should be given as needed during the first 2 or 3 days postoperatively as deemed necessary by the nurse. The patient should not have to ask or have to be asked whether or not he needs it.

Once the colostomy has been opened, it is of paramount importance that the nurse provide meticulous care to the skin area surrounding the stoma. Various ointments are available that may be used to prevent excoriation.

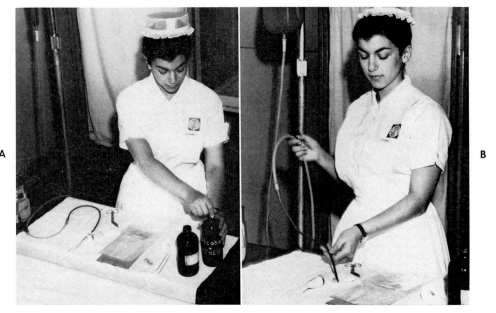

Fig. 11-7. A, Nurse prepares equipment for colostomy irrigation. **B,** Nurse lubricates catheter prior to irrigation.

These should be applied each and every time the dressing is changed. Tincture of benzoin around the stoma will serve to protect the skin as well as to adhere a temporary plastic bag over the opening. This temporary plastic bag can be changed as often as is necessary and will allow for ambulation accompanied by fewer accidents.

If an abdominoperineal resection has been performed, the perineal wound will require irrigation following the initial stage of healing. This can be accomplished by using a one-half strength solution of hydrogen peroxide at first. At a later stage, sitz baths will promote drainage, cleanliness, and wound healing by increasing circulation as a result of the water temperature.

The extent to which the patient can adjust to a colostomy is frequently determined by the degree to which he can get it under control. This will vary according to the anatomical location of the colostomy. The patient must also be taught that proper diet, adequate fluid intake, regularity as to time of irrigation, and emotional status are factors that may affect the functioning and control of his colostomy. Referral to the visiting nurse is usually essential so that she can evaluate his understanding of the care of the colostomy and assist him with any further adjustments that he or his family need to plan. This entails a well-prepared and detailed interagency referral to ensure continuity of care. In this way, too, the visiting nurse in the home can contact the hospital nurse or physician to discuss whatever problems she encounters in providing guidance and assistance to the patient and his family.

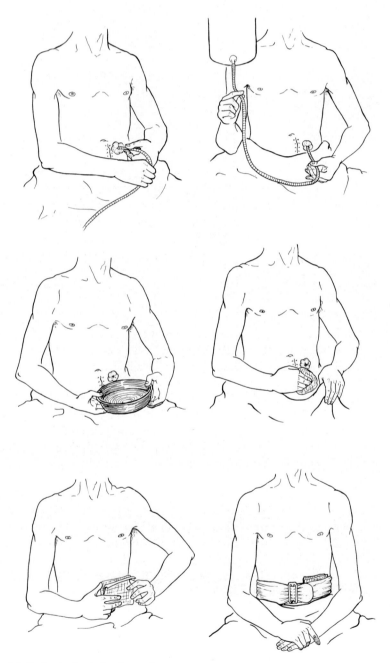

Fig. 11-8. Steps for irrigation colostomy.

PHYSIOLOGY OF ACCESSORY STRUCTURES OF THE GASTROINTESTINAL TRACT

Several glands share an important function in the digestive process, and for this reason it would seem appropriate to consider them at this time. Both the liver and the pancreas are derivatives of the digestive tract in their embryonic development and are connected by their ducts to its wall. The salivary glands produce secretions essential to the digestive process and are, therefore, considered to be accessory structures. Cancer can affect any of these structures either as a primary lesion or as a result of metastasis.

Salivary gland·

Three pairs of salivary glands open into the oral cavity and are named according to their location. They are the parotid, the submaxillary, and the sublingual. These glands secrete saliva into the oral cavity when sensory nerve endings in the oral mucous membrane are stimulated by sight, smell, or taste of food or other substances. The saliva helps prepare the food for digestion in the stomach and small intestine. Many smaller glands (buccal glands) continually secrete saliva, which keeps the mucous membrane of the mouth and pharynx moist and lubricated at all times.

Saliva is a colorless, viscous fluid composed of water, various salts, some protein (chiefly mucin) with small amounts of albumin and globulin, and the enzyme ptyalin. It has a pH ranging from 6.0 to 7.9. The quantity and quality

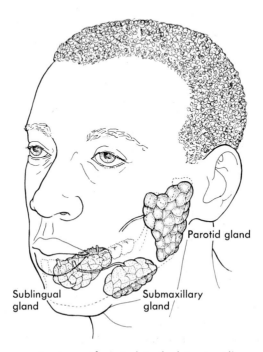

Fig. 11-9. Accessory structures of gastrointestinal tract, salivary glands.

of salivary secretion will vary according to type of stimulation, time of day, age, dietary intake, and so forth. On an average, however, between 1,000 and 1,500 ml. are secreted each day. Salivary secretion is governed by the anatomical nervous system since the glands are innervated by both the sympathetic and the parasympathetic systems.

When a mass occurs in the cheek or upper neck adjacent to the ear, one should certainly consider the possibility of a tumor of the parotid gland. This salivary gland is one of the most frequently involved in terms of malignant disease. If such a mass is slow growing, freely movable, and of long duration, it can be predicted that this will no doubt be a benign lesion. When such a lesion enlarges rapidly, is fixed or adherent to adjacent structures, and is accompanied by pain or dysfunction of the facial nerve, it is almost certain to be a malignant tumor of the gland.

Since all lesions of the parotid gland (benign and malignant) are radioresistant, surgery is the treatment of choice. Ideally, the tumor along with a surrounding margin of normal tissue must be removed if a cure is to be anticipated. While parotid tumors are relatively uncommon, they may occur at any age.

Malignant lesions occur most frequently in middle age and beyond, and males are more often affected than females.

The parotid gland is the largest of the three major salivary glands. It lies on the masseter muscle and extends backward toward the external ear. The carotid artery, jugular vein, and facial nerve are in close proximity to the gland. The patient with a tumor of the parotid gland is usually admitted to the hospital one day prior to surgery for a careful history and physical examination. Routine laboratory studies, including a roentgenogram of the chest, are essential to rule out possible mediastinal or pulmonary metastases. Blood typing and cross matching are of paramount importance since many major blood vessels are in close proximity to the area involved. The hair should be washed the night before surgery, and, if necessary, the hair around the ear should be shaved (particularly if radical surgery is anticipated).

The patient is usually anxious and apprehensive, and the nurse can often assist him to verbalize his fears and clarify any questions he might have. She will of necessity have to ascertain what the physician has told the patient in order to reinforce the physician's explanation. This is especially true when radical surgery is planned, since the patient will require a tracheotomy. Careful planning preoperatively will enhance the patient's adjustment in the early postoperative period. Since the patient will be unable to speak postoperatively, the nurse will need to determine the best method whereby he can communicate with other people. In some instances, the patient may not read or write, or he may not speak English. The nurse, by obtaining such information, can procure the appropriate equipment prior to surgery. On occasion, it may be necessary to develop some simple hand motions that will provide the means of communicating after surgery.

It is important, too, that the nurse demonstrate the suction equipment and how it is used. She should teach the patient how to do his own suctioning as well, since this will provide him with a feeling of security and promote self-confidence. Prior to surgery, all equipment is placed at the bedside.

Following radical surgery, tracheotomy care is extremely important. Some type of inhalator is placed at the bedside to prevent drying and crusting of the tracheal secretions. Usually a moistened 4 by 4 inch gauze compress is kept over the tracheal stoma, and the patient can be taught to change this for himself. Tracheal suctioning should be carried out as often as necessary to prevent accumulation of secretions.

When a mandibulectomy has been performed, a nasal feeding tube is passed and tested by the doctor on the first postoperative day. If possible, the patient should receive an explanation of this prior to surgery. Water is used for the first feeding, after which time formula is given about six times daily. Fruit juice or coffee may be substituted, if the patient wishes, for one or two formula feedings.

As soon as the feeding tube is removed, the patient can be given small amounts of food including gruel, Jell-o, and custard. Since the patient may experience some pain on chewing for the first few days, the nurse should plan to be available at meal times to offer support and encouragement. Gradually semisolid foods, baby foods, and ground meats can be offered, and when he can swallow these without difficulty, he will be ready to go home.

Patients who have had head and neck surgery usually do not experience severe pain, and usually buffered aspirin or Darvon will suffice to alleviate discomfort. This can be given through the nasal feeding tube at first, but oral forms should be introduced as soon as possible to encourage swallowing.

When it has been necessary to sacrifice the facial nerve, the patient may have difficulty in controlling facial movements. Salivation may also present a problem for the first few days. This can be overcome by tucking a small gauze tampon into the side of the mouth and changing it whenever necessary.

Since our culture places great emphasis on physical fitness and beauty, the patient with a facial deformity may have a difficult time in adjusting to the surgery. The nurse is in a position to help the patient overcome the fear of surgery and cope with the facial deformity if she is alert to his needs. Patience and understanding are essential throughout the postoperative period, along with constant encouragement.

Liver

The liver is the largest gland in the body. It is an irregular, wedge-shaped organ weighing between 1,450 and 1,750 grams in the adult. The organ occupies the upper right hypochondriac and epigastric regions directly beneath the diaphragm. The largest and thickest portion fits snugly under the right dome of the diaphragm while the thinner portion extends across the epigastrium into the left subdiaphragmatic region. The liver is divided into four lobes, namely, the right, left, caudate, and quadrate. However, both the caudate and the quadrate lobes are really subdivisions of the right lobe. The organ is anchored in place by five peritoneal folds or ligaments: the coronary ligament, the right triangular ligament, the left triangular ligament, the falciform ligament, and the lesser omentum (hepatoduodenal and gastrohepatic ligaments).

The stroma is described as consisting of four elements: (1) the hepatic capsule, which is a dense network of collagenous fibers containing blood vessels and lymphatic channels; (2) ramified trabeculae that extend from the capsule into the parenchyma as portal canals; (3) a narrow connective ring in the central canal that surrounds the hepatic veins; and (4) the reticular framework of the liver consisting of fine fibers arranged around the hepatic cells.

Three types of cells are associated with liver tissue. These are the cells of the biliary duct system, the Kupffer cells, and the hepatic cells. The Kupffer cells are important in antibody production and bile formation. They also serve to remove foreign bodies and dead and injured red blood cells from the circulation. The hepatic cells are responsible for the majority of functions of the liver, such as in: (1) carbohydrate, protein, fat, mineral, and vitamin metabolism; (2) heat production; and (3) detoxification of poisons and drugs circulating in the blood. More specifically, some of the more important functions of the liver include:

1. Formation and secretion of bile.
2. Excretion of substances withdrawn from the blood such as drugs and heavy metals.
3. Detoxification by conjugation, methylation, oxidation, and reduction.
4. Protein metabolism:
   a. Forms albumin, globulin, and fibrinogen.
   b. Produces prothrombin.
   c. Forms urea and uric acids and removes ammonia from the blood.
5. Fat metabolism:
   a. Synthesizes cholesterol.
   b. Two thirds of the cholesterol in plasma is esterified with fatty acids (the liver maintains this ratio).
   c. 80% of cholesterol metabolized is transformed by the liver into various bile acids that in turn are excreted in the bile.
6. Carbohydrate metabolism:
   a. Gluconeogenesis—conversion of protein and fat to carbohydrate.
   b. Glycogenesis—conversion of glucose to glycogen.
   c. Conversion of lactic acid to glycogen.
7. Enzyme production—transaminases are enzymes that catalyze the transfer of an amino group from:
   a. Aspartic acid to ketoglutaric acid to form glutamic and oxaloacetic acids (glutamic-oxaloacetic transaminase–GO-T).
   b. Alanine to ketoglutaric acid to form glutamic and pyruvic acids (glutamic-pyruvic transaminase GP-T).
8. Vitamin metabolism:
   a. Forms vitamin A from carotene.
   b. Converts vitamin K to prothrombin.
   c. Stores vitamins A, D, and B complex.

9. Stores iron, copper, and other minerals.
10. Stores the erythrocyte-maturing factor (antipernicious anemia factor).
11. Produces heparin, an anticoagulant.
12. Aids in maintaining body temperature by heat production due to metabolic activities.
13. Plays an important role in immune and defense mechanisms by the activity of the Kupffer cells.

The incidence of primary carcinoma of the liver is exceedingly rare and has been estimated at less than one half of one percent (0.5%) of all forms of carcinoma reported in the United States. Primary hepatomas (carcinoma arising in the liver cells proper) and cholangiocarcinomas (carcinoma arising in the cells lining the bile ducts) are the forms most commonly encountered. The disease occurs more frequently in females than in males.

Once the patient is admitted to the hospital, numerous laboratory tests, roentgenograms, and so forth are performed. These can be extremely trying for the patient—for many of them he must be in a fasting condition. This can be particularly difficult for the patient who has no major symptoms of liver involvement. The nurse will have to develop an extremely good rapport with the patient, explain every test as well as possible, and indicate why these tests and procedures are important (Table 11-5).

Fortunately, for the patient with primary malignant disease there is a good possibility for a cure. For the past ten years there has been an opportunity for surgery if only one lobe of the liver is involved. With improved techniques, it is possible to perform either a right or a left lobe hepatectomy for malignant disease of the liver.

Primary liver tumors are associated with abdominal pain, jaundice, anorexia, and ascites. Fever is frequently a presenting symptom. Weight loss and diarrhea may also be a chief complaint.

When a decision has been made to resect a portion of a diseased liver, the patient is admitted and laboratory tests are carried out (Table 11-5). Patients who are heavy smokers are asked to reduce or even stop smoking to prevent postoperative complications.

The patient suspected of carcinoma of the liver (either primary or metastatic) is frequently emotionally upset and apprehensive. It is of vital importance that the nurse, therefore, be aware of the problems and anxieties that the patient is facing. It is essential that she make herself readily available to both the patient and his family to provide reassurance and to discuss any problems they might have. In this way, she can alleviate apprehension (for the patient and his family) with regard to hospitalization and care.

Once all of the extensive laboratory tests have been completed and the patient has taken numerous medications (especially vitamins), as well as having undergone a daily colonic irrigation, he will be ready for surgery. During the entire preoperative period, the nurse needs to clarify the reasons for all medications as well as to explain that the daily colonic irrigation will help minimize infection postoperatively, especially, should further abdominal exploration and surgery be indicated.

Table 11-5. Liver function tests along with normal values

Test	Normal value
Albumin/globulin ratio	−1.5 + 1.0
Serum albumin	3.2 − 5.6 Gm./100 ml.
Serum globulin	1.3 − 3.2 Gm./100 ml.
Alkaline phosphatase	1.0 − 5.4 Bodansky units
Bromsulphalein (B.S.P.)	Normal retention of the dye is 5% at 30 minutes and no dye at 45 minutes
Cephalin-cholesterol flocculation	Negative − 1+
Galactose tolerance test	3.0 Gm. or less secreted in urine within 3 to 5 hours; blood sugar returns to normal within one hour; I.V., none found
Glucose tolerance test	Peak of not more than 75-minute specimen 150 mg./100 ml. of serum with return to fasting level within 2 hours; intravenous return to fasting level within 1 hour
Hippuric acid test	Intravenous test: 0.7 Gm. of hippuric acid excreted in 1 hour; oral test: 3.0 Gm. in a 4-hour period
Icterus index	4 - 6 units
Plasma cholesterol	Normal total blood cholesterol 150 to 250 mg./100 ml. 60% to 70% esterified
Prothrombin level	11 to 18 seconds—100% of normal
Serum transaminase	40 units
Urine bilirubin content	Normally not found in urine
Gmelin test	
Harrison test	
Huppert-Cole test	
Urobilinogen content	Average—0.64 mg.
Wallace-Diamond test	Normal—4.0 Gm. in 24 hr.
Urobilinogen in feces	50 - 250 mg./day
van den Burgh test	0.1 - 1.0 mg./100 ml.
Indirect reaction—very small amount of bilirubin bound to protein present in blood serum; precipitation of protein in blood serum with alcohol; illness likely to be hemolytic; direct reaction-free bilirubin due to obstruction; alcoholic extract not neccesary	

Since a colonic irrigation is ordered as a daily procedure, the nurse will ascertain that the patient is positioned comfortably on his side with knees flexed. The lubricated rectal tube is inserted approximately 4 inches into the rectum, and fluid is allowed to flow into the rectum slowly until 400 to 500 ml. have been instilled. The return fluid clamp is then released, allowing the rectal drainage to drain into a pail. This procedure is continued until rectal drainage is clear. Results are charted and will include the amount of fluid used, the type and consistency of returns, and how the patient tolerated the procedure.

On the evening prior to surgery, a Levin tube is inserted and attached to suction. Preoperative shaving of the abdomen and chest may be done at the same time or may be done in the morning before the patient is taken to the operating room.

During the preoperative period, the patient is taught deep-breathing exercises and how to cough, so that following surgery these procedures will not be completely new to him. When a recovery room is available, the patient is usually kept there for the first 48 hours, since this is the most crucial period in terms of his ultimate recovery.

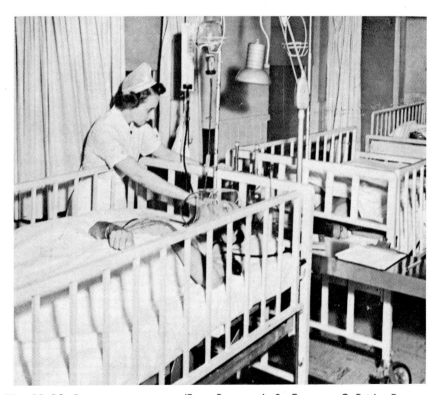

Fig. 11-10. Recovery room care. (From Brunner, L. S., Emerson, C. P., Jr., Ferguson, L. K., and Suddarth, D. S.: Textbook of medical-surgical nursing, Philadelphia, 1964, J. B. Lippincott Co., p. 273.)

The patient is maintained on intravenous fluids, blood transfusions, and constant suctioning through the Levin tube. Because the surgery involves opening of the thoracic cavity, underwater chest drainage tubes are connected to underwater seal drainage bottles (Chapter 13), and nasal oxygen is administered to help the patient regain conciousness as rapidly as possible. Vital signs must be checked every 15 minutes until stable, and then every hour. Dressings must be checked by the nurse at frequent intervals to ascertain whether or not the patient may be bleeding.

Skin care is of utmost importance. Cleansing with sterile saline followed by thorough drying (patting dry with a sterile towel) before redressing will help prevent excoriation and wound infection. On occasion, the doctor will request that all dry and soiled dressings be weighed. This can provide an estimate of body fluid loss so that fluid and electrolyte imbalances are avoided.

Once the patient has regained consciousness, deep breathing and coughing every hour are essential to stimulate normal respiratory and circulatory processes and to prevent complications. The nurse can assist the patient when coughing if she places her hands over the incision, thereby splinting the operative site.

The patient is usually most comfortable in a semi-Fowler's position. It is the nurse's responsibility, however, to ascertain that his position is changed frequently. This will also serve to prevent respiratory and circulatory complications. Small pillows appropriately placed will make the patient more comfortable and will also prevent formation of decubitus ulcers and reddened areas at pressure spots.

It is imperative that the nurse maintain an accurate measure of intake and output. This means keeping a careful record of urinary output, Levin tube, and chest tube drainage. This will minimize any chance of fluid and electrolyte imbalance from occurring.

During the time the Levin tube is in place, the patient will receive nothing by mouth. Since the mucous membrane is under constant irritation from the Levin tube and dry from mouth breathing, a mixture of lemon juice and glycerin as a mouth swab will provide considerable relief. Mineral oil applied to the lips will also prevent cracking and chapping.

The nurse will want to maintain a patent Levin tube in order to control abdominal distention and elimination of gastric contents, thereby minimizing nausea and vomiting. Irrigation of the tube whenever necessary (at least every 3 hours) will keep the tube patent and draining freely.

While the patient has a Levin tube connected to suction, any medications ordered for him are added to the intravenous solution whenever possible. Those medications that cannot be administered intravenously are usually administered intramuscularly until such time as they can be tolerated by mouth. Usually 5 days postoperatively (or when bowel sounds are audible), the Levin tube can be removed, and water and clear liquids can be started. The diet is increased gradually to semisoft, soft, and regular as tolerated.

About 3 days after surgery, the patient is allowed to dangle. Frequently this procedure is carried out after pain medication has been administered.

This will minimize any pain or discomfort the patient may experience at this time.

Further care is similar to that for any other major surgical procedure; that is, the patient is encouraged to carry out as much of his own care as possible as soon as it is feasible. The nurse uses every opportunity to teach him and his family in terms of immediate convalescence following discharge as well as long-range goals including good health measures and follow-up care. Again, referral to the visiting nurse or the public health nurse can reinforce teaching for both the patient and the family and can greatly enhance a more rapid rehabilitation.

Pancreas

The pancreas is a soft, red-gray or yellow-gray gland lying in front of the first and second lumbar vertebrae behind the stomach. Shapewise, it resembles a hammer, having a head, body, and tail. Normally it weighs between 2 and 3 ounces. The organ is a racemose gland composed of lobules each consisting of one of the branches of the main duct that terminates in a cluster of pouches or alveoli. Lobules are joined together in the same manner to form lobes, which in turn comprise the gland. The small ducts from each lobule open into the duct of Wirsung, which runs transversely from the tail to the head through the substance of the gland. The duct of Wirsung and the common bile duct lead into the duodenum. A short tube, formed by the union of these two ducts, is dilated and is referred to as the ampulla of Vater.

Interalveolar cell islets (more commonly referred to as the islands of Langerhans) are surrounded by a rich network of capillaries and furnish the internal secretion (insulin) of the pancreas.

The pancreas has two major functions, mainly: secretion of pancreatic fluid and formation of insulin.

The pancreas can be affected by every possible type of disorder including congenital malformations, inflammatory disease, benign tumors, and cancer. Malignant lesions include islet cell adenoma (may or may not be malignant), islet cell carcinoma, carcinoma of the pancreas and periampullary area, and metastatic disease.

Carcinoma of the pancreas, despite its origin, presents similar problems with regard to diagnosis, treatment, and nursing care. For the most part, initial symptoms are vague, and once diagnosed accurately, the condition is no longer in the early stages of the disease.

Primary carcinoma of the pancreas comprises about 1% to 2% of all carcinomas. It is more prominent in males than in females and can occur anywhere between 30 and 60 years of age. It is more common, however, in the older age group.

Presenting symptoms, again vague, include a steady, dull, midepigastric pain that extends to the lower portion of the back; the pain may be paroxysmal or radiating, or it may present as a colicky pain originating in the right hypochondrium, sometimes extending to the subscapular area. Jaundice is observed in about 75% of the cases. It may be persistent or intermittent depending on the site of the primary lesion (head of pancreas or region of the ampulla of Vater). Weight loss, usually rapid and severe, is a common complaint. Invariably, fatigue is a major complaint. This may well be due to the rapid weight loss as well as to the drain on the metabolism of the body from the malignant neoplasm. Vague digestive symptoms including anorexia, nausea, vomiting, chills, fever, and diarrhea and/or constipation may be expressed. Jaundice, an enlarged liver, and a palpable gallbladder are frequent physical findings.

Metastatic disease may involve any or all organs of the body. In order of frequency, the regional lymph nodes, liver, and lungs may be involved. Involvement of other organs varies.

When the patient's physical status warrants, surgical resection may be undertaken. This will entail Whipple's procedure. Preoperative preparation is extensive and may take 4 to 5 days before surgery can be planned. The patient is usually quite debilitated on admission. For this reason, a high-carbohydrate, high-protein, low-fat diet is prescribed along with oral supplements of vitamins. Intravenous glucose may also be given. With anorexia, nausea, and vomiting as presenting symptoms, the nurse will have to utilize every form of encouragement to get the patient to eat. She will need to explain the importance of such food intake in terms of the surgical procedure planned for him.

Blood transfusions are frequently indicated preoperatively to combat anemia and depleted blood volume. Here, again, this may cause undue anxiety for the patient, who may believe firmly that blood transfusions are given only when death is imminent. Since the liver is frequently involved, vitamin K must be supplemented in order to overcome prothrombin deficiency. Antibiotics are administered to the patient preoperatively to prevent infection and to minimize postoperative complications. A gastric lavage is undertaken prior to surgery, and the tube is left in place to maintain gastric decompression postoperatively for at least 72 hours, or until flatus is passed. This will prevent dilatation of the loop of the jejunum, which is anastomosed to the pancreas.

Pancreaticoduodenectomy (Whipple's procedure) may be carried out in comparatively few cases, since this procedure is performed in one stage. Usually the patient is not in good enough condition (or considered to be a good operative risk) for such radical surgery. In some cases, therefore, the procedure may be undertaken in two stages. In the first stage, obstruction of the biliary tract is relieved so as to permit a free flow of bile into the intestinal tract. This, in turn, will decrease jaundice and provide improvement of the state of nutrition, thus improving liver and kidney function. Therefore, the risk of more extensive surgery is lessened. The time lapse prior to the second stage of surgery should be sufficiently long to permit the patient to become a "good" surgical risk with as near normal laboratory reports as possible. In the second stage, the duodenum and pancreas and, in some instances, a portion of the stomach are dissected. The jejunum is then anastomosed to the cut end of the common bile duct. The remaining portion of the pancreas is also anastomosed to the side of the jejunum a short distance distal to the choledochojejunal anastomosis. The divided end of the stomach is then anastomosed to the jejunum several inches distal to the pancreaticojejunostomy.

Nursing care for these patients is essentially the same as that for the patient with hepatic lobectomy and, for this reason, will not be repeated. These patients, in the majority of instances, are acutely ill and will require ingenuity, creativity, and patience on the part of the nurse who undertakes their care. They do, indeed, present a tremendous challenge for her in terms of technical and imaginative skill, psychological support, and family assistance.

Bibliography

A cancer source book for nurses, New York, 1963, American Cancer Society, Inc.

Ackerman, L. V., and del Regato, J. A.: Cancer: diagnosis, treatment, and prognosis, ed. 3, St. Louis, 1962, The C. V. Mosby Co.

Anderson, R., and Byars, L. T.: Surgery of the parotid gland, St. Louis, 1965, The C. V. Mosby Co.

Anthony, C. P.: Fluid imbalances, formidable foes to survival, Amer. J. Nurs. **63**:75, December, 1963.

Bacon, H. E.: Cancer of the colon, rectum, and anal canal, Philadelphia, 1964, J. B. Lippincott Co.

Bacon, H. E., and Berkley, J. R.: Plea for early diagnosis in cancer of the colon and rectum, Ca **9**:24, 1959.

Beahrs, O. H., et al.: Surgical management of parotid lesions, Arch. Surg. **80:890,** 1960.

Beeson, P. B., and McDermott, W., editors: Cecil-Loeb textbook of medicine, ed. 11, Philadelphia, 1963, W. B. Saunders Co.

Bockus, H. L.: Gastroenterology, ed. 2, Philadelphia, 1963, W. B. Saunders Co., vol. 1.

Bockus, H. L.: Gastroenterology, ed. 2, Philadelphia, 1964, W. B. Saunders Co., vol. 2.

Bockus, H. L.: Gastroenterology, ed. 2, Philadelphia, 1965, W. B. Saunders Co., vol. 3.

Boles, R. S.: Precancerous lesions of the stomach, how to treat them, Postgrad. Med. **27**:359, 1960.

Brubaker, W.: A message to all new ileostomy, colostomy, and ileal bladder patients, United Surgical Supplies Co., Inc., Portchester, N. Y., reprint, 1962.

Brunner, L. S., Emerson, C. P., Jr., Ferguson, L. K., and Suddarth, D. S.: Textbook of medical-surgical nursing, Philadelphia, 1964, J. B. Lippincott Co.

Cabera, A., and Lega, J.: Polyps of rectum and colon in children, Amer. J. Surg. **100**: 551, 1960.

Cancer manual for public health nurses, Washington, D. C., 1963, United States Department of Health, Education and Welfare, Public Health Service, No. 1007.

Ceulemans, G.: Total pelvic exenteration for rectal cancer, Progr. Roy. Soc. Med. **52**:47, 1959.

Collins, J. K.: Care of the colostomy patient, Nurs. World **134**:24, 1960.

Conley, J., and Arena, S.: Parotid gland as a focus of metastasis, Arch. Surg. **87**:757, 1963.

Converse, J. M.: Reconstructive plastic surgery, Philadelphia, 1964, W. B. Saunders Co., vol. 3, Head and neck.

Crumpacker, E. L., and Baker, J.: Proctosigmoidoscopy in periodic health examination, J.A.M.A. **178**:169, 1961.

Davis, L., editor: Christopher's textbook of surgery, ed. 7, Philadelphia, 1960, W. B. Saunders Co.

Davisohn, I., and Wells, B. B.: Todd-Sanford clinical diagnosis by laboratory methods, ed. 13, Philadelphia, 1963, W. B. Saunders Co.

Deddish, M. R., and Whiteley, H. W.: Complications of abdominoperineal resection for cancer of the rectum, Surg. Clin. N. Amer. **44**:449, 1964.

Derricks, V. C.: Rehabilitation of patients with ileostomy, Amer. J. Nurs. **61:**48, May, 1961.

Dockerty, M. B.: Pathologic aspects in the control of colonic carcinoma, Proc. Mayo Clin. **33:**157, 1958.

Drummond, E. E., and Anderson, M. L.: Gastrointestinal suction, Amer. J. Nurs. **63:**109, December, 1963.

Dukes, C. E.: The etiology of cancer of the colon and rectum, Dis. Colon Rectum **2:**27, 1959.

Dyk, R. B., and Sutherland, A. M.: Adaptation of the spouse and other family members to the colostomy patient, Cancer **9:**123, 1956.

Fields, J. B., editor: Cancer: diagnosis and treatment, Boston, 1959, Little, Brown & Co.

Fisher, J. A.: The dumping syndrome, Amer. J. Nurs. **58:**1126, 1958.

Frazell, E. L., Strong, E. W., and Newcombe, B.: Tumors of the parotid, Amer. J. Nurs. **66:**2702, 1966.

Godwin, T. S.: Polyps of the colon and rectum in children, Southern Med. J. **54:**526, 1961.

Gore, D. O., et al.: Tumors of salivary gland origin, Surg. Gynec. Obstet. **119:**1290, 1964.

Grollman, S.: The human body: its structure and physiology, New York, 1964, The Macmillan Co.

Hallberg, J. C.: The patient with surgery of the colon, Amer. J. Nurs. **61:**64, March, 1961.

Hampton, J. M., Meyers, J., and Bacon, H. E.: A simplified method for the diagnosis of cancer of the colon by exfoliative cytology, Dis. Colon Rectum **4:**177, 1961.

Hertz, R.: Rectum and colon, including perianal area, GP **21:**111, 1960.

Horwitz, A., and Rosensweig, J.: Carcinoma of the gallbladder—a real hazard, J.A.M.A. **173:**234, 1960.

Ingles, T., and Campbell, E.: The patient with a colostomy, Amer. J. Nurs. **58:**1544, 1958.

Klug, T. J., Lucinda, et al.: Gastric resection—and nursing care, Amer. J. Nurs. **61:**73, December, 1961.

Krouse, J. M., Eyerly, R. C., and Babcock, J. R.: Tumors of the small bowel, Amer. J. Surg. **101:**121, 1961.

Kurihara, M.: The patient with an intestinal prosthesis, Amer. J. Nurs. **60:**852, 1960.

Lindner, J.: Inexpensive colostomy irrigation equipment, Amer. J. Nurs. **58:**844, 1958.

Lyons, A. S.: Ileostomy—management and complications, Surg. Clin. N. Amer. **35:**1411, 1955.

McHardy, G., editor: Current gastroenterology, New York, 1962, Harper & Brothers.

McNeer, G.: Stomach, small intestine and pancreas, GP **21:**140, 1960.

Magruder, L., and Rauch, M. K.: Nursing care in gastric resection, Amer. J. Nurs. **61:**76, December, 1961.

Maingot, R.: Abdominal operations, New York, 1961, Appleton-Century-Crofts.

Marshall, S. F.: Carcinoma of the stomach, Postgrad. Med. **27:**683, 1960.

Martin, H.: Radical neck dissection, Clin. Sympos. **13:**103, 1961.

Martin, H.: Surgical removal of parotid tumors, Clin. Sympos. **13:**121, 1961.

Maynard, A. de L., and Froix, C. J. L.: Immediate morbidity after thoracotomy for esophageal disease, Surg. Clin. N. Amer. **44:**349, 1964.

Mini-Guide (Catalog No. 21-200), Portchester, New York, 1963, United Surgical Supplies Co., Inc.

Molander, D. W., and Brasfield, R. D.: Liver surgery, Amer. J. Nurs. **61:**72, July, 1961.

Pack, G. T.: The current status of gastric cancer, Ca **11:**239, 1961.

Pack, G. T., and Ariel, I. M., editors: Treatment of cancer and allied diseases, ed. 2, New York, 1962, vol. 5, Tumors of the gastrointestinal tract, pancreas, biliary system, and liver, Paul B. Hoeber, Inc.

Raskin, H. F., Moseley, R. D., Jr., Kirschner, J. B., and Palmer, W. L.: Carcinoma of the pancreas, biliary tract and liver, Ca, pp. 137 and 166, 1961.

Remine, W. H., Priestly, J. T., and Berkson, J.: Cancer of the stomach, Philadelphia, 1964, W. B. Saunders Co.

Rousselot, L. M., and Slattery, J. R.: Immediate complications of surgery of the large intestine, Surg. Clin. N. Amer. **44:**397, 1964.

Rowe, R. J., and Barnett, W. D.: Cancer of the rectum, Dis. Colon Rectum **3:**194, 1960.

Scott, H. T.: The nurse and the ileostomist, Nurs. World **134:**29, 1960.

Secor, S. N.: Colostomy care 1964, Amer. J. Nurs. **64:**127, September, 1964.

Shafer, K. N., Sawyer, J. R., McCluskey, A. M., and Beck, E. L.: Medical-surgical nursing, ed. 3, St. Louis, 1964, The C. V. Mosby Co.

Shahon, D. B., and Wangensteen, O. H.: Early diagnosis of cancer of the gastrointestinal tract, Postgrad. Med. **27:**306, 1960.

Spratt, J. S., Ackerman, L. V., and Moyer, C. A.: Relationship of polyps of colon to cancer, Ann. Surg. **148:**695, 1958.

Stacy, R. W., and Santolucito, J. A.: Modern college physiology, St. Louis, 1966, The C. V. Mosby Co.

Statland, H.: Fluid and electrolytes in practice, ed. 3, Philadelphia, 1963, J. B. Lippincott Co.

Thoma, K. H.: Oral surgery, ed. 4, St. Louis, 1963, The C. V. Mosby Co.

Thomas, W. H., and Coppola, E. D.: Distant metastases from mixed tumors of the salivary glands, Amer. J. Surg. **109:**724, 1965.

Virgadamo, B. T.: Care of the patient with liver disease, Amer. J. Nurs. **61:**74, July, 1961.

Wolfman, E. F., Jr., and Flotte, C. T.: Carcinoma of the colon and rectum, Amer. J. Nurs. **61:**60, March, 1961.

Zuidema, G. D., and Klein, M. K.: A new esophagus, Amer. J. Nurs. **61:**69, September, 1961.

Chapter 12

Management of the patient with a urinary tract or reproductive system disorder

Cancer of the urinary tract comprises 7% of all cancers in the male and 3% of all cancers in the female, while that of the genital organs is considerably higher (12% in the male and 21% in the female).* The American Cancer Society estimates that there will be approximately 31,000 new cases of kidney and bladder lesions diagnosed in 1967, with 15,000 deaths from these lesions.† New cases of prostatic cancer diagnosed are expected to number 34,000 with 16,000 deaths in the same year. Uterine cancer will be diagnosed in 44,000 persons, with 14,000 dying from the disease.†

ANATOMICAL, PHYSIOLOGICAL, AND GENERAL FUNCTIONS OF THE URINARY TRACT

In any discussion of the urinary tract, anatomy and physiology must be considered before any comments can be made regarding pathology.

A brief review of the anatomical features of the tract will suffice. The kidney, on gross appearance, consists of the pelvis (upper expanded end of the ureter), calyces (cuplike cavities of the pelvis), medulla (inner striated portion made up of cone-shaped pyramids), and the cortex (outer portion of the kidney).

The kidneys are located on either side of the spinal column opposite the last thoracic and first three lumbar vertebrae. They are embedded in a fatty capsule called the adipose capsule and are held in place by means of renal fascia, abdominal muscles, and pressure and counterpressure of the neighboring

---

*Cancer incidence by site and sex, 1967 Cancer facts and figures, New York, 1966, American Cancer Society, Inc., p. 5.

†Reference chart: Leading cancer sites, 1967 Cancer facts and figures, New York, 1966, American Cancer Society, Inc., p. 5.

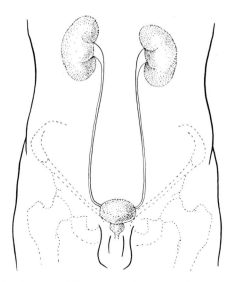

Fig. 12-1. Schematic diagram of kidneys, ureters, and bladder.

organs. The microscopic structure of the kidney reveals the renal tubules, blood vessels surrounding the tubules, lymphatics, nerves, connective tissue, and the renal (malpighian) corpuscles. The nephron, the basic structural unit of the kidney, is a rather complex microorgan composed of many parts, each of which serves a specific function in the process of urine formation. The major functions of the kidney are to keep body fluids at normal constancy by removing waste substances as well as toxic substances from the blood. Another function is the regulation of osmotic pressure of body fluids by adjustment of water elimination. Further, the kidney plays a major role in the regulation of body salt content, blood sugar level, and acid-base balance. These functions are carried out in the process of urine formation and excretion. Normally urine is produced at a rate of 1 to 2 ml. per minute but may reach a maximum of 20 ml. The urine collects in the pelvis of the cavity. The ureters commence as calyces in the pelvis of the kidney and serve as a passageway for the urine from the kidney to the urinary bladder.

The ureters are two tubular ducts consisting of an epithelial lining surrounded by a connective tissue layer. This, in turn, is surrounded by muscular fibers arranged in three layers—inner longitudinal, middle circular, and outer longitudinal.

The urinary bladder is a hollow muscular organ located in the pelvic cavity behind the pubes, in front of the rectum in the male, and in front of the anterior wall of the vagina and neck of the uterus in the female. The organ is held in place by folds of peritoneum and fascia. Its size, shape, and position depend upon age, sex, and the degree of fullness or emptiness. The bladder is lined with mucous membrane. Connecting this mucous membrane to the muscular layers is areolar connective tissue. Like the ureters, the bladder has the same three muscular coats. A serous layer, derived from peritoneum, serves as a partial outer covering. At the base of the bladder the smooth muscle coat passes around the urethral opening to form the internal sphincter. The urethra is a membranous canal that extends from the bladder to the urinary meatus. This canal is approximately 8 inches long in the male but only 1½ inches long in the female. An external sphincter surrounds the urethra a short distance below the inner sphincter. It is composed of striated muscles and is innervated by the pudendal nerves, which are spinal somatic nerves, so that regulation of this sphincter is under voluntary control.

The nephron of the kidney includes Bowman's capsule and the tubules. It is designed to help keep the composition of the blood constant. As the blood passes through Bowman's capsule, all of the substances in the plasma that have small enough molecules filter through the membranes to enter the cavity of the capsule, which is continuous with the tubule. Only proteins fail to be filtered in this manner. As the filtrate flows through the tubule, water and many of the other constituents are reabsorbed by the tubular cells. Sometimes the tubules will actually excrete more of a particular substance into the filtrate instead of absorbing it, in order to maintain the normal blood content. Thus, it can be said that formation of urine involves the filtration through Bowman's capsule where an ultrafiltrate is made of blood plasma; then reabsorption of some of the materials of this ultrafiltrate takes place in the tubules, including necessary amounts of water and salts to maintain the internal environment and, finally, tubular secretion where the end product is urine.

Since the anatomy, physiology, and general functions have been touched upon only briefly, it is suggested that any good textbook on anatomy and physiology be consulted for a more detailed description and discussion.

DISORDERS RESULTING FROM KIDNEY DYSFUNCTION

Ackerman and Regato have indicated that kidney tumors constitute about 2% of all malignant tumors in the adult and 20% of those in children.* Malignant renal tumors occur chiefly in middle life between 40 and 60 years of age with the exception of Wilms' tumor, which is found primarily in children up to 4 years of age (Chapter 9).

The majority of renal tumors are adenocarcinomas or renal cell tumors. They have often been referred to as hypernephromas; however, this gives no indication as to origin or specific structure involved. They are, by far, the commonest type of tumor encountered. They usually arise in the parenchyma of the kidney. On gross examination they appear as rounded or globular masses with an irregular nodular surface quite well differentiated from the normal renal substance. They tend to grow toward the medullary portion of the kidney and its pelvis. On a cut surface, the tumor is a rich yellow color having areas of hemorrhage and necrosis commonly present. On microscopic

---

*Ackerman, L. V., and del Regato, J. A.: Cancer: diagnosis, treatment, and prognosis, St. Louis, 1962, The C. V. Mosby Co., p. 795.

examination, the cells of the tumor are characteristically large, pale, polyhedral in shape, and contain small pyknotic nuclei.

These tumors often grow slowly. Metastasis may develop at any time; however, many authorities are in agreement that the tendency to metastasize is in direct proportion to the size of the lesion. When metastasis does occur, it is predominantly by invasion of the blood vessels. Thus, adenocarcinomas can metastasize to the lung, bones, regional lymph nodes, liver, and other viscera.

Another type of malignant parenchymal tumor is composed of small granular cells with small deep-staining nuclei. These tumors are also adenocarcinomas. They usually are grayish in color and show a marked tendency to infiltrate more rapidly than the hypernephroma since hypernephromas are not encapsulated. For this reason, they are considered to be of a higher grade of malignancy and have a poor prognosis.

Papillary carcinoma of the kidney pelvis is a third distinct type of tumor encountered. These tumors form soft red or gray masses and characteristically have smooth glistening surfaces. They sometimes resemble small pedunculated polyps with irregular surfaces. The main tumor is often surrounded by smaller masses. These usually represent direct invasion of the ureter. Oddly enough, local recurrences are frequent following surgical excision, but distant metastases are rarely observed.

A relatively uncommon tumor is the ulcerating epidermoid carcinoma arising from the kidney pelvis. These tumors are usually associated with pyelonephritis and nephrolithiasis. They tend to metastasize rapidly to the regional lymph nodes, and, at the time of diagnosis, distant metastases are also noted.

Carcinomas of the kidney rarely produce specific symptoms until the tumor mass has attained a considerable size. Usually the earliest and most common complaint is that of painless hematuria. It should be emphasized here that no patient with a history of hematuria should be released from medical supervision until a thorough investigation as to its cause is adequately established. Once in a while, a patient may complain of renal colic. This may result from the passage of long wormlike blood clots down the ureter from hemorrhagic areas within the tumor. Pain is present in about half of the patients seen. It is often dull in character unless it is due to the passage of blood clots, when it is described as "colicky." Since renal tumors rarely produce symptoms until they have reached a considerable size, presence of a palpable mass may be one of the chief complaints of the patient.

Many authorities are in agreement that in the individual who complains of hematuria, pain, and has a palpable mass in the kidney region, a malignant renal tumor should be suspected. Still other authorities maintain that this triad of hematuria, pain, and palpable mass is evidence of advanced disease and a poor prognosis.

When a diagnosis of renal carcinoma is suspected, the patient should be hospitalized at the earliest possible time. A careful and complete history and physical examination are indicated once the patient has been admitted. Intensive diagnostic studies are required before therapy can be appropriately prescribed. A flat plate of the abdomen (commonly referred to as a K.U.B. plate) will determine the size and position of the kidneys, ureters, and bladder. It can also visualize the presence of stones or other gross abnormalities. A retrograde pyelogram, where radiopaque solutions are injected through ureteral catheters, will provide a means of evaluating the bladder, ureters, or kidneys in terms of abnormal findings and neoplastic disease. Cystoscopic examination is also a routine measure in determining the presence of malignant disease.

It is often the responsibility of the nurse to explain these various procedures to the patient. While the physician may have given a brief explanation, the nurse can reinforce his explanation and clarify any questions the patient might have concerning them. Unless such procedures are fully understood, the patient's fears will undoubtedly make him anxious and tense. This entails recommending that the patient drink one to two glasses of water before going for the cystoscopy. The nurse can allay some of his fears by indicating that he will receive a sedative before going for the procedure and that he will receive adequate medication for pain as needed following the treatment. The nurse will do well to force fluids after the patient has returned. If anesthesia has been administered, she will not administer fluids until the patient has fully reacted.

Renal aortography may also be performed as a diagnostic measure particularly when benign cysts or malignant tumors are suspected. This procedure is carried out by the injection of radiopaque material through a long needle introduced through the back into the aorta near the renal arteries while the patient is on the x-ray table.

Many other tests are utilized in the diagnosis of any renal disease including malignant tumors of the kidney. One of the first tests undertaken (whether in the doctor's office or on admission to the hospital, or both) is urinalysis. This consists merely of collecting a voided urine specimen in a bottle. If any abnormal findings occur in this voided specimen, catheterization is usually recommended as a means of differential diagnosis.

Once in a while it is helpful to have separate specimens collected from the same voiding. This is referred to as the multiple glass test. It is frequently a means of determining where the abnormality lies within the urinary tract.

When an order is written to obtain a urine specimen for culture, it may be obtained either by catheterization or as a catch specimen on voiding, depending on the physician's preference.

Many other renal function tests may be ordered depending on what the physician anticipates the final findings and diagnosis may be. The majority of these tests involve urinalysis or blood determinations.

Once a diagnosis of malignant tumor of the kidney has been established, appropriate therapy will be initiated. This may take the form of radical surgery or radiation therapy depending on the extent of invasion of the disease.

Malignant tumors of the kidney are most often treated by radical surgery if the prognosis appears favorable. Radical surgery implies removal of the perinephric fat, the entire Gerota's fascial capsule, the adrenal gland, a major portion of the ureter along with the kidney, as well as removal of the paracaval and paraaortic nodes. This type of procedure is best accomplished by means of a thoracoabdominal approach, which permits a wider exposure of the kidney and allows for exploration of the retroperitoneal space with a minimum of trauma. Findings of distant metastases may contraindicate the extensive procedure initially planned.

In papillary carcinoma of the renal pelvis, radical surgery is also indicated. This will entail removal of the entire kidney and ureter including the intramural portion within the bladder wall in order to minimize local recurrence of the tumor.

If surgical intervention is deemed impossible or impractical, adenocarcinomas of the kidney are, for the most part, radiosensitive. However, since these tumors tend to metastasize to areas in the ureters, radiation therapy can serve only as a means of palliation in inoperable or recurrent cases. It also serves as a means of palliation in the treatment of metastases.

In caring for a patient with a confirmed diagnosis of malignant disease of the kidney (whether he knows his diagnosis or not), it is extremely important that the nurse establish good rapport with him as quickly as possible. In this way, she can anticipate his needs, be aware of the questions in his mind that are probably overwhelming to him, and help the family understand the entire therapeutic regimen as well. Many patients have the impression that losing a kidney means imminent death. Still others are of the opinion that death is preferable to surgery since by removal of a kidney they will die anyway. The astute nurse can help overcome these anxieties and fears by discussing what will take place with both the patient and his family.

Once a malignant renal tumor has definitely been diagnosed, the treatment of choice is radical nephrectomy unless distant metastatic lesions have been noted on roentgen-ray examination. In this event, local excision of the tumor may be indicated to relieve pain from pressure as a result of the size of the lesion. On occasion, the lesion may be a small one that appears localized, and radical surgery will not be necessary.

When the tumor appears to be localized to the kidney, nephrectomy may be performed through a flank incision. This procedure involves special nursing responsibilities due to the operative site as well as to the fact that the kidney is highly vascular.

Preoperatively, the nurse can be most helpful by preparing the patient for various diagnostic procedures that will be carried out. Maintaining open channels of communication with the physician, the nurse is in a good position to reinforce his recommendations with the patient and his family. When the specific surgical procedure has been determined, the nurse can begin to teach the patient regarding his postoperative care. If she knows, for example, that the kidney will be removed through a flank incision, she can teach the patient deep breathing and coughing exercises that will be helpful in the immediate postoperative period when it will be essential that he cough and take deep breaths at least every 2 hours. Deep breathing postoperatively can be quite painful since the incision extends from directly below the diaphragm, and the patient is often reluctant to take deep breaths or move about. He can also be taught how to turn from side to side since this, too, will be expected of him in the postoperative period. All of these measures will minimize possible development of atelectasis or hypostatic pneumonia.

Since pain can be quite severe, narcotics should be given every 4 hours for the first 2 days, after which time they can gradually be decreased. Part of the reason for the patient having severe pain is the result of the hyperextended position required for the surgery. The patient may experience some relief if the nurse uses pillows to support the back while he is on his side.

A common postoperative complication is abdominal distention, which may be the result of paralytic ileus of reflex origin. In some patients who have had ureteral colic prior to surgery, this condition may be quite severe. Because this does occur with such frequency, the patient is usually maintained on intravenous fluids for the first 24 to 48 hours, after which time fluids may be started by mouth.

Various therapeutic measures may be ordered to minimize the amount of discomfort produced by abdominal distention. A heating pad to the abdomen and insertion of a rectal tube may help the patient expel flatus. Neostigmine may be ordered to promote expulsion of flatus. Here, again, insertion of a rectal tube and turning the patient on his side will help the gas to pass along the bowel. If the condition persists, carminative enemas may prove successful in elimination of flatus. Thorough preparation for and clarification of the procedure prior to its administration by the nurse will alleviate tension and anxiety for the patient.

Because of the vascularity of the kidney, the patient should be observed closely for any signs of hemorrhage. This may occur on the day of operation, although the nurse must be alert to the fact that hemorrhage may occur as late as 8 to 10 days postoperatively. This is thought to coincide with the period when tissue sloughing normally occurs in healing. Some physicians will order the patient back on bedrest on the eighth day postoperatively in an effort to prevent hemorrhage from occurring. The patient should be informed by the physician why he is being placed back on bedrest, and the nurse can reinforce, clarify, and interpret this for the patient. The patient may become depressed or anxious believing that his condition has regressed, and the nurse can alleviate this depression and anxiety by making herself available to the patient and his family during this period.

When the kidney is widely resected in an attempt to remove all adjacent tissues involved in the lesion, the surgical procedure may be performed through a transthoracic approach. A catheter is inserted into the thoracic cavity postoperatively and attached to underwater chest drainage. (Nursing care of the patient with underwater chest drainage will be discussed in Chapter 13.)

Occasionally, when radical surgery has been performed, the pleura may accidentally be perforated, and the patient should be observed closely by the nurse for any evidence of spontaneous pneumothorax. Any signs of dyspnea, restlessness, anxiety, increased diaphoresis or symptoms of shock, or complaint from the patient of sudden sharp chest pain should be reported immediately, keeping the patient quiet and in a semi-Fowler's or high Fowler's position until the doctor arrives. In the interim, the nurse should ascertain that oxygen is available for emergency use and that a thoracentesis set is at the bedside. The patient should not be left alone at this time since he will be extremely apprehensive and will need a great deal of emotional support.

DISORDERS RESULTING FROM URINARY BLADDER DYSFUNCTION

Carcinoma of the urinary bladder occurs more frequently in males than in females. The great majority of these tumors occur in individuals between 50 and 69 years of age, although the disease has been reported occasionally in younger individuals.

While the etiology is not known, various theories have been cited as premalignant factors in its onset. Carcinoma of the bladder is known to occur more frequently in workers of the dye industry. Thus, it may be considered an occupational disease for this group. Several authorities have shown a definite association between long-standing smoking habits and the development of cancer of the bladder in men. There is also a definite association noted between leukoplakia and epidermoid carcinoma of the urinary tract.*

Transitional cell carcinoma is the most common type of primary bladder tumor encountered. These tumors appear to arise from the transitional epithelium of mucous membrane. Thus, in all probability the benign papilloma can be considered the precursor to this disease. The lesion may appear as a cauliflowerlike papillary growth or may be flat and invade the wall.

---

*Ackerman, L. V., and del Regato, J. A.: Cancer: diagnosis, treatment, and prognosis, St. Louis, 1962, The C. V. Mosby Co., p. 822.

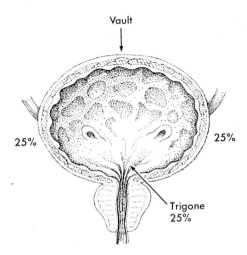

Fig. 12-2. Location of cancer of bladder.

Adenocarcinoma is a rare tumor encountered in the bladder, the incidence being under 2% of all bladder tumors. Malignant tumors arising from the wall of the bladder are even less common, comprising about 1% of the total bladder lesions.

Treatment of carcinoma is dependent upon the size of the lesion and the depth of tissue involvement. Small superficial tumors may be treated by transurethral resection and fulguration, implantation of radon seeds, or, if the tumor involves the dome of the bladder, segmental resection may be the procedure of choice.

Slight variations will result in nursing care, depending on the therapy initiated. The patient who has had a transurethral resection and fulguration of the tumor may or may not have a Foley catheter. The nurse can anticipate that his urine may be slightly tinged due to the operative procedure. The patient will frequently complain of a burning sensation on urination. Knowing that this is a common complaint, the nurse can request that the physician leave appropriate orders to cover her so that she can initiate measures as soon as the symptom appears. Application of a heating pad to the bladder region is often comforting. A sitz bath applies the same principle as the heating pad and can also be soothing for the patient as well as provide early ambulation. The patient can usually be discharged within a few days after operation.

Radon seeds may be implanted around the base of a tumor. This may be accomplished through a cystotomy, or they may be implanted through a cystoscope. The tumor is usually excised and fulgurated before the seeds are implanted. The patient may or may not have a cystotomy tube. It is more likely that only a urethral catheter will be used.

Since radon seeds emit alpha, beta, and gamma rays, the nurse will need to observe principles of time, distance, and shielding in caring for the patient for the first 4 days. The patient is likely to have a severe cystitis caused by the irradiation effects. The nurse should be aware of this problem and offer the patient medication as needed or as ordered by the physician. She can apply a heating pad to the lower part of the abdomen as this can often relieve some of the patient's discomfort. Antispasmodic drugs may offer further relief. Once the urethral catheter has been removed, the patient will be ready for discharge.

Segmental resection of a bladder tumor may be done when the tumor involves the dome of the bladder. This may entail removal of over half of the bladder in order to remove the entire tumor. Immediately postoperatively, the capacity of the remaining bladder may be as little as 60 ml. Within several months, however, the elastic tissue will regenerate to the extent that the patient will be able to retain from 200 to 400 ml. of urine. This factor is of major importance both in the immediate postoperative period and in planning for his discharge.

Following surgery, the patient will have catheters draining the bladder both from a cystotomy opening and from the urethra to prevent possible obstruction and overdistension of the remaining bladder and the suture line.

One or both of these catheters may be connected to a "bubble" suction for drainage. The nurse should be alert to observe the amount and character of this drainage. Bladder spasm occurs in the majority of cases because of the limited bladder capacity and the presence of the catheters. The urethral catheter is usually removed 21 days postoperatively unless the cystotomy wound has not healed completely. At this time, the patient becomes extremely aware of the limited bladder capacity as he will usually need to void at least every 20 minutes. The nurse needs to reassure him that this is only temporary.

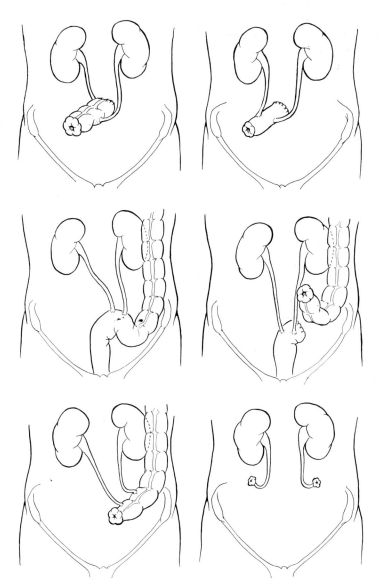

Fig. 12-3. Types of urinary diversion.

At the same time, she can teach him how to regulate his fluid intake so that he can obtain adequate rest and sleep. This can best be accomplished by advising the patient not to drink anything after 6 o'clock in the evening. Another point the nurse needs to make to the patient is that he should drink large quantities of fluid at one time rather than small amounts frequently. In this way, he will not become a "bathroom invalid." She can also instruct the patient to limit fluid intake for several hours before he plans going out.

If the tumor has invaded the entire bladder, a cystectomy may be performed. This type of surgery, wherein the entire bladder is removed, is usually performed when the physician is reasonably sure the tumor can be completely eradicated and that the patient's physical status can withstand this radical procedure. Since this operation requires permanent urinary diversion, the physician will also evaluate the patient's emotional status as well. At the same time he usually informs the patient of what to expect after surgery and obtains the patient's consent for operation.

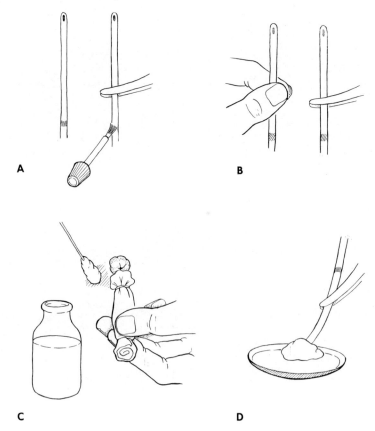

Fig. 12-4. Inserting and positioning of catheter (ureterostomy). **A,** Marking catheter with nail polish for distance to be inserted before sterilizing. **B,** Catheters marked with nail polish. **C,** Cleansing area around stoma. **D,** Dipping tip of sterile catheter into sterile lubricating jelly in sauce dish.

The patient is usually admitted to the hospital several days prior to surgery for a thorough preoperative evaluation and preparation. During this time, nursing personnel have an opportunity to get to know the patient and his family and to form relationships that will continue throughout the entire period of hospitalization. It is most important that the nurse take time to listen to the patient and his family, to allow them to verbalize their fears, and

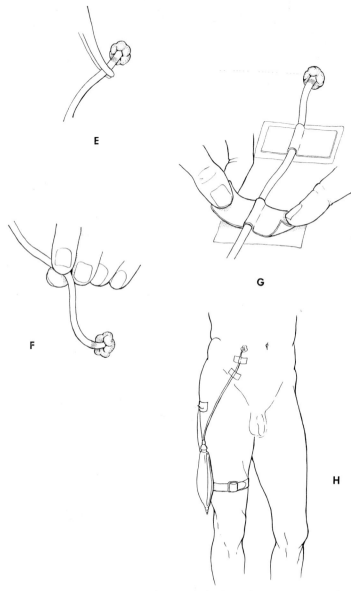

Fig. 12-4, cont'd. E, Inserting catheter gently into the ureterostomy leaving the nail polish marking ¼ to ½ inch from opening. **F,** Allowing catheter to fall into its natural position. **G,** Securing catheter with adhesive tapes (2 inches apart). **H,** Catheter attached to drainage tubing and leg urinal.

to provide emotional support for them. She can also minimize the patient's apprehension by providing simple explanations in preparing him for the diagnostic procedures to be carried out. By including the patient's family in the plan of care, she allays their apprehension and makes this trying period less traumatic.

Urinary diversion may be accomplished in a variety of methods. The ureters may be transplanted into the skin (cutaneous ureterostomies), into the intestine (ureteroenterostomy), into the sigmoid colon (wet colostomy), into an isolated section of ileum (ileal conduit or ileal bladder), or into an isolated segment of the sigmoid colon (colocystoplasty).

The nursing care will differ somewhat depending upon the method employed for the urinary diversion. At the present time, the most common method of urinary diversion is by construction of an ileal conduit or ileal bladder. Briefly, in this operation a loop of ileum is isolated. One end of the loop is closed while the other end is brought through the abdominal wall and sutured to the skin. The remaining ileum is anastomosed to permit normal bowel function. The ureters are severed at a convenient level and are then implanted into the isolated ileal segment. After closure of the abdominal incision, a clear disposable plastic ileostomy appliance is cemented to the skin over the stoma. A Levin tube is usually inserted upon completion of surgery (if not prior to the operation). This tube is attached to Gomco suction to prevent distention of the bowel at the level of anastomosis. It may require irrigation every 2 hours or more frequently with normal saline.

In the immediate postoperative period, the patient is usually acutely ill and will require intensive nursing care. The nurse will check vital signs every 15 minutes until they are stable and as often thereafter as ordered by the physician. This permits prompt recognition of symptoms of hemorrhage, shock, or early atelectasis, any of which demand prompt action if they do occur. A major responsibility of the nurse is to check frequently on the drainage from the incision, the ileal conduit, and the Levin tube with regard to the character, amount, and color of each. At the same time, she will maintain an accurate record of intake and output as a means of determining renal function.

Ace bandages are usually applied to the lower extremities prophylactically to minimize the possibility of thrombophlebitis. To prevent early postoperative complications, the nurse will turn the patient from side to side (or assist him in turning) until he is able to turn by himself. She will encourage deep breathing and coughing at periodic intervals to prevent chest complications.

Since the patient is not permitted anything by mouth, the nurse can offer special oral care at frequent intervals to keep the mucous membrane of the mouth and throat moist and clean. This will also help to prevent formation of lesions in the mouth, on the tongue, or around the lips. As soon as the patient's physical status is satisfactory, the physician will undoubtedly want the patient out of bed. The patient should be encouraged to get out of bed as soon as possible since early ambulation helps to prevent weakness and vascular stasis, which accompany prolonged bed rest. It also lessens the likeli-

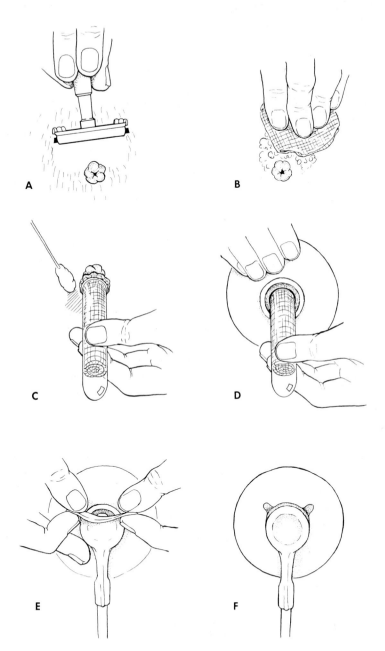

Fig. 12-5. Applying the Whitmore cup. **A,** Shaving area around stoma. **B,** Cleansing skin around stoma. **C,** Painting skin around stoma, placing a tightly rolled ball of absorbent cotton over ureteral opening. **D,** Placement of flange on skin surface. **E,** Attaching cup into position. **F,** Cup fully in place.

hood of ileus, urinary retention, and fecal impaction. Wound healing is accelerated indirectly as a result of improved circulation.

The temporary drainage bag is changed daily by the physician, at which time he dilates the stoma. After the third or fourth day, this may become a nursing procedure. Briefly, a finger cot is slipped onto the finger to be inserted and the cot is well lubricated with a water-soluble jelly. The finger is then inserted gently through the stoma into the conduit. It becomes the nurse's responsibility to teach the patient how to carry out this procedure before he is discharged. One point to be emphasized is that good aseptic technique must be adhered to so that organisms are not introduced into the conduit.

The permanent ileal bladder bag is custom made for each patient. Since it takes approximately 6 weeks for the stoma to shrink to its permanent size, measurements should not be made before this time. It is generally recommended that the patient obtain two bags in order to provide time for the bags to air between use. The nurse will need to reinforce teaching the patient to apply the ileal bladder bag, and she may find that writing out the procedure step by step may be extremely beneficial.

These patients need a tremendous amount of emotional support throughout the period of hospitalization. When discharge is imminent, the nurse is in a unique position to offer constructive help and reassurance to both patient and family. In addition, she can serve a useful function in her role as a listener. She can review the importance of special stomal and skin care, observation of good general hygiene, and keeping appointments for medical checkups.

The urinary bladder may be invaded by carcinoma from other organs. Carcinoma of the prostate frequently invades the bladder by direct extension, as may carcinoma of the neighboring rectum and sigmoid. In the female, carcinoma of the uterus and cervix may also invade the bladder by direct extension. This does not necessarily negate surgery as long as the disease is confined within the pelvis. There are three types of procedures that may be performed, namely, total pelvic exenteration, anterior exenteration, or posterior exenteration. (Discussion regarding these procedures and nursing care appears on pp. 196-208 of this chapter.)

PHYSIOLOGY RELATED TO THE ORGANS OF REPRODUCTION

The female organs of generation are anatomically divided into the internal and external organs. External organs consist of the labia majora and minora, the clitoris, the hymen, the urinary meatus, the vulvovaginal glands, and the mucous and sebaceous glands. Internal organs consist of the vagina, uterus, fallopian tubes, and ovaries. In the male, the organ most considered is the prostate gland.

The ovaries are situated deep in the pelvic cavity, one on each side of the uterus. They are connected to the uterus by means of the fallopian tubes and ligaments. Their major function is the production of mature reproductive cells. This begins at puberty (between 12 and 15 years of age) and continues until 40 or 50 years of age or longer. Every 28 to 30 days a mature ovum is developed. Ovulation occurs approximately midway between periods and is said to occur 14 ± 2 days prior to the next menstrual period. Immediately following ovulation, a blood clot is formed at the site of the ruptured follicle. This site closes almost immediately in the human female so that the blood clot may or may not be observed. The remaining granulosal and thecal cells undergo a series of changes and give rise to a definite glandlike spherical organ called the corpus luteum. This body is partly embedded in the cortex of the ovary. The corpus luteum is maintained for about 14 or 15 days, although the period during which it elaborates progestational hormones is somewhat less, being between 7 and 11 days. If fertilization of the ovum takes place, the functional activity of the corpus luteum will continue for 5 to 6 months. However, if the ovum is not fertilized and menstruation occurs, this body undergoes rapid degeneration because of fatty infiltration and is then referred to as the corpus albicans because of its white-appearing fibrous structure.

In addition to producing ova, the ovaries have another major function. This is to produce two hormones, mainly estradiol and progesterone. The estrogens are responsible for maturation and maintenance of secondary sex characteristics and sexual organs. Removal of the ovaries prior to puberty causes the girl to remain in the sexually undifferentiated state since secondary sex characteristics fail to develop. Following the onset of puberty, removal of the ovaries will result in cessation of menstruation, gradual atrophy of the sex organs, suppression of sexual drive, and a gradual change in body configuration toward the masculine form. There may also be hair growth in areas of the body such as the face and chest, which typically occurs in the male.

The primary function of progesterone is to maintain the uterus and its implanted fertilized egg during the early months of pregnancy. To a certain extent, the actions of progesterone are dependent upon the prior action of estrogen.

The menstrual cycle is a complicated series of events associated with the sexually mature uterine lining or endometrium. Characteristically four phases are observed during the typical menstrual cycle. Specifically these are the following: (1) the proliferative or follicular phase, (2) the ovulatory phase, (3) the secretory or luteal phase, and (4) the destructive or menstrual phase.

While regulation of ovarian function and menstruation is dependent on the action of ovarian hormones, it is also influenced by gonadotropic hormones secreted by the anterior portion of the pituitary gland. These hormones are commonly referred to as the follicle-stimulating hormone (FSH), luteinizing hormone (LH), and lactogenic hormone (LTH).

The physiological mechanisms that regulate ovarian function and the phases of the menstrual cycle are controlled by hormonal secretions from the ovary and the pituitary gland.

In the male, the genital organs include the penis, the prostate and Cowper's glands, the testes, the vas deferens, and the seminal vesicles. The testes in the male are the counterpart of the ovaries in the female.

The testes are two small, flattened, oval-shaped glands contained within a musculomembranous pouch (the scrotum) and suspended by the spermatic cords. With the onset of puberty these glands attain adult proportions and structure. The substance of each gland consists of a number of pyramid-shaped lobules. Each lobule has several seminiferous tubules between which are the interstitial cells of Leydig. The testes, like the ovaries, have a dual function of producing mature sperm cells and sex hormone. Spermatogenesis, or the production of mature sperm cells, begins at puberty and continues without interruption throughout life.

The second major function of the testes is to secrete the male sex hormone or androgenic hormone. Five principal androgenic substances are secreted in the adult male body, the most important of which is testosterone. The androgens are metabolized and excreted in the urine in the form of androsterone.

The androgen secreted by the testes functions to bring about the development and maintenance of the male accessory sex organs and genitalia as well as being responsible for the development of the male secondary sexual characteristics. Regulation of testicular function is reliant upon secretions from the anterior pituitary gland as is ovarian function in the female.

Removal of the testes prior to puberty or failure of the testes to descend into the scrotum will result in effeminate characteristics in the male. Castration after puberty lessens sexual desires as in the female.

DISORDERS RESULTING FROM DYSFUNCTION OF THE ORGANS OF REPRODUCTION

Carcinoma can affect any organ in the body as discussed in previous chapters in this book. The reproductive organs affected in the female are the ovaries and the uterus and in the male, the testes and the prostate.

Testis

Cancer of the testis is uncommon and accounts for less than 1% of the cancer mortality rate in males. For the most part, this disease affects young men between 20 and 40 years of age. The largest number of testicular tumors are found in patients 29 to 34 years of age, during which period they are the most common malignant tumors found in men.* Testicular tumors occur most frequently in individuals with undescended testicles.

These tumors vary greatly in size, enlarging the organ at times to ten times its normal size, or they remain very small, not being noticed until metastasis has already occurred. The tumor itself is fairly firm but will vary in consistency depending upon cellularity, bone, cartilage, and connective tissue content. These tumors may be softer in consistency (especially those less differentiated), and areas of hemorrhage and necrosis often develop.

The first sign is usually a painless enlargement of the testis accompanied by a sensation of heaviness and aching in the perineum. Because of the com-

---

*Cancer incidence by site and sex, 1967 Cancer facts and figures, New York, 1966, p. 20.

plicated lymphatic network leading from the testis, metastasis may occur while the primary growth is still small. Metastases may occur anywhere in the body. If the lung becomes the site of metastatic disease, there is a good chance that liver metastases may also be present as a result of invasion through the bloodstream. It is interesting to note that metastasis to bone is relatively rare.

The treatment for all tumors of the testis is surgical excision accompanied by retroperitoneal node dissection or possibly transperitoneal bilateral lymphadenectomy. This procedure is of considerable value in determining evidence of abdominal spread or involvement, in which instance postoperative abdominal irradiation may be instituted. This will, for the most part, enhance the results of the surgery.

Following surgery, especially when a radical node dissection has been carried out, there is danger of hemorrhage since lymph nodes may have been resected from around many of the large abdominal vessels. Vital signs must be observed closely. Deep breathing should be encouraged at hourly intervals. To minimize active movement, which may be contraindicated due to the danger of hemorrhage, a turning sheet and a chest binder are usually helpful. In this way, the patient can be turned from side to side whenever necessary to prevent postoperative pneumonia. Passive leg and arm movements will be of value to prevent postoperative thrombosis.

Radical node dissection involves removal of large amounts of tissue from the groin. The skin sutures are quite taut, which causes a considerable amount of discomfort. Careful positioning in the bed with pillows arranged to eliminate undue pulling and strain on the sutures when the patient moves may be helpful. Narcotic and sedative drugs should not be withheld during the first 2 to 3 weeks (or until the sutures can be removed). Sloughing of the tissues around the inguinal incisions is not uncommon, and healing is a slow process. A heat lamp may provide some comfort. Since the healing process is a long drawn-out one, the patient may become quite discouraged. By providing various forms of diversional therapy, the nurse can keep the patient from thinking too much about himself, thereby minimizing his state of depression. By listening carefully to both the patient and his family, the alert nurse can assess the situation and suggest that help may be obtained from other members of the paramedical team.

Prostate

Carcinoma of the prostate will be diagnosed in approximately 34,000 men during 1967.* The disease affects males between 50 and 75 years of age and increases in frequency with each succeeding decade of life.

The prostate gland is a small gland about the size of a chestnut that weighs between 16 and 24 grams. It consists of 5 lobes: (1) posterior lobe that passes through the ejaculatory ducts; (2) anterior lobe that consists of

---

*Reference chart: Leading cancer sites, 1967 Cancer facts and figures, New York, 1966, American Cancer Society, Inc., p. 5.

the tissue forming the roof of the urethra; two lateral lobes that are formed by the prostatic tissue lying between the anterior and posterior lobes; and (3) median lobe that is formed by the narrow strip of tissue that lies between the internal sphincter and the verumontanum and that forms the floor of the urethra.

Carcinoma of the prostate arises most commonly in the posterior lobe. The anterior lobe may be the site of the disease occasionally, and the median lobe is rarely affected or involved. The lesion is an adenocarcinoma and may vary considerably in appearance.

Early symptoms are rarely present; however, the patient may complain of dysuria. Frequency may also be mentioned by the patient. Later symptoms, usually associated with advanced disease, include the following: (1) pain (referred to the lower back or leg) often suggestive of sciatica; (2) urinary retention resulting from tumor pressure on the urinary bladder; and (3) once in a while, hematuria. Unfortunately, these symptoms are indicative of far-advanced metastatic disease. To effect an early diagnosis, at the time of the annual routine physical examination, a digital rectal examination may verify a small lesion.

The diagnosis of a suspected early lesion may be verified by the carrying out of various procedures. Cystoscopy may prove of value in identifying an early lesion. Biopsy, as with other forms of malignant lesions, will demonstrate the presence of an early lesion. Recently, urethrography has been of some value, although it is not conclusive for accurate diagnosis. Laboratory tests of most significance are the acid and alkaline phosphatase determinations. The adult prostate gland produces acid phosphatase. Serum acid phosphatase is elevated in advanced prostatic cancer. The alkaline phosphatase level is often elevated when bony metastases are present; however, with osteolytic metastases, this determination may be within normal limits.

Treatment of carcinoma of the prostate is dependent upon (1) the stage of tumor growth, (2) the size of the tumor, and (3) the physical status of the patient.

Carcinoma, limited to the prostate gland (early lesion), is best treated by radical perineal prostatectomy, which in all probability will prove curative. This type of surgical procedure entails removal of the entire prostate gland (including the capsule), the seminal vesicles, and adjacent tissue. Anastomosis of the remaining urethra to the bladder neck is required. Incontinence is a frequent sequela to this type of surgery since both the internal and external sphincters of the bladder lie in close proximity to the prostate gland.

Preoperatively, enemas, cathartics, sulfonamides, and/or antibiotics are given to prevent postoperative infection and other complications. The day prior to surgery, a clear liquid diet is commonly ordered. Postoperatively, the patient may be maintained on intravenous feedings, clear liquids by mouth, or a low-residue diet until the perineal wound is practically healed. Drugs that will inhibit bowel action may also be prescribed.

Following this type of surgery, the patient has a urethral catheter to drain the bladder as well as to serve as a splint for the urethral anastomosis. Care must be taken to ascertain that the catheter does not become dislodged or blocked so that postoperative complications can be averted. The catheter is kept in place for 2 or 3 weeks postoperatively.

The patient who undergoes this type of surgery (whether radical or conservative) often becomes extremely depressed when he suddenly realizes the implications of being permanently impotent and perhaps permanently incontinent. This entails constant support and encouragement from the nurse and other members of the health team so that the patient does not withdraw from everyone and become completely asocial. Keeping the patient dry at all times, as well as the use of protective devices so that he is not constantly in fear of wetting himself, will be extremely helpful in averting this withdrawal from family and friends. The nurse should make every effort (when realistic) to help the patient regain control of micturition by observing the amount of fluid intake, checking the time of the day when incontinence occurs, and offering a urinal prior to such periods.

Occasionally, a retropubic prostatectomy will be the surgical procedure of choice. In this procedure, a low abdominal incision is made without opening the bladder, and the lesion is removed through an incision into the anterior prostate capsule. With this type of surgery, the urethral sphincters are not likely to be damaged, and incontinence or urinary fistulas are not likely to be problems. Following surgery, the patient has a large Foley catheter in the urethra. His major complaint, in the majority of cases, is urgency to void. Bladder spasm is uncommon; however, hemorrhage and wound infection are frequent complications. The patient may be able to go home within a week following surgery, and the nurse needs to inform him that if fever, perineal tenderness, or pain on walking develop, he should notify the physician immediately.

When radical surgery for prostatic cancer is contraindicated due to advanced and metastatic disease, various alternative methods of treatment may be utilized. Thus, any of these forms of therapy must be considered as palliative. Surgically, a transurethral resection may be performed. A resectoscope (an instrument similar to a cystoscope but having a cutting and cauterizing attachment) is used to remove tiny pieces of abnormal prostatic tissue so that adequate patency of the urethra is ensured. Following this procedure, a Foley catheter is inserted into the urethra. After the 30-ml. balloon has been inflated, the catheter is pulled down so that the balloon rests in the prostatic fossa. This serves a dual purpose: it provides hemostasis, and it retains the catheter in the urethra. The catheter is then connected to a gravity drainage apparatus. Presence of the catheter causes a mild urethral irritation that in turn produces the sensation of having to void. This can be alleviated by use of mild sedatives or analgesics and reassurance that this sensation is only temporary. If the discomfort persists, however, the nurse should check for patency of the catheter. If the catheter has become plugged, and prescribed irrigations do not dislodge any obstructing plugs, the physician should be notified since this may signify one of several serious complications all of which require immediate medical attention (hemorrhage, unsuspected perforation of bladder or prostate during surgery, etc.).

The urethral catheter may be removed 3 to 7 days postoperatively by the physician. The patient should be taught to keep an accurate account of intake and output. This is essential since either the internal or external sphincter (or both) may have been injured during the surgery, and the patient may experience occasional incontinence or, on the other hand, may be unable to void due to urethral edema. In this event, the catheter may be reinserted for several days longer.

Prior to discharge, the nurse should emphasize the importance of calling the physician if the patient experiences difficulty in voiding or passes any blood. This may occur anytime between 2 and 4 weeks postoperatively and results from sloughing of coagulated prostatic tissue.

Periodic dilatation of the urethra may be required once healing is complete because urethral mucosa has been destroyed by the operative procedure, and stricture may result.

Other palliative procedures include the use of supervoltage radiation equipment, cobalt teletherapy, and orchiectomy followed by administration of estrogen therapy.

Ovary

Most ovarian tumors are benign lesions or simple cysts. Carcinoma of the ovary is relatively rare before the age of 20. The relative frequency of ovarian tumors increases with age, and most cases occur around the fifth decade.

The ovary is an extremely complex structure. It has an intricate embryologic development, many details of which are still not clearly understood. Tumors are generally classified according to their histogenesis, and many, therefore, have been described. Carcinoma of the ovary has an insidious onset and may be difficult to diagnose early. Enlargement or asymmetry of the

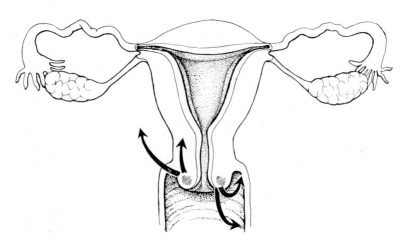

Fig. 12-6. Spread of cervical cancer.

abdomen with increasing girth may be the first symptoms noted. Later in the course of the disease, abdominal pain, weight loss, dysuria, or urinary frequency (results from pressure of the tumor on the bladder), constipation, and occasional vaginal bleeding appear.

Because of the insidious onset, the lesion is rarely if ever diagnosed before it has already metastasized. Surgery is the preferred form of therapy. This may mean oophorectomy, bilateral oophorectomy, or bilateral salpingo-oophorectomy with hysterectomy. Radiation therapy and/or chemotherapy may be utilized to provide palliation in advanced stages of the disease.

Nursing care does not differ essentially from that given for any type of abdominal surgery. The nurse does need to provide emotional support to the patient since removal of any part of the reproductive system poses many problems for her—creation of an artificial menopause, change in the way the patient perceives herself as a woman, and her concern as to how she will be accepted by her husband.

Uterus

Carcinoma of the uterus can affect any part of the organ—the cervix and body of the uterus. Since incidence, symptoms, therapy, and prognosis differ somewhat, each site will be discussed separately.

Cancer of the cervix ranks second in incidence to cancer of the breast in women. The disease is more prevalent in women who have had children, women who have married young, and women in a low socioeconomic group. Jewish women and virgins rarely develop this disease.

Though the disease can now be detected before symptoms appear, it has been estimated that about 44,000 new cases will be diagnosed while some 14,000 women will die of the disease in 1967.* Early detection can be accomplished if every woman in the cancer age group has an annual routine physical checkup that includes a pelvic examination and Papanicolaou smear test.

The Papanicolaou test is based upon examination of vaginal secretions and scraping from the surface of the cervix. These are fixed, stained, and analyzed under the microscope. Any change in the cell from normal alerts the physician to suspect the presence of a malignant lesion even when there is no evidence of disease on examining the cervix during the pelvic examination. Diagnosis can be confirmed by biopsy.

Methods of treatment vary markedly. If the woman is in the childbearing age and wants children, the physician may decide that hysterectomy can be deferred as long as the patient is examined regularly and the mucocutaneous junction containing the entire in situ carcinomatous lesion is excised. When the patient is beyond the childbearing age (or does not want to bear more children), hysterectomy is advocated.

Carcinoma of the cervix, which has become invasive, characteristically appears as either an ulcerated or a fungating growth on the surface of the cervix. The lesion tends to spread in all directions: by direct extension, into the

---

*1967 Cancer facts and figures, New York, 1966, American Cancer Society, Inc., p. 20.

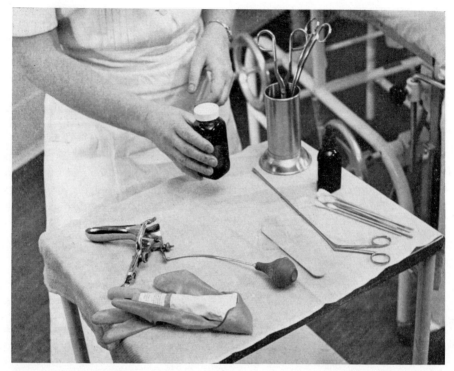

Fig. 12-7. Equipment needed for Papanicolaou smear test. (Courtesy American Cancer Society, Inc., New York, N. Y.)

vaginal wall; laterally, into the parametrium toward the rectum; and by lymphatic metastases, to the pelvic lymph nodes. Distant, blood-borne metastases are far less common; however, with lateral extension, the ureters may become surrounded and compressed, causing urinary retention and uremia.

Invasive carcinoma of the cervix may be treated in a variety of ways. Appropriate therapy is determined by the physician and is dependent on the stage of the disease and the individual patient. Surgery sometimes consists of removal of the entire uterus, fallopian tubes, parametria, and ovaries. The pelvic lymph nodes may or may not be excised.

Occasionally, the patient may be treated with supervoltage roentgen-ray therapy alone, or in combination with intracavitary application of radium, cobalt, or iridium to the cervical lesion within the vagina.

Nursing care is similar to that required for any patient undergoing abdominal surgery, or for the patient receiving radiation therapy (Chapter 5).

Cancer of the body of the uterus arises from the endometrium and is seen most often in women who are postmenopausal. It is less common in younger women. Since the endometrium is a highly vascular area, bleeding is likely to occur early. Any bleeding after the menopause should be considered to be cancer until proved otherwise. A diagnostic dilatation and curettage will confirm the diagnosis.

Treatment may consist of supervoltage roentgen-ray therapy, a combination of irradiation and panhysterectomy, or surgery alone.

Vulva

Carcinoma of the vulva occurs in the older age group of postmenopausal women. The disease ranks third in frequency of all female genital cancers. The lesion is commonly preceded by leukoplakic changes lasting many years. Pruritis is a common complaint.

The lesion is removed surgically, and the procedure will in all likelihood be radical. This involves the removal of several very vital structures and includes an en bloc vulvectomy, excision of the lower portion of the vagina, and excision of the inguinal lymph nodes.

Over and above routine preoperative and postoperative care, the patient who has had a vulvectomy will have other special nursing needs. She will have a Foley catheter to provide for urinary drainage. This will help to prevent contamination of the vulval wound. She will, no doubt, be placed on a low-residue diet in order to minimize the need for straining to defecate.

Since the extensive surgery involves removal of large amounts of tissue from the vulva and the groins, the sutures are usually quite taut, thereby causing severe discomfort. Pillows should be used in positioning the patient to prevent undue pulling on the sutures when the patient moves. Medication to relieve pain should be given at frequent intervals during the first 2 to 3 weeks postoperatively and until such time as the sutures are removed.

The vulva wound should be cleansed twice a day. Hydrogen peroxide, normal saline, pHisoHex, or other antiseptic solutions may be used unless a specific solution has been ordered by the physician.

It is not unusual for the wound to be left exposed; however, if a dressing is used, it should be held in place with a T-binder. Once the wound has been cleansed, a heat lamp is used to dry the area, promote circulation, and stimulate healing. The nurse must ensure complete privacy for the patient at all times. After the sutures have been removed, the use of the heat lamp can be discontinued. Sitz baths replace the use of the heat lamp and are more acceptable to the patient.

The wound heals very slowly, and the patient is likely to become extremely discouraged. She may become quite depressed as well, since some women feel that their femininity has been irreparably damaged. The nurse should encourage the patient to express her feelings with regard to this disfiguring surgery. She can also reassure the married patient that within several weeks to a month after the wound is completely healed, sexual intercourse may be resumed. The nurse should provide diversional activities for the patient. This will help to keep the patient's mind occupied, thereby keeping her from thinking too much about herself. Socializing with other patients when she feels like it will also help to pass the time.

If the wound has not healed and the patient is ready for discharge, the nurse can initiate referral to the visiting nurse service for follow-up care at home. She may also contact social service to assist in obtaining any dressings or medications that the patient may need. She should reinforce the need for continuing the sitz baths at home. It is also advisable to teach the patient how to apply her own dressings if they are needed, even allowing the patient to do these herself for several days before going home.

PELVIC EXENTERATION

It is obvious that tumors of the pelvic viscera may arise in the urinary bladder, rectum, or genital organs. Surgical treatment may involve a single organ or more than one organ as the disease process spreads. The extent and direction of the spread of the disease in addition to the physical condition and age of the patient are factors taken into consideration in order to determine the type of surgery to be undertaken.

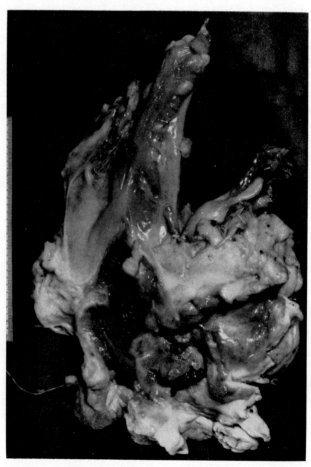

Fig. 12-8. Pathologic specimen from first pelvic exenteration performed in December, 1946. (Courtesy Dr. Alexander Brunschwig, Memorial Center, New York, N. Y.)

Cervical cancer may invade the vaginal vault, the bladder, and the rectum by direct extension. Lymphatic spread involves the parametrial nodes as well as the nodes of the lateral pelvic wall. With prostatic carcinoma, characteristically the spread is local and to bones. Infrequently, the rectum may be encroached upon or invaded. The periaortic and iliac nodes and even the tracheobronchial nodes may be involved. Metastatic lesions may also be found in the liver, lungs, and brain.

Total pelvic exenteration may be performed when carcinoma has invaded widely within the pelvic brim. This procedure usually includes a panhysterectomy, pelvic node dissection, cystectomy, vaginectomy (prostatectomy), and removal of the rectum, along with the fat and soft tissues surrounding these organs. This results in the formation of a permanent colostomy with one or another form of urinary diversion such as: (1) transplantation of the ureters into the skin, or cutaneous ureterostomies; (2) transplantation of the ureters into the sigmoid colon with subsequent formation of a wet colostomy; (3) transplantation of the ureters into the lower bowel, or anal bladder; (4) construction of an ileal bladder for the conduction of urine to the skin, or ileal conduit; and (5) construction of a colosigmoid bladder from an isolated segment of sigmoid colon.

When carcinomatous invasion does not involve all of the pelvic viscera, a partial exenteration may be performed. Depending upon the organs invaded, this may result in either anterior or posterior exenteration.

Anterior pelvic exenteration consists of removal of the bladder, panhysterectomy (prostatectomy), and aortic node dissection. This necessitates one or another form of urinary diversion.

Posterior pelvic exenteration consists of resection of the rectum, panhysterectomy (prostatectomy), and pelvic node dissection. Since the urinary tract remains intact, the patient will have a dry colostomy.

Preparation for surgery. Thoroughness in establishing the diagnosis and preparing the patient for this extensive radical surgery usually entails several days of hospitalization before such a procedure can be carried out. This period is extremely important for testing and evaluating the patient physically as well as emotionally prior to surgery. It provides an opportunity for the patient to become adjusted to hospital routines. It also allows time for the patient to become acquainted with the nursing personnel who will share in the rehabilitative processes required for full recovery and return to his family and community.

On admission, the patient is likely to be in a state of panic. The decision to submit to surgery is often difficult. The patient is afraid to have the surgery and equally afraid to risk the consequences if she refuses the treatment. While the final decision must be made by the patient, the nurse can be of considerable assistance if she allows the patient to articulate her fears.

By providing simple, clear explanations and reasons for the numerous tests and procedures, the nurse can alleviate anxiety and provide reassurance. Intravenous pyelogram and cystoscopy may be performed to determine kidney function and to ascertain the appropriate management of urinary diversion at the

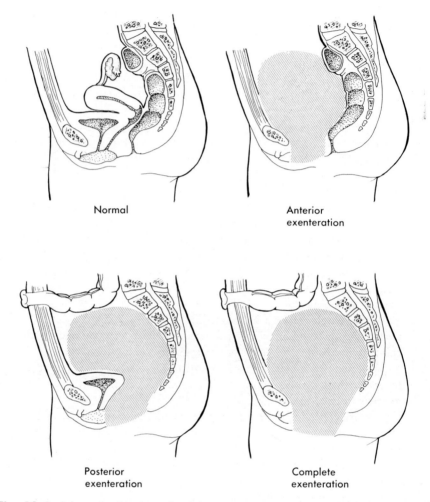

Normal

Anterior
exenteration

Posterior
exenteration

Complete
exenteration

Fig. 12-9. Schematic drawing of pelvic exenteration (anterior, posterior, and complete).

time of surgery. Fluid and electrolyte determinations and blood tests will serve as an indication of the patient's metabolic condition and will allow for sufficient time to make up any deficiencies. They will also serve as a base line for treatment during and after surgery. The patient's potential recuperative powers must be built up to a maximum level to withstand the extensive surgical procedure.

Once all preoperative tests and procedures have been completed, the final preoperative preparations are usually initiated. These may entail 48 to 72 hours prior to surgery. These preparations may vary from one hospital to another, from one service to another, or even from one physician to another on the same service or in the same hospital. This will probably include a low-residue diet, saline cathartics, cleansing enemas, and rectal aspirations to cleanse the bowel of feces, gas, excess mucus, bacteria, and bacterial products. Drug therapy is usually instituted at least 3 to 5 days preoperatively and is continued, to decrease the bacterial flora in the colon. Such drugs as oral neomycin, Terramycin, or one of the sulfonamides may be ordered for this purpose. These drugs are poorly absorbed from the gastrointestinal tract, and thus their concentration in the bloodstream is low. After the abdominal preparation has been completed, the projected site for the ileal stoma is mapped out on the skin in the right lower quadrant. Care must be taken to determine the most appropriate site, for encroachment on the crest of the ileum, umbilicus, or fold of the groin and symphysis must be avoided. Close proximity to the colostomy stoma (if one is contemplated) must also be avoided.

Even though the patient has been completely informed of most factors concerning the exact nature of the surgery and the subsequent adjustments that will have to be made, fear and apprehension may be so overwhelming that she really does not hear or understand. The nurse needs to be fully aware of what the doctor has told the patient in order to reinforce and clarify this information with the patient. Here, again, allowing the patient to verbalize her fears and answering her questions in a matter-of-fact way will enable the patient to become more accepting of what is to be done.

Postoperative care. Following surgery, it is the nurse's responsibility to be well prepared to assume the care of the patient and to provide the most expert, comprehensive nursing care possible. The nurse must recognize that the major changes in physical structure resulting from the surgery will present physiological alterations primarily related to kidney function and urinary output as well as to excretory processes from the gastrointestinal tract. With the extensive node dissection and stripping of perivesical fat and surrounding tissues, both denuded areas remain in the pelvic cavity, which causes a continued loss of protein postoperatively. This leads to the development of hypoproteinemia and a state of negative nitrogen balance, which results in excretion from the adrenal cortex of glucocorticoids that have a marked catabolic effect, thus preventing the buildup of proteins. In the first days postoperatively, intravenous therapy with dextrose and saline as well as Amigen (or some other protein hydrolysate) will be required to combat this condition. When the patient can tolerate food by mouth, a high-protein, high-carbohydrate diet with frequent protein supplements will be essential in the treatment of this condition and to prevent further complications.

Another major area of consideration concerns maintenance of adequate fluid and electrolyte balance. Preoperative determinations of nonprotein nitrogen, total protein, albumin-globulin ratio, and electrolyte determinations for sodium, potassium, and chlorides serve as the base line for treatment both during and after surgery. Postoperatively, ileostomy, colostomy, and Levin tube drainage must be measured accurately in order that fluid and electrolyte replacement be initiated promptly. Constant gastric suction, urinary output, daily irrigation of the pelvic cavity, and the pelvic transudate are responsible for enormous losses of sodium and chloride ion, and these must be replaced if metabolic acidosis is to be avoided. It must also be recognized that with this loss of electrolytes, there is also a loss of considerable amounts of potassium ion as well. This is due to the shift in balance between the intracellular and extracellular fluids. Fluid therapy will include administration of dextrose and saline, with hypertonic saline as well, to replace the sodium and chloride depletion. Potassium may be added, if indicated, to avoid the resulting metabolic alkalosis. Here, again, after the gastric suction has been discontinued and the patient can tolerate liquids and food by mouth, it is advisable to increase the amount of salt ingested to aid in maintenance of fluid and electrolyte balance. An accurate record of intake and output will be extremely valuable in maintaining this balance.

Occasionally the patient returns from the operating room having a wet colostomy. These patients have had an abdominoperineal dissection and the terminal bowel has been brought out through the abdomen to form a colostomy. The ureters have been transplanted into the bowel so that both urine and feces drain from the colostomy. It is essential for the nurse to recognize that a wet colostomy, or any type of urinary diversion to the colon, must *never be irrigated*.

In the immediate postoperative period, the nurse should check the abdominal and perineal dressings at frequent intervals since perineal drainage occurs as a result of the large perineal defect. Dressings should be changed whenever necessary and reinforced with sterile 4 by 8 inch gauze sponges and abdominal pads. A scultetus binder should be applied to the abdomen, and a T binder should be firmly applied to support the perineal dressings. These will be of special value in helping to control bleeding.

Since the colostomy will drain urine as well as feces, the output is measured by counting the number of 4 by 8 inch sponges and abdominal pads soiled or by weighing the dressings before they are applied and again when they are removed. This will assist the physician in terms of fluid and electrolyte replacement. Intake and output must be measured accurately and charted to serve as a guide to the physician in ordering intravenous fluids.

Skin care is extremely important in the patient with a wet colostomy, since excoriation may develop easily if dressings are not changed at frequent intervals. Aluminum powder is ordered frequently to dry excoriated areas. This can be dusted on the skin around the colostomy stoma before the compound tincture of benzoin has dried. It can enhance healing of the excoriated area. Mineral oil or castor oil will remove this coating with ease.

Once the colostomy has begun to function, sterile dressings are no longer required; rather, surgically clean dressings are used.

Perineal wound packing is usually removed 48 to 72 hours postoperatively. Since this may be extremely painful, it is often removed with the patient under sodium pentothal anesthesia. The nurse must be alert to signs of hemorrhage since removal of the packing releases pressure in the perineal wound.

Within 5 to 7 days postoperatively, a Pierce bag can usually be applied. At this stage, the colostomy bud is usually still edematous, and the first bag will require a larger opening than subsequent ones after a maximum shrinkage has occurred. Maximum shrinkage should take place within 2 to 3 weeks postoperatively. Further teaching, in terms of application of the Pierce bag and its care, will involve principles similar to those for use of Singer cups. In teaching the patient to care for his wet colostomy, the nurse must emphasize that he must *never take an enema*. If he has difficulty with bowel evacuation, a mild cathartic may be taken.

Postoperative complications. The ileal conduit serves as a passageway for urine from the ureters to the outside. With this form of urinary diversion, there should be less difficulty with electrolyte imbalance than in procedures in which ureters are transplanted into the large bowel, since urine is in contact with the mucosa for a short time. Thus, absorption of sodium and chloride ions is minimized, and renal potassium losses are lessened. Patients, however, may manifest a mild hyperchloremia for a short time in the early postoperative period. A permanent hyperchloremic acidosis is unusual and, when seen, is generally associated with severe renal damage.

While there are many advantages to this form of urinary diversion, there still exist certain inherent complications that are more or less peculiar to the diversion itself. Leakage may follow inaccurate suturing or inadvertent perforation of the ileac loop. It may also occur as a result of necrosis of the loop due to interference with the blood supply. Such interference may be caused by direct surgical injury or by traction on the mesentery of the isolated segment due to intestinal distention. A slow leak may ultimately result in an external urinary fistula. Suture lines may be disrupted if the collecting bag is not emptied before it becomes filled and pressure is transmitted directly back to the ileac loop. Swelling about the stoma or the ureteroileal anastomosis may also prevent adequate function of the conduit. Once in a while, especially in thin patients, the belt of the Perry bag is applied tightly enough that it compresses the isolated segment, or the edge of the plastic collar may slide, thereby occluding the stoma. Regardless of the cause, distention can cause injury to the kidney and can produce increased tension on the suture line, causing disruption leading to fatal peritonitis. Close observation of the bag and frequent emptying are essential. These are preventable complications and fall within the realm of nursing responsibility.

Leakage of fecal material about the intestinal anastomosis or leakage of urine into the peritoneal cavity from the ureteroileal anastomosis may cause pain in the lower abdomen, decreased urinary output, and fever. Any of these symptoms should be reported at once, since they may be an indication of peritonitis. Emergency surgical intervention is required to repair the leak.

Stenosis of the ileal stoma may occur as a late complication as a result of excessive tissue in the abdominal wall around the emerging ileum. Consequently, the patient is supplied with a dilator while he is still in the hospital, and the nurse teaches him to use this before he is discharged. Neglected stenosis causes accumulation of urine within the ileal segment, eventually resulting in a marked renal acidosis. If the situation is not corrected, uremia will ensue.

A basic principle in the postoperative care of the patient with an ileal conduit is to keep the intestines absolutely quiet until the ileal anastomosis has healed sufficiently. This can be accomplished by keeping the patient on nothing by mouth and initiating intermittent gastric suction, which keeps the stomach empty of secretions and swallowed air that could lead to distention and tension on the suture line. Sometimes the physician will prefer to use an enterostomy tube that will lie in the small bowel, extending from the proximal jejunum to the terminal ileum. These tubes must be irrigated about every 2 hours to ensure patency. Isotonic saline should be used for irrigation of indwelling tubes.

Production of edema and subsequent obstruction of the intestines may result from a decrease in nerve stimulation to the bowel or a decrease or lack of all peristalsis. If the edges of mesentery of the isolated segment have not been secured snugly, a loop of bowel may slip between them and become kinked. Likewise, the same thing may happen in a space between the mesentery of the segment and the posterior abdominal wall. Generalized ileus may also be responsible for distention of the isolated segment.

Paralytic ileus is a common complication following extensive abdominal procedures, and for this reason suction is continued for some time following surgery. This condition is due to a failure of the bowel to maintain its normal motor functions and, more specifically, its tone. Trauma to the intestines resulting from construction of the ileal conduit causes an excessive neurogenic interference of sympathetic inhibitory impulses. With a deficit of potassium ion, this condition may also result.

Although movement of the bowel has ceased, secretions of proteolytic enzymes continue, and the lumen of the bowel remains filled with fluid. As the condition progresses, breakdown of tissue frees potassium ion from the intracellular compartment. Further electrolyte imbalance occurs, and the patient may develop a hypopotassemia. This condition increases gastric secretions so that more electrolytes are lost when gastric intubation is instituted (if it is not already in effect), thereby causing a hypochloremic alkalosis since loss of chloride and potassium produces a compensatory increase of base bicarbonate. Inasmuch as chloride is most rapidly excreted as a potassium salt, there is a depletion of chloride levels as well. Since kidney function is closely related to a stasis of intestinal movement with the accumulation of fluids within the lumen of the bowel along with seepage of protein containing transudate into the peritoneum, electrolyte balance may be further affected.

Hormone secretion. Many workers have verified the fact that in response to any stress there is a release of ACTH from the pituitary gland. This hormone stimulates the adrenal cortex that in turn secretes several types of steroids affecting the electrolyte changes: mineralocorticoids, or aldosterone, and glucocorticoids. Although these both act differently, the essential result is the loss of potassium and retention of sodium.

Aldosterone, or mineralocorticoids, causes diminished sodium excretion, both by the kidney and the sweat glands, and indirectly increases the loss of potassium. It is not yet clear to what extent aldosterone secretion is influenced by the pituitary gland, although some reports indicate a twofold increase following injections of ACTH. Others have also suggested direct action of this hormone on the individual body cells, resulting in potassium loss and a partial replacement of this cellular electrolyte by sodium.

A second hormone secreted by the adrenal gland has a mineral hormonelike action that likewise causes sodium retention and potassium loss. This hormone also has a marked catabolic effect that prevents the buildup of proteins. Thus, amino acids are made available at the site of injury for tissue repair and for conversion of glucose. It has been suggested that the salt retention and potassium loss (releasing cell water) were designed purposely to maintain the blood volume in time of stress, as well as to supply the elements for healing to the area of damage at the expense of the general body mass.

The duration of the sodium retention and potassium loss will depend to a great extent on the severity of the trauma. The immediate posttraumatic period is followed by a repair period in which there is sodium diuresis and potassium retention.

Hormonal balance. The ability of man to respond and adapt successfully to his changing environment is made possible mainly by the successful coordinative activities of the two great integrating mechanisms, the nervous and endocrine systems. The ultimate end of all endocrine activity with regard to any aspect of metabolism is to maintain and adjust the internal environment to the body needs at the moment. The endocrine glands are governed both by hormonal and nonhormonal stimuli; the former travel to them exclusively through the blood, the latter through either this medium or through nerve pathways.

Removal of the reproductive organs results necessarily in alteration of the normal interrelationship between the endocrine glands and ultimately produces hormonal imbalances of varying degrees. So far, there has been no evidence that the symptoms are sufficiently severe to require replacement therapy.

The female patient is faced with the onset of an artificial menopause with its usual symptoms such as flushing of the head, neck, and thorax; sweats, concurrent with or following flushing, so-called "hot flashes," composed of hot tingling sensations and reactions of a systemic nature including atrophy of the genital tract, breasts, and skeletal structures. Other symptoms commonly associated with the onset of menopause and believed to be of psychological origin include headache, fatigue, nervousness, irritability, vertigo, and depression. Awareness on the part of the nurse that such changes may occur or exist will be helpful in interpreting the patient's response to therapy and her reactions to nursing personnel.

In the male patient, since hormonal balance is not affected appreciably, changes of any degree are difficult to predict. Naturally, removal of the seminal vesicles produces sterility. Likewise, any surgical procedure that damages both the nerves and the vascular supply to the organ of copulation can, and usually does, result in impotence. Sexual desires will be decreased but not totally lost provided sexual activities have been practiced prior to surgery.

Psychological effects. After surgery, the patient has the work of repair and convalescence. He is faced with the damage done to his body and, more important, with the damage done to his pattern of living. It is almost impossible to predict how the patient will react postoperatively since the enormity of the procedure is difficult to grasp and may not cause an emotional impact for 3 or 4 days following the surgery. At this point, the hospital may be representative of an alien and threatening situation, or, due to the results of the mutilating surgery, may represent security against rejection and fear of facing family and friends. At this time, the nurse has many responsibilities to the patient. She needs to learn as much about him and his family as possible if she has not had the opportunity before surgery. She needs to know her own attitudes concerning this radical procedure and be aware that verbal and non-verbal communications are recognized by the patient. These will most certainly affect the total recovery process.

There is no blueprint or set of rules that will tell the nurse how to deal with or handle the psychological problems involved in the care of the patient. Understanding him means to visualize him within the home, family, and community. In our society, with the tremendous emphasis on physical fitness, attitudes of disapproval, revulsion, and rejection toward the person with a physical disfigurement are commonplace. Mindful of this, the nurse can be instrumental in assisting the patient and his family to accept the physical deformity by answering their never-ending questions and by providing reassurance within realistic limits.

When the patient is faced with the need for extensive and radical surgery, he needs help in planning for this new phase of his life. This is not always feasible prior to surgery, but, whenever possible, planning should begin soon after admission to the hospital. By cooperative planning, the nurse can assist both the patient and his family to make a smooth adjustment to a new pattern in his life routine. This entails balancing sympathy and objectivity on the part of the nurse in meeting the needs of the patient.

Teaching self-care. While emotional support is essential, the physical aspects must take precedence in order to restore body function to its maximum physiological state. The nurse has a major role in this phase of care of the patient so that his rehabilitation can bring him to his optimal level of functioning.

It is not easy to motivate a patient to work toward his own recovery; however, this is a primary objective that the nurse must meet. The nurse needs to recognize that teaching self-care and independence in such care is a slow process, and that the patient must be ready to assume this responsibility if the rehabilitative process is to be effective. If the nurse proceeds in a calm, efficient manner and shows a sincere interest in the patient, he will feel that he is in good hands. It is important that she be skilled in carrying out any and all procedures, as any minor slipup may be traumatic for the patient.

As the patient regains strength, the nurse has a major responsibility for teaching him how to care for himself. This involves care of the colostomy and the ileal bladder (or other forms of urinary diversion). The nurse must avoid teaching too much at any one time since this can be overwhelming and can result in his refusal to learn or cooperate. Making him responsible for a small part at a time allows him to progress at his own pace. Even when the patient assumes major responsibility for his own care, the nurse should continue to do some part of the procedure occasionally, so that he will not feel that a distasteful assignment has been completed. By providing constant encouragement, the patient will become more receptive to instruction that he will carry out after discharge.

The patient with an ileal conduit (or cutaneous ureterostomies) needs special teaching since the skin area almost always becomes irritated and excoriated during the early postoperative period. It will usually take anywhere from 6 to 10 weeks for the skin to toughen and gain tolerance for the appliance and cement. Tincture of benzoin is usually most effective for protecting the skin in most patients. Prior to its application, cleansing with soap and water along with meticulous drying of the area will keep this problem to a minimum. The patient should be encouraged to try various adhesive materials postoperatively until he is satisfied by one particular type. The temporary ileostomy bag should be changed as often as necessary, especially when it pulls away from the skin and permits leakage. The permanent device can be applied after all sutures are removed, or about the eighth or ninth day postoperatively.

The patient who has cutaneous ureterostomies or an ileal conduit returns from the operating room with polyethylene, polyvinyl, rubber, or latex catheters threaded into each ureter to provide optimum urinary drainage in the immediate postoperative period. These are usually left in place until the anastomosis is firmly fixed, at which time, if there are no complications, they are removed and Singer cups are applied.

The patient needs to be taught appropriate skin care, proper method for applying the Singer cups and leg urinals, care of the equipment, and signs or symptoms that may be indicative of obstruction or infection. All of these must be taught slowly and not before the patient is ready to help himself.

In teaching skin care, it is important that all hair around the area of the stoma be shaved off within a 2-inch radius. This is probably more essential for the male patient than for the female patient. The skin and stoma are then cleansed with soap and water and wiped dry. The skin should then be painted with two or three coats of compound tincture of benzoin and allowed to dry completely. While this is being done, a 4 by 8 inch gauze compress rolled in cigarette fashion (with a rubber band on each end) should be held over the stoma to absorb the urine, which flows continuously, thus keeping the surrounding skin dry.

In applying the Singer cups, the patient is taught to spread a thin coating of cement evenly on the flange of the cup and on the skin surrounding the stoma. When the cement is set, the rolled 4 by 8 inch gauze can be removed from over the stoma. Some urine may flow over the cement on the skin, and it should be wiped dry with the opposite end of the gauze roll before applying the Singer cups. The Singer cup should be held firmly against the skin for approximately 5 minutes to be certain that the cement is fixed. The leg urinal is then attached.

When the Singer cup needs changing, it can be peeled off in the same manner as removing adhesive tape. If necessary, a drop of benzine can be placed on the edge of the flange to facilitate removal. This should be washed off im-

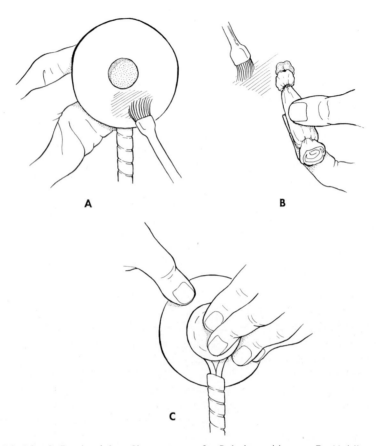

Fig. 12-10. A-D, Applying Singer cups. **A,** Painting phlange. **B,** Holding gauze pledget over ileal stoma and painting skin with tincture of benzoin. **C,** Placing Singer cup in place until it adheres to skin.

mediately to prevent skin irritation. When benzine has been used, the cups should be washed immediately since benzine softens the rubber and hastens deterioration. Cups and bags should be washed carefully with soap and water and rinsed well in a vinegar solution to remove odors. They should then be hung in a cool, dry area. The same principles apply to care of the ileal conduit.

There are many problems involved in daily living with a patient who has a colostomy. There may be strong feelings of disgust or revulsion toward a colostomy. Home life may be completely disrupted, and severe reactions may cause the patient to become completely withdrawn from society.

While in the hospital, nothing by mouth is offered for at least 48 hours. After this time one ounce of water may be given every hour if tolerated. There is a gradual progression in diet until the patient can tolerate regular food.

The patient needs to be taught how to care for his colostomy and gain independence and security in carrying out the irrigation. Teaching must take place gradually, adapting the procedure to the individual needs of the patient.

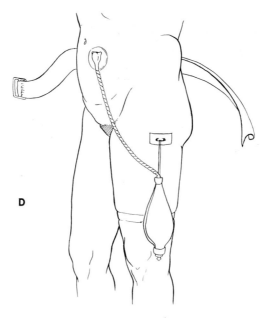

Fig. 12-10, cont'd. D, Belt to secure cup in place.

It should be recognized that it is never easy for anyone to accept a colostomy and that the attitude of the doctor, nurse, and others caring for the patient can have a profound effect on his acceptance or rejection.

For the most part, management of the different types of colostomies will vary with each physician. The purpose of the colostomy irrigation is to evacuate the colon at specified intervals in order to control the passage of feces and to prevent soiling. The procedure is no different than that for any patient who has undergone a colostomy regardless of diagnosis. The first irrigation is given on the fifth or sixth postoperative day with the patient in bed and turned on his left side after the irrigating cup has been properly positioned over the stoma. The patient should be encouraged to hold his hand over the plastic cup at the time of this first irrigation so that he begins to participate in his care from the very beginning. While the patient is hospitalized, irrigations are ordered on a daily basis. This serves a dual purpose: to regulate the colostomy as quickly as possible and to teach the patient self-care quickly and efficiently, since his period of hospitalization is of a comparatively short duration. The nurse needs to recognize that while it is easier for her (and less time-consuming) to perform the irrigation, this will prolong the period of rehabilitation for the patient. She must also remember in teaching that the patient can learn only one step at a time. Constant reassurance and patience are essential characteristics that the nurse must possess throughout this period.

Preparation for discharge. When the patient is ready for discharge, irrigations are usually ordered every other day, and a routine dietary regime is prescribed. As time progresses, however, the patient learns what he can or cannot eat in terms of colostomy control as well as to establish his own irrigating routine. The nurse needs to emphasize and constantly reinforce the fact that "the colostomy should not rule or regulate the patient" but, rather, "the patient will rule and regulate his colostomy."

Once the nurse is aware that the patient may go home within a few days, it is advisable that a referral be sent to the visiting nurse or public health nurse for follow-up care to ascertain that the patient has carried over principles and techniques of colostomy care from the hospital to the home. This may mean obtaining approval from the physician, contacting social service, requesting referral through the outpatient department, or direct referral. Forms, of necessity, will need to include the type and amount of teaching while the patient was hospitalized, his degree of acceptance, cooperation, and learning, and recommended therapy after discharge. Referral reports are, in many instances, ineffectual since they contain inadequate information to provide for continuity of care.

By the time the patient is ready for discharge, he should feel secure enough to take care of his colostomy and ileal bladder, or whatever type of urinary diversion he may have.

Summary. In summary, it is obvious that continuity of care is an essential factor in the successful rehabilitation of the patient. This starts in the doctor's office, continues throughout the period of hospitalization, and carries over into the home, which is the most important and often neglected phase in rehabilitation. In many instances, the nurse may make or break rehabilitation for the patient. The care of the patient who undergoes pelvic exenteration is probably the most challenging and most rewarding of experiences if the patient is to be adequately rehabilitated. Finally, alert, accurate observation based on scientific knowledge and recognition of symptoms resulting from altered physiological processes will greatly enhance the early and uncomplicated recovery for the patient who has undergone pelvic exenteration.

Bibliography

A cancer source book for nurses, New York, 1963, American Cancer Society, Inc.

Ackerman, L. V., and del Regato, J. A.: Cancer: diagnosis, treatment, and prognosis, ed. 3, St. Louis, 1962, The C. V. Mosby Co.

Alpenfels, E. J.: Cancer in situ of the cervix: cultural clues to reactions in society, Amer. J. Nurs. 64:83, April, 1964.

Bard, P., editor: Medical physiology, ed. 11, St. Louis, 1961, The C. V. Mosby Co.

Beeson, P. B., and McDermott, W., editors: Cecil-Loeb textbook of medicine, ed. 11, Philadelphia, 1963, W. B. Saunders Co.

Bricker, E. M.: Substitution for a urinary bladder by the use of isolated ileal segment, Surg. Clin. N. Amer. 36:1117, 1956.

Bricker, E. M., Butcher, H. R., Jr., and McAfee, C. A.: Surgical treatment of advanced and recurrent cancer of the pelvic viscera, Ann. Surg. 152:388, 1961.

Brunner, L. S., Emerson, C. P., Ferguson, L. K., and Suddarth, D. S.: Textbook of medical-surgical nursing, Philadelphia, 1964, J. B. Lippincott Co.

Brunschwig, A., and Brockunier, A.: Postoperative rupture of the major blood vessels after radical pelvic operation, Amer. J. Obstet. Gynec. 80:485, 1960.

Brunschwig, A., and Daniel, W.: Pelvic exenteration operations, Ann. Surg. 151:571, April, 1960.

Burnham, J., and Farrer, J.: Urinary diversion, J. Urol. **83**:622, 1960.

Burns, R. O., Henderson, L. W., Hager, E. B., and Merrill, J. P.: Peritoneal dialysis: clinical experience, New Eng. J. Med. **267**:1060, 1962.

Campbell, M., editor: Urology, ed. 2, Philadelphia, 1963, W. B. Saunders Co.

Cancer manual for public health nurses, Washington, D. C., 1963, U. S. Department of Health, Education and Welfare, Public Health Division of Chronic Diseases, Cancer Control Branch.

1967 Cancer facts and figures, New York, 1966, American Cancer Society, Inc.

Ceccarell, F. E., and Smith, P. C.: Studies on fluid and electrolyte alterations during transurethral prostatectomy, J. Urol. **86**:434, 1963.

Chiappa, S., et al.: Considerations on the restoration of the lymphatic circulation after pelvic lymphadenectomy, Surg. Gynec. Obstet. **120**:323, 1965.

Cordonnier, J., and Nicolai, C. H.: An evaluation of the use of an isolated segment of ileum as a means of urinary diversion, J. Urol. **83**:834, 1960.

Creevy, C. D., and Tollefson, D. M.: Iliac diversion of the urine and nursing care of the patient with iliac diversion of the urine, Amer. J. Nurs. **59**:530, 1959.

de Vries, J. K.: Permanent diversion of urinary stream, J. Urol. **73**:217, 1955.

De Weerd, J. H.: Urinary diversion via an ileal segment, Surg. Clin. N. Amer. **39**:907, 1959.

Dyk, R. B., and Sutherland, A. M.: Adaptation of the spouse and other family members to the colostomy patient, Cancer **9**:123, 1956.

Field, J. B., editor: Cancer: diagnosis and treatment, Boston, 1959, Little, Brown & Co.

Fitzpatrick, G. M., and Shotkin, J. M.: Pelvic perfusion, Amer. J. Nurs. **61**:79, June, 1961.

Frenay, Sister M. Agnes Clare: A dynamic approach to the ileal conduit patient, Amer. J. Nurs. **64**:80, January, 1964.

Funnell, J. W., and Roof, B.: Before and after hysterectomy, Amer. J. Nurs. **64**:120, October, 1964.

Geist, D. I.: Round the clock specimens, Amer. J. Nurs. **60**:1300, 1960.

Geist, R. W., and Ansell, J. S.: Total body potassium in patients after ureteroileostomy, Surg. Gynec. Obstet. **113**:585, 1961.

Giebisch, G.: Kidney, water and electrolyte metabolism, Ann. Rev. Physiol. **24**:357, 1962.

Gilmer, R., and Hassels, A.: Cancer in situ of the cervix: nurses' practices and attitudes towards cancer, Amer. J. Nurs. **64**:84, April, 1964.

Grollman, S.: The human body: its structure and physiology, New York, 1964, The Macmillan Co.

Gusberg, S. B.: Cancer in situ of the cervix: treatment as preventive medicine, Amer. J. Nurs. **64**:80, April, 1964.

Guyton, A. C.: Textbook of medical physiology, Philadelphia, 1961, W. B. Saunders Co.

Hofmeister, F. J., Reik, R. P., and Anderson, N. J.: Vulvectomy—surgical treatment and nursing care, Amer. J. Nurs. **60**:666, 1960.

Horgan, P. D.: The artificial kidney, RN **22**:39, September, 1959.

Huffman, J. W.: Gynecology and obstetrics, Philadelphia, 1962, W. B. Saunders Co.

Jewett, H., and Eversole, S.: Carcinoma of the bladder: characteristic modes of local invasion, J. Urol. **83**:383, 1960.

Leadbetter, W. F., and Clarke, B. G.: Five years experience with ureteroenterostomy by "combined" technique, J. Urol. **73**:67, 1955.

Lewis, G. C., Jr.: Cancer in situ of the cervix: screening and diagnosis, Amer. J. Nurs. **64**:72, April, 1964.

Mikuta, J. J., and Murphy, J.: The team approach of pelvic exenteration for cervical cancer, Amer. J. Obstet. Gynec. **80**:795, 1960.

Miller, O.: Nursing care after pelvic exenteration, Amer. J. Nurs. **62**:106, 1962.

Miller, O. M.: When radical surgery saves a life, RN **24**:29, 1961.

Moore, C., Atherton, D., and Haynes, D. M.: Modified pelvic exenteration, Surg. Gynec. Obstet. **118:**59, 1964.

Mossholder, I. B.: When the patient has a radical retropubic prostatectomy, Amer. J. Nurs. **62:**101, July, 1962.

Murphy, J., and Mikuta, J. J.: Urinary diversion in pelvic exenteration, Surg. Gynec. Obstet. **112:**743, 1961.

Nesbit, R. M.: Your prostate gland, Springfield, 1961, Charles C Thomas, Publisher.

Newton, K.: Geriatric nursing, ed. 3, St. Louis, 1960, The C. V. Mosby Co.

Pack, G. T., and Ariel, I. M., editors: Treatment of cancer and allied diseases; vol. 6, Tumors of the female genitalia, ed. 2, New York, 1961, Harper & Row, Publishers.

Pack, G. T., and Ariel, I. M., editors: Treatment of cancer and allied diseases; vol. 7, Tumors of the male genitalia and the urinary system, ed. 2, New York, 1962, Harper & Row, Publishers.

Parkhurst, E., and Leadbetter, W.: A report on 93 ileal loop urinary diversions, J. Urol. **83:**398, 1960.

Parsons, L., and Sheldon, C. S.: Gynecology, Philadelphia, 1962, W. B. Saunders Co.

Paull, D. P., and Hodges, C. V.: The rectosigmoid colon as a bladder substitute, J. Urol. **74:**360, 1955.

Price, J. M., Wear, J. B., Brown, R. R., Satter, E. J., and Olson, C.: Studies on etiology of carcinoma of the urinary bladder, J. Urol. **83:**376, 1960.

Robbins, L. C., and Walker, E.: Cancer in situ of the cervix: problems of control, Amer. J. Nurs. **64:**80, April, 1964.

Sawyer, J. R.: Nursing care of patients with urologic diseases, St. Louis, 1963, The C. V. Mosby Co.

Secor, S. N.: Colostomy care 1964, Amer. J. Nurs. **64:**127, September, 1964.

Senescu, R. A.: The development of emotional complications in the patient with cancer, J. Chron. Dis. **18:**813, 1963.

Shafer, K. N., Sawyer, J. R., McCluskey, A. M., and Beck, E. L.: Medical-surgical nursing, ed. 3., St. Louis, 1964, The C. V. Mosby Co.

Silva, T. F., Friedell, G. H., and Parsons, L.: Pelvic exenteration of cancer of the cervix, New Eng. J. Med. **260:**519, 1955.

Smith, G. I., and Hinmann, F.: The rectal bladder (colostomy with ureterosigmoidostomy); experimental and clinical aspects, J. Urol. **74:**354, 1955.

Spellman, R., and Swanwick, M.: The management of cutaneous ureterostomies, Amer. J. Nurs. **55:**800, 1955.

Stacy, R. W., and Santolucito, J. A.: Modern college physiology, St. Louis, 1966, The C. V. Mosby Co.

Statland, H.: Fluid and electrolytes in practice, ed. 3, Philadelphia, 1963, J. B. Lippincott Co.

Straffon, R. A.: Cancer chemotherapy in the urologic patient, J. Urol. **86:**259, 1961.

Sutherland, A. M.: The impact of cancer: Part II, Postoperative responses, State of Mind, August-September, 1958.

Taylor, E. S.: Essentials of gynecology, ed. 2, Philadelphia, 1962, Lea & Febiger.

Te Linde, R. W.: Operative gynecology, ed. 3, Philadelphia, 1962, J. B. Lippincott Co.

The Travenol twin-coil artificial kidney, Morton Grove, Ill., 1962, Travenol Laboratories, Inc.

Thompson, G.: After renal surgery, Amer. J. Nurs. **61:**106, September, 1961.

Thompson, H. T.: The use of isolated loops of bowels in urologic surgery, Surg. Gynec. Obstet. **108:**683, 1959.

Thompson, P.: Let's take a look at the aging, Amer. J. Nurs. **61:**76, March, 1961.

Titchner, J., and Levine, M.: Surgery as a human experience, New York, 1960, Oxford University Press.

Trail, I. D., and Monke, J. V.: Psyche sequellae of surgical change in body structure, Nurs. Forum **2:**14, 1963.

Walsh, M. A., Ebner, M., and Casey, J. W.: Neo-bladder, Amer. J. Nurs. **63:**107, April, 1963.

Whitmore, W. F., Jr.: The rationale and results of ablative surgery for prostatic cancer, Cancer **9:**1119, 1963.

Whitmore, W. F., Jr., and Bongart, T.: A device for the management of cutaneous ureterostomy, J. Urol. **74:**603, 1955.

Chapter 13

Management of the patient with a disorder affecting the respiratory system

One very important phase of homeostasis is the maintenance of a constant, adequate supply of oxygen for the body tissues. The major function of the respiratory system is the intake of an adequate oxygen supply and the elimination of carbon dioxide produced in metabolism. Other functions associated with this system include maintenance of acid-base balance, control of water content, warming of inhaled air, and evaporating of water to saturate this air.

The respiratory passages by which air is transported from the environment to the lungs include a network of tubular structures, mainly, the nasal cavity, nasopharynx, pharynx, larynx, trachea, bronchi, bronchioles, and alveoli.

The great majority of primary tumors arising in the head and neck are readily accessible; they may draw early attention because of impairment of some common function such as speech, voice, swallowing, or breathing. If the significance of these early manifestations were recognized, this might lead to early diagnosis and prompt treatment. Early treatment is especially important in head and neck cancer to permit adequate excision that will forestall the development of metastases and yet avoid excessive disfigurement.

Treatment of the primary lesion is of greatest importance. Detailed and explicit information regarding the biological characteristics of each tumor including variation in cell morphology, rapidity of growth, predictable spread to regional lymph nodes or contiguous tissues, and incidence of extension by hematogenous route is essential to ensure successful therapy.

An accurate and correct diagnosis can be obtained by means of a detailed history, physical examination, and biopsy. A careful history may elicit the mode of onset and duration of symptoms. It may also provide a means of differential diagnosis such as inflammatory process in the case of a cervical mass of short duration, or a congenital or benign tumor if the lesion has been

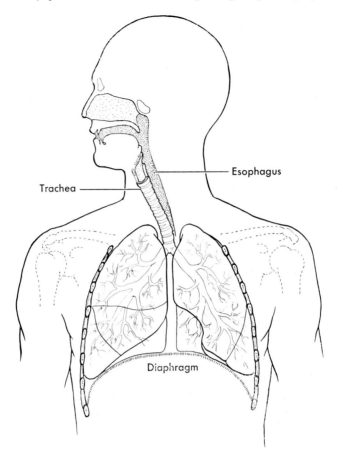

Fig. 13-1. Schematic drawing of the respiratory system.

present for many years. History of dental treatment is often important in arriving at a correct diagnosis, such as Ludwig's angina following a recent extraction of a lower molar. Any difficulty in talking, chewing, swallowing, or breathing should be elicited with specific notation of presence or absence of pain. This may further pinpoint whether the lesion is benign or malignant and may even indicate the primary site.

Examination of the head and neck should follow a definite pattern. It should include meticulous observation for any deformities in the skin or in the contour of the region, as well as careful visualization of the nasal and oral cavities, the external auditory canal, the pharynx, and the larynx. Presence of any swelling, ulceration, or exudate should be noted. Palpation may elicit a cervical mass that may have been overlooked during inspection. Location of such a mass along with its consistency, mobility, or degree of fixation to surrounding tissue is of extreme importance in evaluation; for example, solitary supraclavicular masses may represent metastasis from a primary lesion below the clavicle, whereas masses in the upper cervical region are more often indicative of a primary lesion in the head and neck. Roentgenograms may be useful in determining fractures or foreign bodies and may provide essential information with regard to metastatic lesions. A chest plate should always be a part of the roentgenographic study of the head and neck patient.

Biopsy of lesions of the head and neck is a relatively simple procedure since most of them are readily accessible. This is essential to making a definite diagnosis and should be carried out prior to initiating therapy. Exceptions to utilization of this procedure include small skin lesions that may be completely excised without disfigurement, or those lesions suspected of being malignant melanomas. In the case of cervical node enlargement, biopsy should be one of the last diagnostic procedures to be employed, since this most often is indicative of a metastatic lesion, and biopsy will only complicate matters when therapy is initiated.

DYSFUNCTIONS RESULTING IN SURGERY TO THE HEAD AND NECK REGION

Primary cancer of the head and neck region occurs mainly in the mouth, pharynx, larynx, or thyroid gland. Cancer of the mouth is the term commonly used to define those malignant tumors that arise in the mucous membranes of the oral cavity beginning anteriorly at the mucocutaneous junction of the lips and extending to the soft palate, the tonsil, and the base of the tongue posteriorly. It is of utmost importance that the primary site of origin of the tumor be definitely determined before therapy is initiated, since growths arising in these different areas present distinct clinical problems.

Clinical manifestations of oral cancer will vary according to site and according to whether the lesion is localized or advanced. Symptoms may be

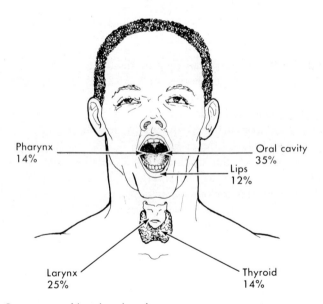

Fig. 13-2. Occurrence of head and neck cancer.

absent in the case of a localized lesion in oral cancer. Often the patient may see the lesion in the mirror or may feel an abnormality with his tongue. On occasion, dentures may cause an irritation, especially if they come in contact with the lesion. Bleeding may result. A small indurated and/or ulcerated, coarsely granular lesion may be palpable with the examining finger. Leukoplakia is often associated with the lesion. Occasionally, despite a very small primary lesion, cervical node involvement, as a result of metastasis, is demonstrable. This may be the first clue to the presence of cancer. With advanced lesions, pain is usually present. This may be due to secondary infection, bone invasion, or nerve involvement. Salivation and drooling may occur due to hypersecretion and inability to swallow properly as a result of pain or obstruction. A foul breath is often present. This may be due to necrosis or secondary infection of the tumor. Symptoms, secondary to bulky disease in the neck and posteriorly, may include respiratory obstruction, dysphagia, and hoarseness. The primary tumor may reach a great size, especially if it is situated posteriorly. Necrosis and secondary infection are usually noted. Hemorrhage may occur. Metastatic node involvement is frequently present and may be bilateral, especially if the primary lesion has developed near the midline. Signs of cancer cachexia develop often, as a result of the tumor proper, or due to near starvation.

Malignant tumors arising in the walls of the pharynx (which anatomically is a funnel-shaped, hollow tube extending from the base of the skull to the level of the lower border of the cricoid cartilage) above the level of the soft palate posterior to the nasal cavity are properly classified as cancer of the nasopharynx. Those tumors that arise in the pharyngeal mucosa below the level of the soft palate but above the lower border of the cricoid cartilage (excluding the palatine tonsil, base of the tongue, and extrinsic larynx) are properly referred to as cancer of the pharyngeal wall. A localized or early lesion may not produce any symptoms. A tumor arising in the region of the orifice of the eustachian tube may produce symptoms referable to the ear. These patients complain of a "lump in the neck" (cervical metastasis), or of "stuffiness in the ear" (unilateral deafness or tinnitus). Other signs and symptoms are similar to those cited in terms of oral cancer. The sixth cranial nerve may become involved as the disease progresses, as a result of extension of the growth in the nasopharynx, which tends to erode into the base of the skull. This may also lead to a diplopia due to a paralysis of the external rectus muscle of the eye. Later, the growth may extend into the base of the skull and invade the third, fourth, and fifth cranial nerves. Tumors in this region tend to be either highly anaplastic epidermoid carcinoma or lymphosarcoma. For this reason, systemic metastases are common.

Cancer of the head and neck spreads mainly through the lymphatic pathways. Malignant tumor cells enter lymphatic vessels by direct invasion. They are then carried to regional lymph nodes that act as a filter and as a nidus for further growth. Gradually the node is completely replaced by tumor, at which time lymphatic flow becomes blocked.

Surgical procedures for head and neck tumors are tolerated surprisingly

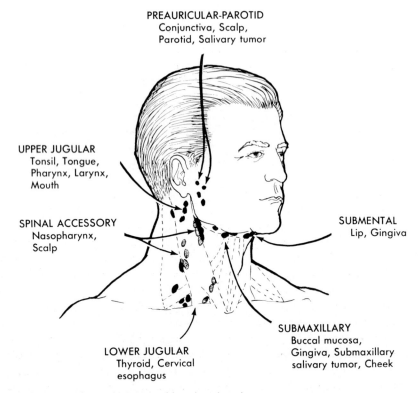

PREAURICULAR-PAROTID
Conjunctiva, Scalp,
Parotid, Salivary tumor

UPPER JUGULAR
Tonsil, Tongue,
Pharynx, Larynx,
Mouth

SPINAL ACCESSORY
Nasopharynx,
Scalp

SUBMENTAL
Lip, Gingiva

SUBMAXILLARY
Buccal mucosa,
Gingiva, Submaxillary
salivary tumor, Cheek

LOWER JUGULAR
Thyroid, Cervical
esophagus

Fig. 13-3. Lymphatic drainage of head and neck.

well. Mortality is extremely low, even in older patients and in patients with complicating cardiovascular or pulmonary disease. Careful evaluation of the patient's general status and management of cardiovascular or respiratory conditions is necessary if surgery is contemplated. Nutritional status must be established and vigorous replacement therapy of vitamins, electrolytes, and fluids given as indicated prior to surgery. Local infection is a problem commonly encountered in the patient with head and neck disease, and every effort must be made to eradicate such infections preoperatively. Use of gargles, sprays, and irrigations as well as administration of antibiotics will frequently reduce inflammation and clear up the local infection. Psychological preparation is imperative for the patient contemplating a major head and neck operation, since all kinds of fears develop—fear of disfigurement, inability to swallow or talk—and these fears can produce near panic in the patient.

Cancer of the mouth occurs predominantly in men. The greatest number of cases is observed between the ages of 50 and 60 years, although it has been diagnosed in patients from early youth to advanced age. While the etiology is not known specifically, several forms of chronic irritation are considered to be possible contributing factors. Long-time use of alcohol and tobacco are admitted to by the majority of patients who develop this form of disease. Excessive exposure to sunlight, chewing of the betel nut, and sharp, jagged teeth or prolonged use of ill-fitting dentures may also be contributing factors. Leukoplakia may or may not be present prior to the onset or finding of a malignant tumor. Treatment of these tumors may be surgery or irradiation, alone or in combination. Chemotherapy, at present, is of little or no value in the treatment of these lesions and is considered purely experimental.

Cancer of the tongue, a highly lethal disease, is the most common form of mouth cancer. Depending on whether the lesion occurs in the anterior or posterior portion of this organ, symptoms may or may not be suggestive of a malignant tumor, and such a diagnosis may not even be suspected. Tumors arising in the anterior region many times are discovered by the patient himself by the presence of a lump or sore, or an area of irregularity that is usually painless. Lesions that arise on the base of the tongue are relatively inaccessible and are rarely detected by the patient. Pain is the most frequent complaint, but this is often attributed to a sore throat. Oftentimes it is aggravated by talking or swallowing and may be referred to the side of the head or ear. In many instances, the patient does not seek medical advice until the primary lesion is extremely bulky, or cervical lymphadenopathy occurs.

In treating carcinoma of the tongue, many factors are involved in terms of its management: the extent of the lesion, the possible degree of metastasis, and the physical status of the patient. In some cases, radical surgery is the only treatment of choice; if the tumor is radiosensitive, irradiation may be the treatment of choice; in other situations, a combination of surgery and irradiation may be indicated.

Carcinoma may also arise on the lip, in the tonsil, and in the nasopharynx or hypopharynx. Cancer arising in the hypopharynx carries a grave prognosis, since it forms a common passageway for both the upper alimentary and respiratory tracts. This may give rise to severe interference with respiration, or deglutition, or both. Radical surgery, including laryngectomy, is the preferred method of treatment.

Carcinoma of the nasal cavity and paranasal sinuses is most frequently encountered in the male sex between the ages of 50 and 70 years. It may occur, however, from early childhood to advanced age. Treatment of these lesions has, for the most part, been considered difficult since aggressive therapy is likely to result in mutilation, protracted morbidity, and ultimate dysfunction. There is, furthermore, considerable hazard to the patient when the lesion is excised or destroyed by irradiation due to the close proximity of other vital organs.

Nursing care

Nursing care of the patient with cancer in the head and neck region will vary according to the degree of involvement and the site of the primary lesion. Since these patients have many complications when the diagnosis is made, they are frequently admitted several days prior to surgery. They are (in many instances) extremely apprehensive, since head and neck surgery is mutilating. Providing time for the patient to express his fears and ask questions may

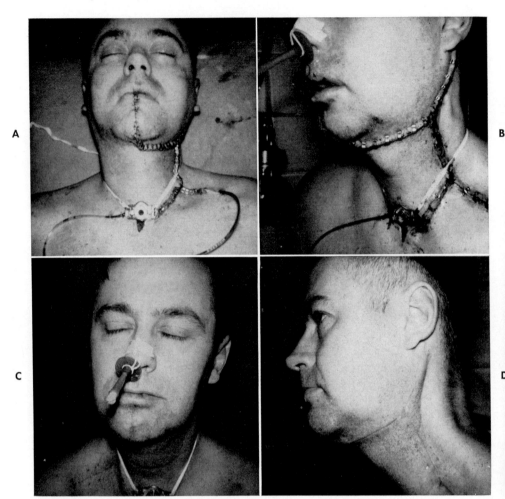

Fig. 13-4. A, Patient postoperatively showing tracheotomy tube in place and Hemovac tubing inserted in neck wound. **B,** Same patient showing suture line of radical neck dissection. **C,** Same patient showing nasogastric feeding tube in place. **D,** Same patient showing healed suture line of radical neck dissection. (Courtesy Dr. Charles C. Harrold, New York, N. Y.)

greatly enhance his acceptance for the needed surgery. Honest, straightforward answers given sincerely are essential.

Mouth care is extremely important prior to surgery, and especially if infection is present. Mouthwash, gargles, sprays, and/or irrigations may be ordered. The patient can be taught how to carry out these procedures for himself. This saves the nurse's time for other important activities and also helps the patient to be as independent as possible.

If an oral irrigation is ordered, the nurse will explain the procedure to the patient and teach him how to carry this out for himself. She will probably do the first irrigation herself, teaching as she goes along. The patient should demonstrate the procedure for the nurse. Whenever necessary, the nurse may provide assistance until such time as the patient feels secure and is capable of self-care. The patient is instructed to sit with the head bent forward and his mouth over a basin. After filling the irrigating bag with the solution ordered and allowing it to fill the tube, it is clamped off. The bag should be hung about a foot above the patient's shoulder.

The patient is then instructed to hold the emesis basin under the chin with one hand, while using the other hand to hold the tube. The rate of flow of the solution is controlled by using the finger. The patient is instructed to irrigate during exhalation but to pinch off the tube at the time of inhalation. He should also be taught to direct the stream to all parts of the mouth.

When the irrigation is completed, the nurse shows the patient how to care for the equipment. This entails washing the set with soap and water thoroughly and then rinsing and drying it.

Many of these patients are undernourished. The nurse can encourage frequent small feedings or try to elicit food preferences and, when feasible, obtain them from the dietary department. Patients with lesions involving the floor of the mouth, salivary glands, or the tongue may have feeding problems. The patient may be offered a paper or plastic straw or a teaspoon if these will minimize this difficulty. Sometimes a Breck feeder may be used. Foods should be served attractively to tempt the patient. They should be soft or liquid and should not be highly seasoned or served too hot or too cold.

Patients who cannot take anything by mouth are usually fed through a nasogastric tube. Before feedings are given, the position of the tube should be checked to be certain it is in the esophagus and not in the trachea. The nurse can determine this by slowly injecting 1 or 2 ml. of saline or Dakin's solution, which will cause violent coughing if the tube is in the trachea. If this occurs, the tube should be removed and, after the patient has had a chance to rest, reinserted. In some agencies, this can be done by the nurse, but it is important that she know the policy in the situation where she is employed.

The physician passes the tube the first time to ascertain that no obstruction exists. A No. 16 French catheter with a nasal stop is recommended. The tip of the catheter is lubricated with a water-soluble lubricant prior to insertion. Holding the catheter approximately 4 inches from the tip, with the patient in a sitting position, the nurse instructs the patient to take a deep breath. At this time, the tube is gently inserted into the nostril, pointing it directly backward in the horizontal plane. The patient is told to close his mouth and swallow repeatedly as the tube is advanced. If the catheter curls or enters the mouth or trachea, it should be partially withdrawn before attempting to readvance it. It is then checked for proper placement before feeding is administered.

The patient should be taught to administer his own feeding as soon as possible. The cork is removed from the nasal catheter, and the connecting

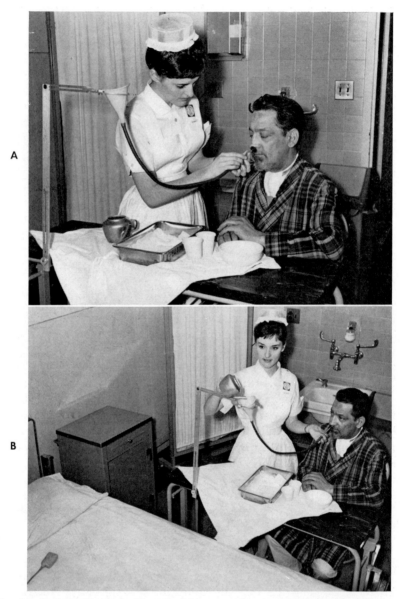

Fig. 13-5. A-C, Nasal feeding. **A,** Nurse attaches funnel and tubing to nasogastric tube prior to feeding patient. **B,** Nurse pours tube feeding through funnel.

tip is attached. The feeding is poured slowly into the funnel, which is held at eye level. Raising or lowering the funnel will control the rate of flow of the feeding. The patient should be instructed not to let the funnel empty completely, to minimize swallowing air. The feeding is followed with a small amount of water to rinse the tube. The tubing is then pinched off and removed, and the cork is replaced.

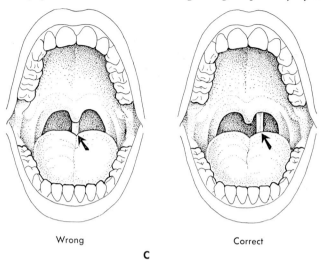

Wrong   Correct

C

Fig. 13-5, cont'd. C, Placement of tube.

Prior to surgery, the patient may experience severe pain. Medication should be offered whenever necessary to alleviate this condition.

Immediate preoperative care will not differ greatly from that given for any form of surgery. The patient needs constant emotional support as does his family. Any procedures should be explained prior to their being carried out. Medications, as ordered, are given to provide sleep. Preoperative sedation is given as ordered, and, if a recovery room is available, the patient should be informed that he will stay there for a while after the operation has been completed.

In the immediate postoperative period, the patient should be observed closely for signs of bleeding and/or respiratory distress. If the surgical procedure has been extensive, the patient may have a tracheotomy. Suctioning should be carried out as often as necessary to maintain a patent airway. The catheter should be inserted approximately 5 inches into the inner tube with the diagonal edge against the wall of the tube. The catheter should be rotated to clear all surfaces as well as the lumen of the tube. Suctioning should be employed intermittently, for no longer than 5 seconds at any one time, because the patient's airway is occluded while the catheter is in the tube. The inner tube should be cleaned at least every 1 to 2 hours, and oftener if necessary. The tube is cleansed well with cool running water using a brush. A sterile 4 by 4 inch dressing (without cotton filler) is slit at the top and is placed under the tube next to the skin. This becomes soiled easily and should, therefore, be replaced whenever necessary. Care must be taken, however, to prevent dislodging of the outer tube. A gauze bit or apron is placed over the tube to protect the airway against dust and foreign particles. A steam inhalator, or cool mist humidifier, will keep the air moistened and will keep the mucous membrane from becoming dry.

The patient who has had surgery of the head and neck area does not

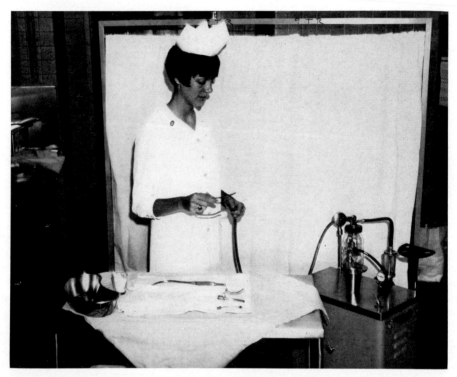

Fig. 13-6. Nurse preparing to suction the tracheotomy tube.

usually experience acute pain. Codeine and aspirin or Darvon will usually alleviate pain. Morphine sulfate is contraindicated in these patients since it depresses the cough center and respiratory center as well.

The patient is usually placed in a semi-Fowler's position following surgery. This may minimize edema and will make suctioning easier and more effective.

The nurse has a major responsibility to both the patient and his family to allay apprehension. Explanation of the reason for the tracheotomy tube and teaching the patient how to suction his own tube as soon as possible are helpful in this respect.

Since the majority of these patients are in an older age group, they must be ambulated as soon as possible. In some instances, this may mean on the day of operation; in the remainder, it means on the following day unless there are unusual and overwhelming reasons that contraindicate it.

Although most of these patients experience a fairly smooth recovery, certain complications may arise not only in the immediate postoperative period but at any time after the patient has been discharged from the hospital.

Bleeding may occur from the operative wound or from the tracheal tube (or around it). This may be observed as a persistent oozing or on occasion may occur suddenly when the dressing or the tube is being changed. When there is a possibility of hemorrhage from a large artery, such as one of the carotids, the doctor will place the patient on "carotid precautions." Hemorrhage may occur as a result of erosion of the vessel by disease or radiation. Deep erosion or slough may interrupt one of the major branches of the external carotid artery. When warning about a possible rupture has been given, the patient is placed on the critical list until the danger period is over. An emergency set, along with sterile gloves and dressings, are kept at the bedside at all times. The patient is typed and cross matched and the blood bank is alerted to keep blood on hand for such an emergency. It is essential that the suction apparatus is attached and in good working order. The patient should be placed in a room close to the nursing station where he can be observed more closely.

If the artery should actually rupture, the nurse should apply continuous pressure to the area and reassure the patient. She should have someone put in an emergency page for the doctor. A second nurse should see that oxygen is available as well as a dressing cart, emergency drug tray, and blood. An intravenous infusion should be started as soon as possible, preparatory to giving blood. She should prepare a hypodermic solution of morphine sulfate, 0.015 Gm., so that it can be given when the doctor arrives if it is needed.

Tracheal obstruction may occur due to plugs in the tube. This manifests itself by labored breathing, cyanosis, or stridor. It is particularly important for the nurse to watch for these signs of respiratory distress and act immediately. The patient will need reassurance as the nurse proceeds. She will first remove the inner cannula of the tube and instruct the patient to cough. This may dislodge the plug and clear the airway. Sometimes slapping the patient on the back as he coughs will dislodge the plug. The tracheotomy tube should be suctioned deeply to remove any other plugs that may be present. If the patient still shows signs of respiratory distress, the doctor should be called. Sometimes a plug is larger than the opening of the tube, in which case the doctor will remove the tube and use forceps (or other instruments of choice) to remove the plug.

Tracheitis sicca can occur at any time but usually not until after the second postoperative day. This is a common and persistent crusting of the tracheobronchial tree. It is frequently seen in patients with recent tracheotomies especially during winter months. The condition is treated by maintaining a high degree of humidity in the patient's room. Cold steam vaporizers will keep the air moist and minimize chances of occurrence of this complication. Recently, pancreatic digestive enzymes such as dornase have been used successfully in treating this condition.

Drainage of saliva into the neck wound is indicative of a salivary fistula. This is a result of faulty healing of the oral suture line. A fistula of this type greatly increases the danger of cellulitis, dehiscence, and hemorrhage. If this occurs, the surgeon may open the neck wound widely to permit drainage. Closure of the fistula, if extensive, may require plastic procedures. A small fistula may close spontaneously.

DYSFUNCTIONS RESULTING IN LARYNGECTOMY

Air enters the body through the nose and mouth, both of which are lined with mucous membrane. The mucous membranes help to filter out foreign materials and warm and moisten the air as it passes through. The nasal cavities open into the nasopharynx by way of the two posterior nares. These, in turn, open into the pharynx, which serves as a common passageway for air entering from both the nose and the mouth. The pharynx transmits air

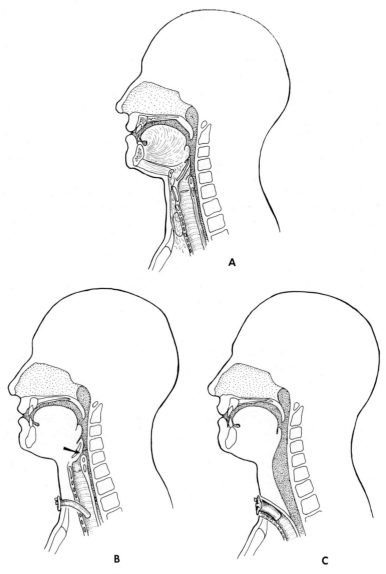

Fig. 13-7. Schematic drawing showing normal respiratory passageway, **A,** alterations due to tracheostomy, **B,** and laryngectomy, **C.**

to the larynx and, from here, to the trachea, bronchi, bronchioles, and alveoli of the lungs.

The larynx is a fairly rigid organ due to the cartilages that form it. The vocal cords are lodged within this box. Muscles act on the cartilages and ligaments to modify its opening, while the mucous membrane lining with its special folds plays an important function in producing sound.

The trachea is a large tube measuring about 2 cm. in diameter in the adult. It is ringed with transverse bands of cartilage that extend about three fourths of the way around the organ and are often referred to as "signet ring formation." The organ is several inches long and leads directly into the thoracic cavity. All passages are lined with cilia, which tend to eject foreign particles. The bronchi, bronchioles, and alveoli are found progressively as the trachea divides. It is through the alveoli that gaseous exchange occurs.

Cancer of the larynx accounts for approximately 2% to 3% of all human cancers. It affects males more frequently than females, and appears commonly between the ages of 55 and 70 years. While the etiology is unknown, there is considerable evidence that chronic irritation plays an important role. Many of the patients who develop the disease have been heavy smokers for a long period of time; a history of chronic laryngitis, vocal abuse, and familial predisposition to cancer are commonly reported.

Cancer of the larynx, if treated early, is one of the most curable of all malignancies since its earliest symptom is hoarseness or alteration in voice. Certainly, hoarseness that persists longer than 10 days to 2 weeks should be thoroughly investigated. Hoarseness may occur as a result of acute or chronic inflammation of the larynx. It may also result from paralysis of the vocal cords. Benign or malignant tumors cause hoarseness because of pressure of the tumor on or between the vocal cords, mechanically preventing their approximation and, therefore, their ability to vibrate against each other.

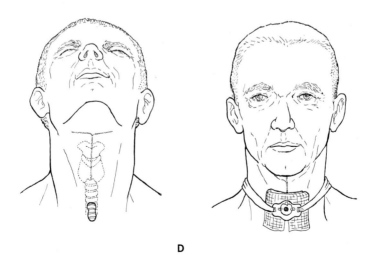

D

Fig. 13-7, cont'd. D, Anterior view with tracheostomy tube in place.

Late symptoms of cancer of the larynx include: pain generally located within or around the "Adam's apple," which radiates to the ear on the affected side; difficulty and pain upon swallowing; increasing dyspnea; enlarged cervical nodes due to metastasis; and cough. If ulceration of the lesion occurs, the cough may be productive of purulent blood-stained sputum, and frank hemorrhage may also be experienced.

A mass in the neck, indicative of cervical node metastasis, may be the first symptom that causes the individual to see the doctor. When such a mass is present, it is always evidence of advanced disease. This may often occur when the individual has ignored the early hoarseness or a persistent slight tickle in the throat.

The diagnosis of cancer of the larynx is made by means of a detailed history and physical examination, followed by roentgenographic studies of the head, neck, and chest and routine laboratory investigations. Visual examination of the larynx includes both direct and indirect methods. Indirect laryngeal examination makes use of a laryngeal mirror. In this method, the tongue is pulled forward and held out of the mouth with one hand, while the laryngeal mirror is passed over the tongue with the posterior portion of the mirror raising the uvulva and soft palate. Direct visualization through a laryngoscope is essential so that a biopsy of the lesion may be obtained for microscopic examination and verification of the diagnosis.

Treatment of cancer of the larynx may vary according to the exact site of the lesion, its size, and degree or extent of metastasis. External radiation therapy, implantation of radioactive seeds, and/or surgery may be employed. If the disease is localized to one vocal cord, is freely movable, and does not extend to the anterior commissure or posteriorly to the vocal process, external radiation may be utilized as a curative measure. On occasion, a laryngofissure or thyrotomy may be the procedure of choice. In this procedure, the thyroid cartilage is split, and the involved vocal cord and tumor are removed. The patient may have a temporary tracheotomy to facilitate breathing during the immediate postoperative period, or until edema in the surrounding tissue subsides. This may be needed only for the first 48 hours following surgery. Nourishment during this period may be provided intravenously or by nasogastric tube. As the suture line heals, a band of scar tissue, at the site from which the cord was removed, is formed. This band then becomes a vibrating surface for production of husky but acceptable speech. The patient is usually instructed not to speak for at least 72 hours postoperatively and then to whisper only until complete healing has occurred.

If the disease has progressed to involve an entire vocal cord or to extend to the opposite side, a total laryngectomy becomes necessary. This involves complete removal of the larynx, the vocal cords, and the thyroid cartilage or Adam's apple. Usually the upper part of the trachea is also resected, and the open end of the remaining portion is brought out to the anterior portion of the neck and sutured. This, then, becomes the permanent stoma through which the patient will breathe for the rest of his life. This type of surgery removes many structures essential to the production of voice and interferes with both olfactory and taste mechanisms. These patients will be unable to speak and will also have difficulty in detecting odors and tasting certain foods.

Where there are known or suspected metastatic cervical nodes, even more radical surgery is imperative. This consists of an en bloc radical neck dissection combined with total laryngectomy in an attempt to remove all evidence of disease. Surgery for the radical neck dissection* extends from the lower edge of the mandible to the clavicle and from the anterior edge of the trapezius muscle to the midline. All tissues between the platysma and the deep fascial layer are removed, with the exception of the common, the internal, and the external carotid arteries, the vagus and phrenic nerves, and the trunks of the brachial plexus. The sternocleidomastoid muscle, omohyoid muscle, internal jugular vein, accessory nerve, and submaxillary salivary gland are structures removed routinely. In specific instances, when indicated, the external carotid artery, a lobe of the thyroid gland, the strap muscles, the tenth and twelfth nerves, and the lingual branch of the fifth nerve, as well as a portion or all of the mandible, may be sacrificed.

It can easily be seen that the physiological alterations resulting from this surgery will present many nursing problems as well as functional disabilities. In addition to specific localized functional disturbances that may result, a number of general complications following major head and neck surgery may occur.

Injury or necessary resection of the facial nerve may result in facial asymmetry. The occurrence of Horner's syndrome following neck dissection is fairly frequent. This may be only temporary, although in patients who have extensive metastases, it may be permanent. This results in ptosis, miosis, and enophthalmos and is manifested clinically by inequality in the size of the pupils.

With such extensive and major head and neck surgery, complications concerned with blood loss, interference with the vital functions of breathing and swallowing, wound infection, and delayed wound healing may result. The classic picture of surgical shock, characterized by an anxious, apprehensive patient with a cold clammy skin of dusky color, a rapid pulse, and low blood pressure can be prevented in head and neck surgery by correct blood replacement at the time of surgery. In some instances in which operative wounds extend from the tissues of the neck into the oral cavity and/or pharynx, wound surfaces are unavoidably and grossly contaminated, thereby inhibiting wound healing. Antibiotic therapy minimizes this complication today. Other conditions that may inhibit wound healing and promote gross infection and breakdown in wounds include diabetes mellitus and disturbances of liver function and protein metabolism frequently encountered in the chronic alcoholic.

Since total laryngectomy results in inability to communicate verbally, the surgeon informs the patient completely about the proposed surgery. The nurse may have to reinforce this information and clear up any misconceptions. The patient will be worried for many reasons and may face his operation with

---

*Martin, Hayes: Radical neck dissection, Clin. Sympos. **13:**116, 1961.

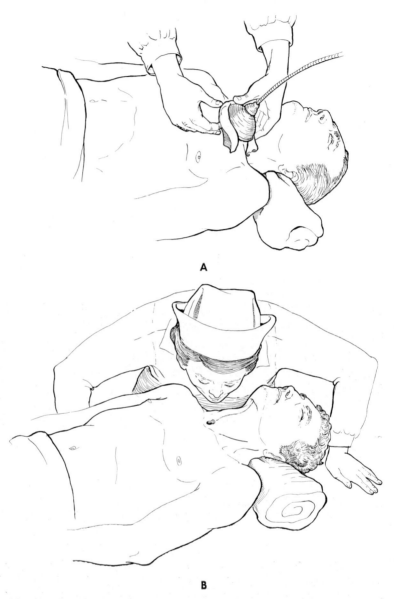

Fig. 13-8. A-D, First aid for neck breathers. **A,** Small rubber funnel to deliver oxygen after surgery. **B,** Mouth-to-stoma breathing.

terror and despair. The nurse, who understands the emotional strain he is undergoing, can do much to allay his fears and provide answers to his many questions regarding his future. The patient may fear asphyxiation. The nurse can reassure him that his respirations will not be impeded by the surgery and that she will assist him with the care of his tracheostomy until he is capable of self-care. He may fear disfigurement. Many questions arise with regard to

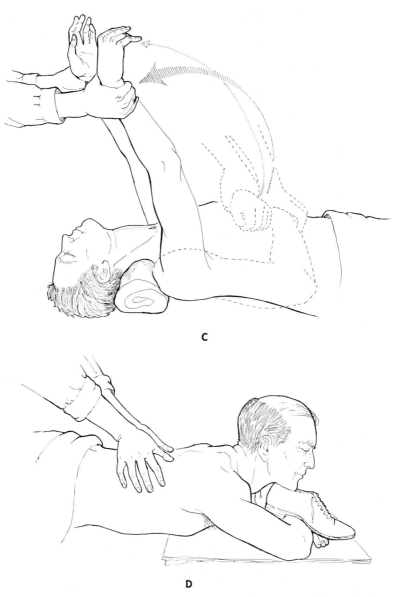

Fig. 13-8, cont'd. C, Arm-chest method of resuscitation. **D,** Head (chin) resting on shoe to maintain a patent stoma.

physical appearance: How will I look? How will my friends accept me? Can I face my wife? The nurse is the greatest help to the patient when she listens to him. Listening with a minimal amount of comment develops within the patient the ability to verbalize his fears and cope with his anxieties. The patient is often concerned as to how he will support his family. What can I do for a living? Will I be able to go back to my old job? Will my employer take me back? These are some of the fears that the patient may raise. The nurse can refer the patient to social service who may provide interim assistance. Obviously, psychological preparation is as important as physical care for the patient.

Undergoing such surgery is a traumatic experience, and the patient is often depressed when the full impact of the operation is recognized. In some cases it may be helpful to have another patient who has undergone the same operation and who has made a successful rehabilitation visit the patient about to undergo surgery. No one else can reassure the patient as effectively as a fellow patient.

Nursing care

Physical care of the patient does not differ from that described for the patient with a tracheotomy for surgery of the head and neck region (p. 221). Additional precautions are necessary for the patient with a permanent tracheal stoma. The nurse is usually responsible for telling the patient that he cannot go swimming or take a shower, since he may get water into the stoma and aspirate it. He needs to be extremely careful when shaving to keep the stoma covered so that hair or other matter does not enter. He should keep the stoma covered at all times to protect the opening from dust, lint, insects, or cold air.

DYSFUNCTIONS RESULTING IN PNEUMONECTOMY

The respiratory apparatus is responsible for the exchange of air between the atmosphere and the lungs, where gaseous exchange takes place, and the air is then expelled back into the atmosphere. While for the most part the process of breathing is quite automatic, the forces essential for the movement of air are primarily derived from contraction of skeletal muscles.

The thorax consists of the two major bronchi, the lungs, the side walls, or ribs, the intercostal muscles (between each rib), and the diaphragm, which forms the floor of the thoracic cavity.

The lungs are large, spongy, pulpy masses. In the individual who lives in a rural area where air is clean and fresh, the lungs are a bright pink color; however, in highly populated cities, they may be almost black due to soot that has penetrated them over the years.

"An ancient military adage states that there is a defense for every offense. It is indeed fortunate that a defense is available to combat pulmonary cancer inasmuch as this form of cancer has increased in incidence to an extent that has assumed pandemic significance. No other noninfectious disease has increased at such an alarming rate."*

Primary bronchogenic carcinoma, although once considered a rare condition, is now the most frequent type of carcinoma in men, and second only to

*Pack, G. T., and Ariel, I. M.: Treatment of cancer and allied diseases, ed. 2, New York, 1960, Paul B. Hoeber, Inc., vol. 4, Tumors of the breast, chest and esophagus, p. 323.

coronary heart disease with respect to mortality. Both problems are on the increase. In the early 1900's, primary lung cancer was a rare disease; by 1933, the annual death rate for males was reported at 3,410; in 1943, this had risen to 9,750; in 1953, once again a fantastic increase in deaths to 21,582, and in 1963 still a further increase to 35,300. The estimated mortality for 1967 stands at an all-time high of 44,000 men and 8,000 women.*

Although the disease may occur in any age group, approximately 80% appear between the ages of 40 and 70, and it is significantly more frequent in males than in females. The lesion may originate in the epithelial lining of any part of the tracheobronchial tree, although it appears more commonly in the larger bronchi. The right lung seems to be involved more frequently than the left.

To date, there is no specific etiological factor in the formation of pulmonary neoplasms. There are many hypotheses under consideration such as greater longevity, exposure to carcinogenic agents including radioactive gases, and/or atmospheric pollution incident to modern civilization, excessive use of cigarettes, and so forth.

The most important functions of the lungs are oxygenation of the blood and removal of carbon dioxide. Adequate movement of gases into and out of the lungs and a proper perfusion of the pulmonary capillaries are essential for the normal respiratory process.

"Adequate ventilation of the lungs requires a chest cage with sufficient mobility to permit (1) a satisfactory bellows mechanism for gas exchange with the outside atmosphere, (2) pulmonary tissue with reasonable elasticity, (3) the absence of obstruction in the tracheobronchial tree, (4) alveoli that are free of transudate or exudate, (5) the avoidance of interference with pulmonary ventilation by air and fluid in the pleural cavity, (6) a normal respiratory drive, and (7) a proper flow of blood through the pulmonary capillaries."† Needless to say, any lesion will interfere with these functions and cause respiratory embarrassment.

No tumor is more pleomorphic than is bronchogenic carcinoma.‡ Three main types are seen, however. These are the (1) squamous cell, (2) anaplastic, undifferentiated, round cell, or oat cell, and (3) adenocarcinoma. The gross appearance of these lesions varies considerably. In some instances the lesion is hard and finely nodular, while in others it is soft and friable. The margins may be sharp or indistinct with a pink, gray, or white color. The squamous cell tumor, in some instances, may show epidermoid characteristics such as cornification and the formation of epithelial pearls. Metastasis is more likely to be found in the brain and almost never to the cervical lymph nodes. With

---

*1967 Cancer facts and figures, New York, 1966, American Cancer Society, Inc., p. 28.

†Pack, G. T., and Ariel, I. M.: Treatment of cancer and allied diseases, ed. 2, New York, 1960, Paul B. Hoeber, Inc., vol. 4, Tumors of the breast, chest and esophagus, p. 266.

‡Pack, G. T., and Ariel, I. M.: Treatment of cancer and allied diseases, ed. 2, New York, 1960, Paul B. Hoeber, Inc., vol. 4, Tumors of the breast, chest and esophagus, p. 252.

the anaplastic type tumor, the cells are likely to be small and spindle-shaped or oat-shaped, although on occasion they appear round. This type lesion most commonly metastasizes to the lymph nodes. Columnar cells, sometimes distended with mucin and surrounding gland spaces, are characteristic of adenocarcinoma. Thus, it is obvious there is a great diversity in clinicopathologic changes with this disease.

There are no symptoms of early lung cancer. Oftentimes when symptoms become evident, the disease is in an advanced stage. Many procedures are available in the diagnosis of bronchogenic cancer. Various techniques may be utilized to obtain a definite diagnosis, as well as to determine resectability of the lesion by the surgeon. Bronchoscopy is the surgeon's principal technique in the armamentarium of diagnostic measures. This permits direct visualization and biopsy of many lesions, and also assists the surgeon in determining the resectability. The finding of involvement of the tracheal wall or carina by a tumor will preclude a curative resection. Also to be interpreted as signs of nonresectability will be immobility and rigidity of a main stem bronchus and also widening and fixation of the carina.

Biopsy of lymph nodes in the supraclavicular fossa is the next most frequently employed technique.* This may also preclude resection unless hemorrhage or uncontrolled infection is present. Biopsy of palpable scalene nodes has been generally accepted; however, whether or not nonpalpable nodes should be biopsied is a matter of opinion, according to the literature of the past ten years. Needle biopsy, at the present time, is the least frequently employed technique in diagnosis. If all other methods fail, or if undiagnosed pleural effusions and peripheral bronchogenic tumors (which are fixed to or invading the chest wall) are found, this method is of value. Angiocardiography may demonstrate involvement of the vena cava and/or fixation and distortion of the esophagus. These may preclude resectability.

Whatever therapy is advocated will be entirely dependent upon the patient, his age, the stage of his disease, his prognosis, and the surgeon. A large number of patients with bronchogenic carcinoma come to surgery without a histological diagnosis despite the many techniques available. In these instances, exploratory thoracotomy is in order and becomes one of the most efficient means for diagnosis, especially in those patients who have a resectable tumor. This procedure, however, is contraindicated if it is felt that the individual shows evidence of a nonresectable lesion. This is particularly true of the person who is elderly, or who shows signs and evidence of becoming a respiratory cripple.

Various procedures have been utilized in an attempt for either cure or palliation. The procedure of choice will be dependent upon the operative risk of the individual so diagnosed. Whether this be pneumonectomy, lobectomy, segmental resection, radical pneumonectomy or radical lobectomy, or one or another of the surgical procedures in combination with radiation therapy

*Shields, T. W.: Current concepts in the surgical diagnosis and treatment of bronchogenic cancer, Surg. Clin. N. Amer. **43:**110, 1963.

and/or chemotherapy will be determined according to the patient's physical condition as well as his mental, physiological, and psychological status.

Before looking at the physiological alterations resulting from therapy, it is advantageous to consider the changes that occur with tumor formation. The clinicopathology of any primary lung tumor is largely dependent on (1) histological character of the disease, (2) site of origin, and (3) mode and rate of dissemination (bronchial, contiguous, regional, lymphogenous, or hematogenous). Examination of patient histories reveals that over 50% have had complaints of a nonspecific nature for as long as 9 to 12 months. Patterns of pulmonary dysfunction associated with lung cancer include the following: (1) perhaps an audible wheeze or a slight cough; (2) symptoms of infection (fever, purulent sputum); (3) obstruction (wheezing, dyspnea); or (4) ulceration of bronchial mucosa (hemoptysis).

Although the lesion arises in the bronchial wall, the main mass may project into the bronchial lumen or infiltrate widely into surrounding normal tissue with limited intrabronchial extension. Through local extension, the tumor eventually transgresses the pleural planes, extending into blood vessels large and small, or extending medially into the trachea, either directly or by way of lymph node metastases. It is easy to see, therefore, why the symptoms mentioned may occur.

Cough is described by most patients as the first symptom noted. Since many of these individuals are heavy smokers, they attribute this symptom to "my cigarette cough." The act of coughing is a normal reflex and serves to prevent obstruction of the airway due to thermal, chemical, or mechanical stimuli. Several types of coughs have been recognized, and any or all of them may be present in the person with lung cancer. A dry, hacking cough results from bronchial stimulation, while the harsh, brassy cough is heard when there is either narrowing or compression of the passageway. When infections or necrotic exudates are present, the cough is productive of excessive amounts of sputum that may or may not be purulent.

Hemoptysis in lung cancer may be the result of extension of the tumor along the peribronchial and perivascular lymphatics that penetrate the walls of the veins. Likewise, the tumor mass may encroach upon the major vessels, causing irregularity and displacement, or disease process may obstruct passage of blood through the pulmonary vessels to such an extent that a collateral pattern of circulation becomes established. Growth of the tumor cells along the vessels eventually leads to erosion of the vessel with subsequent expectoration of blood-tinged sputum. Massive hemorrhage under any circumstances of lung cancer is rare, even in terminal stages. It is the person with persistent blood-stained specimens who is of greatest concern—one of every four lung cancer patients has this symptom.

"Tumor may cause hemoptysis by:

"1. Necrosis or ulceration of the tumor itself, resulting in bleeding.

"2. Invasion of neighboring structures and erosion of their blood vessels by the tumor.

"3. The rupture of blood vessels in the respiratory tract that have become greatly distended by the pressure exerted by a tumor mass on the tissues that contain them."*

"Pneumonia may be regarded as a symptomatic diagnosis, for there are many causes of pulmonary infection with consolidation of lung tissue and the appropriate acute symptoms of pulmonary inflammation."† Bronchial obstruction, commonly caused by bronchial cancer, is one of the predisposing causes of pneumonia. Blockage of secretions due to bronchogenic carcinoma may be designated frequently as viral pneumonia. In many instances, antibiotic therapy resolves the pneumonia, and the patient develops a confidence that all is well. It has been recommended that every male adult patient with pneumonia should be reexamined within a few weeks of clinical recovery. A chest plate should be part of this reexamination, as time is of the essence if lung cancer is to be discovered early.

Chest discomfort or real pain, a common complaint of the lung cancer patient, may occur at any stage of the disease. The symptom occurs because of (1) malignancy in the tissues or (2) pressure and irritation of the growth on adjacent organs. The pain may first manifest itself as an ill-defined sensation of fullness in the chest, a general feeling of discomfort. Over a period of weeks or months, the pain may become real or severe. Due to involvement of the mediastinum, the pleura, or nerves, sharp axillary, shoulder and subscapular pain of severe intensity may develop. The pain radiates along the medial aspect of the arm on the affected side.

Dyspnea, although rarely if ever an initial complaint, does present a problem to the patient. The problem is indicative of bronchial obstruction or pressure on the carina, mediastinum, or trachea. It may also be a symptom of complication from emphysema, atelectasis, or pleural effusion. The extent of dyspnea varies according to the degree of obstruction or pressure exerted. In some instances, the patient may not even be aware of being dyspneic (especially if the lesion is slow-growing); in other cases, the patient may describe the situation as "feeling wheezy, like with an asthmatic attack"; while the patient with advanced lung disease will frequently complain of "feeling short of breath even when at rest."

A primary tumor may remain small and silent long after there are widespread metastases that may dominate the clinical picture. Unfortunately, the methods of spread are multiform as is the microscopic picture. Although any organ may be involved by metastases, there are six sites that are predominant, namely: the lymph nodes (via the lymphatics), liver, brain, bones, adrenal glands, and kidney. Less frequent sites for metastases are the pancreas, thyroid, heart, and spleen. Of the bones, the vertebrae, ribs, and sternum are most frequently affected. Special attention has been drawn to metastases in the brain and adrenal gland since 31.4% of all cases develop metastases to

---

*MacBryde, C. M.: Signs and symptoms, ed. 3, Philadelphia, 1957, J. B. Lippincott Co., p. 347.

†Hinshaw, H. C., and Garland, L. H.: Diseases of the chest, Philadelphia, 1963, W. B. Saunders Co., p. 305.

the brain, while 21.8% metastasize to the adrenal glands. The figures for other forms of cancer are 0.9% and 1.9% respectively.*

The physiological problems of metastasis may be due to primary lung cancer or secondary to a lesion elsewhere in the body. Metastatic spread by direct extension of a malignant growth is well known. The tumor may invade the surrounding tissue, extending principally along the peribronchial and perivascular lymphatics, setting up secondary centers of growth throughout the lobe, the entire lung, and even the opposite lobe. Hematogenous spread results from invasion of the veins rather than the arteries. This is because the walls of the veins are penetrated by lymphatics. When the cancer cells enter the lumen of the vein, a thrombus is formed. In turn, this is carried by the pulmonary veins as a tumor embolus to the left side of the heart and, thence, by the systemic arteries to distant sites. Metastatic lesions in the lung from other organ tumors are more common than primary lung cancer. The close circulatory relationship between the lungs, the heart, and the lymphatic channels leads to the statistical fact that the lung is a common organ for metastatic disease.

Pulmonary complications from bronchial obstruction are many. Among those most frequently encountered are emphysema, pneumonitis, atelectasis, bronchiectasis, and abscess formation. Others, which occur less often, are malignant pleural effusion, Pancoast syndrome, and cor pulmonale and/or respiratory failure resulting from progressive replacement of normal lung tissue. In emphysema, inspired air becomes trapped behind the occluded bronchus; if it is expelled, it is with considerable difficulty and results in long, labored expiration on the part of the patient. With atelectasis, the lung tissues distal to the obstructing tumor become filled not only with trapped air but also with secretions. As the air is slowly absorbed, the lung collapses. Both bronchiectasis and lung abscess can occur as a further complication from the atelectasis. These conditions are severe, and treatment is prolonged. In some instances, there is such severe distortion and irregularity in the shape of the normal airways as to cause occlusion.

As was stated previously, the choice of therapy hinges on many factors: the age of the patient, the stage of his disease, his prognosis, and the surgeon. Suffice it to say that the more extensive the surgical procedure undertaken, the greater will be the physiological alterations encountered. Furthermore, the physical status of the patient must be considered before undertaking extensive surgery, since pulmonary complications previously mentioned may result in a respiratory cripple if there is too extensive an involvement of the lung tissues.

Pneumonectomy results in the displacement of the mediastinum toward the side of operation with an associated overexpansion of the remaining lung. The anatomical and physiological adjustment is more satisfactory following left pneumonectomy since the left lung is smaller than the right lung. Also,

*Pack, G. T., and Ariel, I. M.: Treatment of cancer and allied diseases, ed. 2, New York, 1960, Paul B. Hoeber, Inc., vol. 4, Tumors of the breast, chest and esophagus, pp. 253 and 254.

due to the smaller size, there is less reduction in the vascular bed; therefore, the heart makes a more satisfactory adjustment. Both the age of the patient and the status of the remaining lung must be considered and evaluated prior to undertaking this procedure. In the older age group (past 70 years) undergoing pneumonectomy for cancer, the frequent presence of emphysema requires a careful consideration of the undesirable features of mediastinal shift and hyperinflation of the remaining lung, which may result in considerable morbidity and mortality from right-sided heart failure and pulmonary insufficiency.

In the first few days following pneumonectomy, there is usually a slight drop in the arterial oxygen saturation. Oxygen therapy will correct this early postoperative hypoxia if the remaining lung is comparatively normal. Immediately postoperatively, it is essential that the intrapleural pressure be adjusted to a slightly negative level to minimize mediastinal shift. If this is not undertaken, a positive intrapleural pressure may interfere with cardiac filling and result in circulatory failure. If the mediastinal shift can be minimal in the first few days postoperatively, there will be a marked reduction in the incidence of cardiac arrhythmia and failure, pulmonary edema, and other respiratory complications.

Lobectomy leads to fewer physiological alterations. Frequently, following resection of a lobe, there will be a moderate drop in the arterial oxygen saturation for a few days. Here, again, oxygen therapy for the first few days will correct this condition. This drop is due to a temporary imbalance between ventilation and circulation in the remaining lobe (or lobes) resulting from splinting of the side of the operation. The effects of resection will vary according to the amount of lung tissue removed. When no more than half of one lung is excised, the remaining portion hyperventilates to occupy a volume only slightly less than that of the entire lung. In some cases in which the lobe excised was markedly diseased, there may be little or no alteration from the preoperative stage.

While pneumonectomy is considered by many as the standard procedure for the patient with a resectable bronchogenic lesion, lobectomy, on the other hand, is frequently utilized in poor-risk patients. However, in recent times, lobectomy may be considered as an adequate operation for cancer in certain circumstances.*

Nursing care

Nursing care for the patient who is to have surgery for lung cancer presents many challenges. His problems are multiple and varied. Prior to surgery, the nurse can help the patient to accept the numerous diagnostic procedures by explaining the reason for each test as well as what he can expect in terms of discomfort (if any). Sometimes, these diagnostic procedures are carried out in the clinic or in the doctor's office. It then becomes the responsibility of

---

*Shields, T. W.: Current concepts in the surgical diagnosis and treatment of bronchogenic cancer, Surg. Clin. N. Amer. **43**:113, 1963.

the clinic nurse or the office nurse to ascertain that the patient understands all directions and that he is informed regarding the reason for the procedure and what he can expect.

Once the physician has indicated the type of surgery to be anticipated, the nurse can begin teaching the patient how to cough correctly so that he will be able to cough more effectively after surgery. Exercises are begun in the preoperative period to preserve symmetrical body alignment, full range of motion of the shoulder, and maximum pulmonary function. These exercises are continued postoperatively. In many hospitals, the responsibility for teaching these exercises lies in the realm of the physical therapist; however, the nurse is responsible for following up on seeing that the patient is doing the exercises correctly.

One of the problems following thoracic surgery is to establish and maintain conditions that will provide normal intrapleural pressure and permit full expansion of the lungs. If optimum conditions are provided, the remaining portion of lung (following lobectomy) may be expanded to fill the thoracic cavity. Because of the nature of the surgery, collapse of the lung on the op-

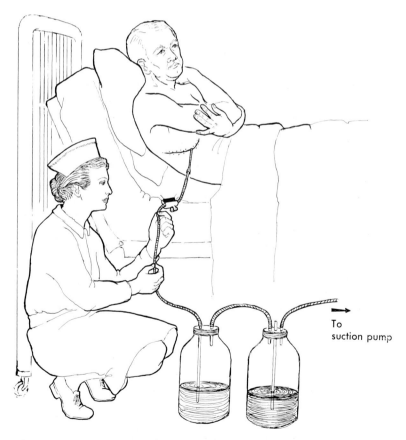

To
suction pump

Fig. 13-9. Schematic diagram showing underwater (water seal or closed) drainage.

erative side is inevitable as it is open to the atmospheric pressure during the procedure. Upon completion of surgery, expansion is attempted by use of positive pressure oxygen through the endotracheal airway used during anesthesia and surgery. In addition, a thoracotomy tube is inserted within the intrapleural space and is attached to underwater drainage (water seal or closed drainage).

When a pneumonectomy is required, the surgery entails resection of the entire lung and regional lymph nodes, ligation and transection of the pulmonary artery and pulmonary veins, bronchial artery and vein, and the main bronchus on the affected side. The problem, here, is one of keeping the mediastinum in the midline and of allowing the remaining lung full expansion despite the defect on the operative side, which exists until healing occurs. Until healing occurs, air must be used to obliterate this defect in order to equalize the pressure between the right and left pleural cavities. In any case, too little or too much air present in the pleural defect will manifest itself in mediastinal shift and resultant cardiac and respiratory distress.

Symptoms of mediastinal shift include: (1) rapid respirations, dyspnea; (2) restlessness, accompanied by an anxious expression if the patient is conscious; (3) cyanosis; (4) rapid and/or irregular pulse; and (5) if severe, shock and death may result.

The patient who has had thoracic surgery will usually be receiving oxygen therapy via the tent. Vital signs should be checked every 15 minutes until stable, then every half hour to hour (or as ordered). Abnormalities may be indicative of hemorrhage or of cardiac and/or respiratory embarrassment. The nurse needs to observe closely for any evidence of subcutaneous emphysema since this may suggest a leaking, non-airtight wound. This may be determined by measuring the size of the neck at the level of the thyroid cartilage. Dressings should be checked frequently for any evidence of bleeding. Patients should be suctioned periodically, especially if they are unable to cough or during the period in which they have not recovered from anesthesia.

When the patient returns to the floor with a thoracotomy tube attached to underwater drainage, the nurse has a major responsibility for close observation to ascertain that it is functioning properly. This means that it is essential to: (1) avoid kinking of the tubing; (2) note the character and amount of drainage—if profuse and bloody, this may be indicative of hemorrhage and the doctor should be notified immediately; (3) notify the doctor when the drainage bottle needs changing; (4) observe for fluctuation of fluid in the bottle, which should continue until the lung is completely expanded unless the drainage tube becomes plugged; and (5) note whether bubbling occurs in the drainage bottle, which may be due to air being expelled from the intrapleural space or may be due to a bronchopleural fistula, tear in the lung, or leakage at the wound site. A hemostat should be available at all times to clamp the tube, if necessary, and to make certain that the drainage bottle is not raised above the level of the bed as fluid may drain back into the intrapleural space. If the bottle must be raised, the tube should be clamped off until the bottle is once again lowered.

The patient should be turned from the operative side to his back hourly

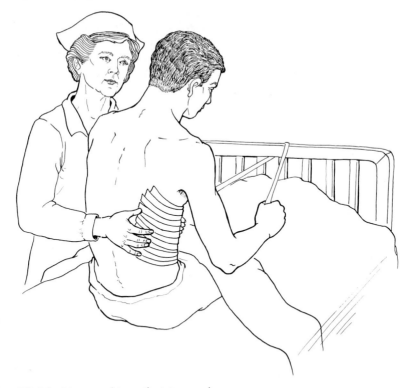

Fig. 13-10. Nurse assists patient to cough.

unless otherwise ordered, to prevent pulmonary complications. Once he has reacted from anesthesia, he should be positioned in a semigatch position. The knee gatch should never be raised. Accurate intake and output must be recorded by the nurse in order to maintain proper fluid and electrolyte balance. Sedation is limited since respiration is impaired. Opiates are contraindicated because they depress respirations; however, these patients experience considerable pain, and medication should be given as needed. The patient is ambulated as soon as possible to prevent further respiratory complications.

When the patient is ready to be discharged from the hospital, it is advisable that a referral be made for follow-up care in the home so that exercises will be continued and his condition is under constant surveillance.

Bibliography

A cancer source book for nurses, New York, 1963, American Cancer Society, Inc.
Ackerman, L. V., and del Regato, J. A.: Cancer: diagnosis, treatment, and prognosis, ed. 3, St. Louis, 1962, The C. V. Mosby Co.
Anderson, H. A., and Bernatz, P. E.: Extrathoracic manifestations of bronchogenic carcinoma, Med. Clin. N. Amer. 48:921, 1964.
Belcher, J. R.: Lobectomy for bronchial carcinoma, Lancet 2:637, 1959.
Berkson, J.: Smoking and cancer of the lung, Proc. Staff Meet. Mayo Clin. 35:367, 1960.

Bloedorn, F. G., and Cowley, R. A.: Irradiation and surgery in the treatment of bronchogenic carcinoma, Surg. Gynec. Obstet. **111**:141, 1960.

Bornstein, P., Nolan, J. P., and Bernake, D.: Adrenocortical hyperfunction in association with anaplastic carcinoma of respiratory tract, New Eng. J. Med. **264**:363, 1961.

Boyd, D. P.: Choice of operation for bronchogenic carcinoma, Surg. Clin. N. Amer. **41**: 755, 1961.

Boyd, D. P., Souders, C. R., and Smedal, M. I.: Surgery and supervoltage therapy in carcinoma of the lung, J.A.M.A. **179**:253, 1962.

Brown, A. L., Jr.: The pathology of dyspnea, Med. Clin. N. Amer. **48**:839, 1964.

Brown, J. B., and McDonnell, F.: Neck dissections, Springfield, Ill., 1954, Charles C Thomas, Publisher.

Burrows, B., et al.: The postpneumonectomy state. Clinical and physiologic observations in thirty-six cases, Amer. J. Med. **28**:281, 1962.

Cahan, W. G.: Radical lobectomy, J. Thorac. Cardiov. Surg. **39**:555, 1960.

1967 Cancer facts and figures, New York, 1966, American Cancer Society, Inc.

Cancer manual for public health nurses, U. S. Department of Health, Education, and Welfare, Public Health Service, 1963.

Chamberlain, J. M., McNeill, T. M., Parnassa, P., and Edsall, J. R.: Bronchogenic carcinoma, an aggressive surgical attitude, J. Thorac. Cardiov. Surg. **38**:727, 1959.

Cherniak, R. M., and Cherniak, L.: Respiration in health and disease, Philadelphia, 1961, W. B. Saunders Co.

Clagett, O. T., and Woolner, L. B.: Surgical treatment of solitary metastatic pulmonary lesion, Med. Clin. N. Amer. **48**:939, 1964.

Clowes, G. H., Jr., Alichniewicz, A., Del Guercio, L. R., and Gillespie, D.: The relationship of postoperative acidosis to pulmonary and cardiovascular function, J. Thorac. Cardiov. Surg. **39**:1, 1960.

Comroe, J. H., Jr.: The lung. Clinical physiology and pulmonary function tests, ed. 2, Chicago, 1962, Year Book Medical Publishers, Inc.

Davies, D. F., and Davies, A. H.: Lung cancer, cigarette smoking as a cause, Amer. J. Nurs. **61**:65, 68, April, 1961.

Farber, S. M.: Clinical appraisal of pulmonary cytology, J.A.M.A. **175**:345, 1961.

Fontana, R. S., Olsen, A. M., and Woolner, L. B.: Recent advances in the diagnosis of bronchogenic carcinoma, Med. Clin. N. Amer. **48**:911, 1964.

Frazell, E. L., and Martin, H.: Cancer of the head and neck, Ca **12**:27, 1962.

Gordon, B. L.: Clinical cardiopulmonary physiology, ed. 2, New York, 1960, Grune & Stratton, Inc.

Grollman, S.: The human body: its structure and physiology, New York, 1964, The Macmillan Co.

Hellwig, C. A., Dreese, W. C., Welch, J. W., and McCusker, E. N.: How useful is biopsy of supraclavicular lymph nodes? Surgery **51**:592, 1962.

Hepper, N. G., and Bernatz, P. E.: Thoracic surgery in the aged, Dis. Chest. **37**:298, 1960.

Hinshaw, H. C., and Garland, L. H.: Diseases of the chest, Philadelphia, 1963, W. B. Saunders Co.

Holford, F. D., and Mithoefer, J. C.: The effect of morphine on respiration in the aged, Surg. Clin. N. Amer. **40**:907, 1960.

Hueper, W. C.: Lung cancer, air pollutants as a cause, Amer. J. Nurs. **61**:64, 66, April, 1961.

Hughes, F. A., and Higgins, G.: Veterans administration surgical adjuvant lung cancer chemotherapy study: present status, J. Thorac. Cardiov. Surg. **44**:295, 1962.

Jackson, C. L., and Norris, C. M.: Cancer of the larynx, New York, 1962, American Cancer Society, Inc.

Kinsella, T. J.: Tumors of the chest, Springfield, Ill., 1963, Charles C Thomas, Publisher.

Knowles, J. H.: Respiratory physiology and its clinical application, Cambridge, Mass., 1959, Harvard University Press.

Knowles, L. N.: How our behavior affects patient care, Canad. Nurse, vol. 58, no. 1, January, 1962.

Kroeker, E. J.: Pulmonary function testing: an approach to the thoracic surgical patient, Surg. Clin. N. Amer. **41:**557, 1961.

MacBryde, C. M.: Signs and symptoms, ed. 3, Philadelphia, 1957, J. B. Lippincott Co.

MacVicar, J.: Exercises before and after thoracic surgery, Amer. J. Nurs. **62:**61, January, 1962.

Marks, L. J., Anderson, A. E., and Lieberman, H.: Carcinoma of lung associated with marked adrenocortical hyperplasia and adrenal hyperresponsiveness to ACTH in the absence of Cushing's syndrome, Ann. Intern. Med. **54:**1234, 1961.

Martin, H.: Cancer of the head and neck: a monograph for the physician, New York, 1949, American Cancer Society, Inc.

Martin, H.: Surgery of head and neck tumors, New York, 1957, Paul B. Hoeber, Inc., Medical Book Department of Harper & Row, Publishers.

Martin, H.: Untimely lymph node biopsy, Amer. J. Surg. **102:**17, 1961.

Monteiro, L.: The patient had difficulty communicating, Amer. J. Nurs. **62:**78, January, 1962.

Moore, C.: Smoking and mouth-throat cancer, Amer. J. Surg. **108:**565, 1964.

Moore, G. E., Sandberg, A. A., and Watne, A. L.: Spread of cancer cells and its relationship to chemotherapy, J.A.M.A. **172:**1729, 1960.

Nealon, T. F., Jr., editor: Management of the patient with cancer, Philadelphia, 1965, W. B. Saunders Co.

Ochsner, A., Ochsner, A., Jr., H'Doubler, C., and Blalock, J.: Bronchogenic carcinoma, Dis. Chest **37:**1, 1960.

O'Donnell, W. E., Day, E., and Venet, L.: Early detection and diagnosis of cancer, St. Louis, 1962, The C. V. Mosby Co.

Pack, G. T., and Ariel, I. M.: Treatment of cancer and allied diseases, ed. 2, New York, 1960, Paul B. Hoeber, Inc., vol. 4, Tumors of the breast, chest, and esophagus.

Paulson, D. L., Shaw, R. R., Kee, J. L., Collier, R. E., and Mallams, J. T.: Combined preoperative irradiation and resection for bronchogenic carcinoma, J. Thorac. Cardiov. Surg. **44:**281, 1961.

Pickrell, K., Woodhall, B., Georgiade, N., Matton, G., and Mahaley, M.: Cancer of the head and neck with reference to perfusion with anti-cancer agents, Surg. Clin. N. Amer. **42:**469, April, 1962.

Pollack, R. S.: Tumor surgery of the head and neck, Philadelphia, 1957, Lea & Febiger.

Rosenblatt, M. B., and Lisa, J. R.: Cancer of the lung: pathology, diagnosis, and treatment, New York, 1956, Oxford University Press.

Shields, T. W.: Current concepts in the surgical diagnosis and treatment of bronchogenic cancer, Surg. Clin. N. Amer. **43:**109, 1963.

Souders, R.: The clinical evaluation of the patient for thoracic surgery, Surg. Clin. N. Amer. **41:**545, 1961.

Souders, C. R., and Smedal, M. I.: The selection of the patient with bronchogenic carcinoma for x-ray therapy, Surg. Clin. N. Amer. **41:**761, 1961.

Spain, D. M., editor: Diagnosis and treatment of tumors of the chest, New York, 1960, Grune & Stratton, Inc.

Special head and neck issue, Clin. Sympos., vol. 13, no. 4, October-December, 1961, Summit, N. J., Ciba Pharmaceutical Products, Inc.

Stacey, R. W., and Santolucito, J. A.: Modern college physiology, St. Louis, 1966, The C. V. Mosby Co.

Stark, R. B.: Immediate complications of head and neck surgery, Surg. Clin. N. Amer. **44:**305, 1964.

Sykes, E. M.: No time for silence, Amer. J. Nurs. **66:**1040, May, 1966.

Vogel, M. D., Keating, F. R., Jr., and Bahn, R. C.: Acute Cushing's syndrome associated with bronchogenic carcinoma, Proc. Staff Meet. Mayo Clin. **36:**387, 1961.

Watkins, E., Jr.: Principles of postoperative management in thoracic surgery, Surg. Clin. N. Amer. **41:**603, 1961.

Williams, M. J., and Sommers, S. C.: Endocrine and certain other changes in men with cancer of the lung, Cancer **15:**109, January-February, 1962.

Wise, R. A., and Baker, H. W.: Surgery of the head and neck, ed. 2, Chicago, 1962, Year Book Medical Publishers, Inc.

Wise, R. E., Johnston, D. O., and Hackett, T. R.: Diagnostic radiology as related to thoracic surgery, Surg. Clin. N. Amer. **41:**573, 1961.

Wylie, R. H., and Bowman, F. O., Jr.: Immediate complications following thoracotomy for pulmonary disease, Surg. Clin. N. Amer. **44:**325, 1964.

Chapter 14

Management of the patient with advanced disease

Once a diagnosis of cancer has been established, the patient who knows his diagnosis lives in constant fear that his disease will recur. Unfortunately, he is probably right since, even with many symptomless years, the disease may recur or a new primary lesion may be discovered. While it has not been proved statistically, there is considerable evidence that the individual who has had cancer once is more likely to develop recurrence or even a second primary lesion.

Although not every patient with cancer can be cured, there is usually something that can be done for almost everyone. Due to scientific advances in the fields of diagnosis, surgery, radiation therapy, and chemotherapy, many patients are now alive and comfortable for longer and longer periods of time despite advanced disease.

Cancer, heart disease, and stroke have been named by the President's Commission on Health as chronic diseases. Somehow, perhaps due to the connotation of the word *cancer,* these patients often seem to have special social, emotional, physical, and economic problems. The magnitude of the problem will vary according to the degree of emotional and psychological stability of the individual patient. Other factors that may contribute to the extensiveness of the problems will be dependent upon how much the patient knows about his condition, his previous experiences with cancer in friends or family, and his family responsibilities.

Whether or not the patient with advanced disease will accept or reject his physical status is often dependent on the attitudes of the physician, nurse, and other paramedical members of the health team as well as those of his family and friends. Nursing care of the patient with advanced disease is time-consuming, especially if the nurse is willing to permit the patient to maintain as much independence in his care as his physical condition permits. The nurse needs to remember that any hint of help grudgingly given will be recognized by the patient who, in turn, will exhibit emotional response that may be in-

243

dicative that he feels worthless or rejected. Not only is physical care time-consuming, but the nurse will also have to allocate sufficient time to listen to the patient's complaints. Nursing care for these patients is often colored or inhibited by the nurse's previous experiences with cancer patients. Job satisfaction is often difficult to gain in caring for the patient with a long-term incurable illness, and the nurse may have to readjust her own thinking in terms of goals to be achieved—planning ways to keep the patient more comfortable for the duration of his illness, rather than planning for total rehabilitation for maximum health.

There are many problems that arise in relation to the care of the patient with advanced disease. For the most part, many of these problems can be resolved by the ingenious and understanding nurse who is willing to spend time teaching the patient and his family and who has insight into the problems, anxieties, and fears of the patient with advanced disease.

In general, these problems involve: (1) ambulation, (2) recreation, (3) skin care, (4) relief of pain, (5) control of odors, (6) metastases to bones, (7) hypercalcemia, (8) nausea and vomiting, (9) nutrition and hydration, (10) elimination, and (11) emotional and psychological aspects of care. Further, extensive, and radical surgery also presents grave problems for the patient and his family as well as for the nurse herself. Here, the nurse needs to examine her own feelings and attitudes toward radical surgery for the patient with advanced disease, since her feelings are readily communicated to the patient whether they are verbally or nonverbally expressed.

AMBULATION

Patients with advanced disease should be kept active as long as possible. This may sound particularly cruel, especially when the patient complains of pain on ambulation or feels that he is "just too weak and too tired to get up." For this reason, it is often difficult for the nurse to maintain objectivity, since she may identify with the patient. If she can remember that prolonged bed rest may result in increased bone destruction, thrombophlebitis, and hypercalcemia, the nurse will be firm in insisting that the patient move about, even if it is in a wheelchair or using a walker. While frequent ambulation is essential, periodic rest periods are necessary so that the patient does not become overfatigued.

RECREATION

When the patient has advanced disease, he is extremely likely to become severely depressed. It is essential, therefore, that the nurse provide a variety of activities that will assist the patient to keep busy so that he will not continue to worry about himself and his condition. While he is still in bed, radio and television may be helpful. Leather making, painting, knitting, crocheting, embroidery, or even sewing may serve as diversional activities. For some patients, following discharge from the hospital, community organizations or clubs are available to provide recreational activities—that is, local branches of the International Association of Laryngectomees, ileostomy clubs, colostomy clubs, and so forth. Former hobbies may be utilized as the patient's condition permits. Many patients, however, resent being forced into recreational activities. In these instances, these activities should not be forced upon the patient, since this may prove more frustrating than doing nothing to pass the time.

The nurse needs to watch the family for increasing tension due to the progression of disease in the patient. This is particularly important in terms of the person who is most involved in giving care to the patient and who is accepting major responsibility for the other family members as well. When the patient remains hospitalized and is ill for a long period of time, the nurse needs to help the family to accept and recognize the need for taking occasional rest periods as well as accepting outside recreational opportunities.

SKIN CARE

The patient who is bedridden for long periods of time due to advanced disease needs meticulous skin care, particularly in areas subject to pressure (bony prominences including the extremities, the buttocks, the hip bones, the shoulders, and the ears, often forgotten). Use of alcohol should be avoided since this tends to increase drying of the skin. Bed patients should be turned

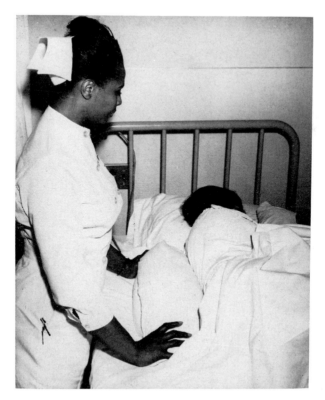

Fig. 14-1. Positioning patient with use of pillows to provide comfort.

hourly, and back rubs with compounds having a cream base should be utilized to give back care to prevent decubitus formation. When skeletal metastases are present, back rubs may be contraindicated. When redness of the skin is suggestive of possible decubitus ulcer formation, the nurse may apply tincture of benzoin compound or thymol iodide powder to the reddened area without a physician's order. If multiple decubiti are present, use of an air mattress or an alternating pressure mattress may prove helpful.

RELIEF OF PAIN

All people experience pain, and all people experience death. Misconceptions about cancer indicate that pain and death are synonymous with such a diagnosis. Only when obstruction of an organ (or system) and bone or nerve involvement occur does the patient with cancer actually experience pain. Open or infected wounds may produce pain (even as nonmalignant lesions do), and treatment with antibiotics and/or narcotics may relieve these conditions. Aspirin or Darvon is usually effective in reducing pain as are combinations of aspirin and codeine. More potent narcotics are withheld until late in the patient's illness when no other medications prove effective.

Once narcotics are started, both the nurse and the physician need to constantly assess the degree of pain the patient is experiencing before administering these drugs in order to minimize development of tolerance to the drug and/or addiction. Any or all nursing measures such as back rubs, changing of position, use of extra pillows to support the patient in a comfortable position, and listening to the patient may lessen the need for narcotics. For many patients, the psychological support he receives has a direct bearing on his need for narcotics. It should be emphasized, however, that medication should not be withheld when the patient really needs it to alleviate his pain. Many times, the nurse is reluctant to administer narcotics as often as necessary due to the fact that they can cause addiction. The management of pain in the advanced and terminal stages of malignancy, however, is often the greatest problem faced by the patient, his family, and nursing personnel. For these patients, the nurse needs to recognize that addiction is not important since there is no chance for cure or rehabilitation, and the patient should be kept as comfortable as possible in the last stages of his illness. Intractable pain may be relieved on occasion by alcohol injections, nerve blocks with phenol or alcohol, or by cordotomy or rhizotomy. Regional perfusion is sometimes beneficial in alleviating intractable pain as well.

Cancer produces pain through a variety of mechanisms. In invading surrounding structures, cancer may cause distortion and destruction of tissue, which may serve as a stimulus for activating pain fibers. Direct extension of the tumor, with infiltration into the surrounding tissues, may result in compression and destruction of adjacent nerves, nerve roots, and nerve trunks, thereby producing pain. Permeation of regional lymphatics and obstruction of venous return or occlusion of an artery often give rise to pain as a result of distention of the vessel or compression of the artery, leading to ischemia or gangrene. Inflammation, infection, and necrosis are known to lower markedly the threshold for pain. Pathological fractures due to primary or metastatic disease in bone may cause pain by injury to the periosteum or distortion of adjacent pain-sensitive structures.

The physical effects of pain depend to a great extent on the severity, duration, and quality and on the mentation, attitude, and mood of the individual. In general, pain alters the pulse rate. Superficial pain usually results in a tachycardia and increase in pulse rate. Severe deep pain causes a slowing of the pulse rate and may, on occasion, cause cardiac arrest. Respirations may be affected as a result of pain; that is, if pain involves the chest wall, breathing is principally abdominal in character, since the patient tends to splint the chest; where abdominal pain exists, a costal type of respiration is observed. Respiratory rate, as a rule, increases during severe pain. Respirations tend to be more rapid and shallow. Pain is frequently accompanied by an increase in the metabolic rate and temperature of the individual. In turn, sensitivity to noxious stimuli increases, thereby intensifying the pain. Reflex irritability and oxygen demand are generally increased, leading to further intensification of pain. Severe pain is often accompanied by nausea and occasionally by vomiting. It may also decrease or completely inhibit gastrointestinal functions, thereby slowing digestion and prolonging emptying time of the stomach.

CONTROL OF ODORS

Scrupulous cleanliness is essential in order to minimize odors. Irrigations, douches, frequent baths, and changing of soiled dressings may also be helpful in keeping odors at a minimum. Spray deodorants may help to eliminate room odors. Adequate ventilation of the room is of utmost importance. These measures will not only add to the patient's comfort but will also save embarrassment when friends or relatives visit.

METASTASES TO BONES

When patients have metastatic disease to bones, osteoporosis, or a primary bone tumor, it is important that they be supported carefully when turned or moved. This will minimize discomfort as well as decrease the possibility of pathological fracture. The patient with skeletal involvement should have a firm mattress. Proper positioning in bed with support at the back will alleviate pain. Small pillows at the nape of the neck, under an elbow, or between the legs are often comforting for the patient as well. Since frequent changes of position are essential to promote circulation and prevent formation of decubiti, a turning sheet will give added support for the patient. When skeletal metastases are present, pain is an ever-constant problem. Before bathing the patient and making his bed, giving him his pain medication may make the ordeal easier for him to tolerate. If the patient can turn by himself, allowing him to do so may very well minimize his discomfort.

NAUSEA AND VOMITING

Nausea and vomiting, if prolonged, can cause serious electrolyte imbalance and affect the nutritional status of the patient. Sometimes, small frequent feedings will control the sensation of nausea. Small sips of ginger ale or other carbonated beverages may be helpful. Occasionally, changing the patient's position will provide some relief. Use of tranquilizing drugs may be extremely beneficial in controlling nausea and vomiting.

NUTRITION AND HYDRATION

Patients with advanced cancer may sustain severe weight losses, which eventually result in malnutrition. Vitamin deficiencies and anemia occur frequently. Anorexia, as a result of nausea and vomiting, is common. The patient's diet should not only provide the daily metabolic requirements but also replacement of previous nutritional losses. The diet should be high in proteins and carbohydrates. Every effort should be made to maintain nutrition and proper hydration. This is oftentimes extremely difficult and will require considerable ingenuity on the part of the nurse. Small, frequent feedings of familiar foods served attractively may tempt the patient. Constant encouragement may serve to motivate the patient to try "just a little more." Sometimes feeding the patient will conserve his energy, thereby making it easier for him to eat more. Praising the patient when he manages to eat fairly well may also prove to be an incentive for him to continue trying. Allowing the family to bring in food from home may also be helpful.

ELIMINATION

Patients with advanced disease often become incontinent of urine or feces, or both. Urinary incontinence may be handled by the use of an indwelling catheter that will drain into a collection bottle. The bed should be protected with rubber sheeting to prevent soilage. Use of disposable Chux pads will be helpful in keeping the bed dry and in preventing breakdown of the skin. These should be changed as often as necessary even when they have not become wet, especially if they are wrinkled. Fecal incontinence presents an even more difficult nursing problem. This may necessitate diapering the patient to protect the bed and/or chair. The patient needs to be observed at frequent intervals so that excoriation of the skin does not develop as a result of fecal incontinence or diarrhea. Frequent bathing, powdering of the skin, and change of clothing are essential to control odors.

PALLIATIVE THERAPY

There are many forms of therapy available today that are useful adjuncts to keeping the patient with advanced inoperable or incurable cancer more comfortable. Specific chemotherapeutic agents are providing considerable improvement in a variety of lymphomas and leukemias and in multiple myeloma. Judicious use of these drugs produces periods of remission and allows for extension of normal life functioning for these patients.

For the patient with metastatic breast cancer, many forms of therapy are available that may keep the patient alive and living in comfort. It has long been known that some breast cancers are hormone dependent. Thus, various surgical procedures that will alter the hormone balance may produce remis-

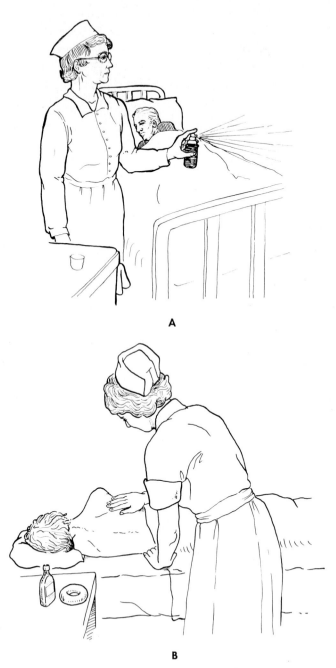

A

B

Fig. 14-2. A and **B,** Needs of advanced cancer patient. **A,** Nurse spraying room to eliminate odors. **B,** Skin care and use of doughnut to prevent decubiti.

sions for some of these women. These procedures include bilateral oophorectomy, bilateral adrenalectomy, and hypophysectomy. There is considerable variation in opinion regarding which method is best and when it should be used. Some physicians advocate bilateral oophorectomy prophylactically at the time cancer of the breast has been diagnosed and mastectomy has been performed. Other physicians are of the opinion that this procedure should be withheld until such time as the patient exhibits symptoms of reactivation of her disease. Bilateral oophorectomy is usually considered the procedure of choice for women who are premenopausal. For the patient who refuses to undergo surgery, similar results can be obtained by radiation therapy. The disadvantage here is that the physician cannot be absolutely certain that castration has been totally accomplished. Another disadvantage is that a longer period of time is necessary to obtain castration effects. When metastases are widespread, some of these patients benefit from chemotherapy with androgens. While this is a useful palliative procedure, the side effects are often very annoying. In some patients, the masculinizing effects are so distressing that treatment has to be discontinued. The most beneficial effect derived from androgen therapy is relief of pain, especially in patients with skeletal metastases. A serious complication of androgen therapy is hypercalcemia. This occurs in approximately 10% of the patients with metastatic bone disease. If undetected and left untreated, sudden death may ensue.

For the patient who is 5 or more years postmenopausal, or in whom vaginal smears show absence of ovarian function, the estrogens are the agents of choice for obtaining palliation. An exception to their use is the presence of extensive bone metastases, which respond somewhat better to androgens. Side effects associated with estrogen therapy include anorexia, nausea, and vomiting. Other side effects that may occur are the following: (1) pigmentation of the areola and nipples, the axillary folds, and the perineum; (2) tenderness and enlargement of the breasts; (3) vaginal bleeding; and (4) retention of body fluids. These symptoms often prove less distressing for the patient, and therapy can usually be continued.

When the patient obtains a remission from her disease by bilateral oophorectomy and/or androgen therapy, the chances are good that her tumor is "hormone dependent." Thus, it is likely that further ablative surgery will be beneficial when recurrence of disease occurs again. Whether this will take the form of bilateral adrenalectomy or hypophysectomy is dependent upon the philosophy of the physician, the type of facilities available, and the patient herself.

There is still considerable variation among physicians as to whether hypophysectomy should be performed (bypassing bilateral adrenalectomy) or whether hypophysectomy should be withheld for further recurrence of disease.

It is known that the adrenal cortex is the chief source of estrogen production once ovarian function has been destroyed or suppressed. This forms the basis for use of adrenalectomy in the management of advanced breast cancer. However, it has also been shown that while adrenalectomy reduces estrogen excretion, it does not always abolish it. This may also be a reason for indecision as to whether the procedure of choice is adrenalectomy or hypophysectomy.

There is considerable evidence that hormones other than estrogens are associated with the growth of mammary cancer. Herein lies the basis for hypophysectomy. As was stated previously, the premenopausal patient who has responded to bilateral oophorectomy is more likely to respond to further ablative surgery including hypophysectomy. It may also be expected that the postmenopausal patient who has responded favorably to estrogen therapy may anticipate a favorable response to hypophysectomy as well.

Whether the operative procedure is adrenalectomy or hypophysectomy, the patient will require large doses of cortisone during and immediately after surgery to control adrenal insufficiency. This dosage can usually be decreased to a maintenance dose of 37.5 mg. per day at the end of the first week. It must be emphasized that the patient will be required to take the cortisone for the rest of her life and that dosage must be altered during periods of stress, including intercurrent illness, severe stress as with further surgery, and so forth.

After hypophysectomy, thyroid replacement will be required, since thyroid-stimulating hormone from the pituitary gland has been removed. Other hormonal replacements may also be necessary. Despite these hormonal replacements, many patients are able to maintain good health for a number of years (at times).

Since the patient who consents to hypophysectomy has undergone surgery and extended treatment previously, it is assumed that this patient needs little or no explanation because she is "used to things." This is indeed a fallacy, since every new admission to the hospital requires interpretation. Furthermore, an explanation can mean much more than interpreting to the patient what will be done; it ensures or instills in her that the nurse will be available to help, that she understands what she is going through, and that she will not be left alone to cope with her problems.

The patient who is contemplating hypophysectomy has many fears: (1) fear of impending death; (2) fear of facial disfigurement because of the incision; and (3) fear of possible brain injury. Fear of death is a common occurrence, regardless of the type of procedure to be undertaken. The nurse can utilize reflective counseling techniques to permit the patient to express these fears. She can also reassure the patient about the many advances and successes in neurosurgery. Frequently, a clergyman may be able to help the patient overcome these fears better than the nurse can, and, for this reason, such a visit should be offered.

For the most part, fear of disfigurement is an extremely traumatizing experience. The nurse can suggest a new hair style (wearing bangs) or, in this day and age, the use of a wig, since these are now extremely popular. When surgery of the brain is involved, there is a natural fear of brain injury along with loss of intellectual capacity and personality characteristics. With careful explanation, geared to the sophistication of the patient, these fears can be overcome. Hormonal replacement therapy should be explained carefully prior to surgery.

Preoperatively, the patient should be informed of the fact that she will probably be excessively thirsty following surgery but that this is usually a temporary condition. She can be taught to assist with accurate intake and output measurement so that she can help with this procedure after surgery.

Following surgery, these patients do extremely well. The patient is usually able to be ambulatory after the first or second postoperative day. She should be advised that there will be little or no discomfort following this type of surgery and that, as a matter of fact, she will feel extremely well. Since pain has been considerably decreased or even absent, her appetite usually increases.

Because the sense of smell is impaired or often totally lost, the patient who had nutrition problems prior to surgery may continue to have a poor appetite following the operation. Offering small, frequent feedings of foods the patient particularly liked prior to surgery may help to ensure an adequate intake. A female patient about to be discharged should be told that she cannot rely on her sense of smell for determining when foods are done, since olfactory sensation is usually almost completely lost due to the surgical procedure.

If cortisone replacement is inadequate, the nurse should watch for anorexia, progressive weakness, lethargy, nausea and vomiting, and eventual prostration. The patient should also be taught to observe for these symptoms because they may occur following discharge in the event of any stress situation (no matter how minor). Large doses of cortisone, however, may lead to signs of Cushing's disease—puffiness of the face, masculinization, hypertension, a buffalo torso, and an elevated serum glucose that may be insulin resistant. Such symptoms will require a reduction in cortisone dosage.

The time required for observable hypothyroidism varies from 6 weeks to 6 months. It is usually evidenced, however, 2 months postoperatively. Dryness of the skin is the first symptom indicative of this condition. Since patients are rarely hospitalized long enough for myxedema to develop, the nurse is responsible for teaching the patient and her family that cold intolerance, constipation, lassitude, mental apathy, and dryness or thickening of the skin mean that the patient is in need of additional thyroid medication.

Following surgery, the nurse should observe for signs indicative of cerebral edema. Although cortisone therapy should prevent this complication, it must still be considered a possibility. In the immediate postoperative period, nasal suctioning is contraindicated since this may cause pressure on the operative suture line, especially if the transsphenoidal approach has been utilized.

Accurate intake and output are essential in the immediate postoperative period, since profound polyuria may develop within a few hours following surgery. This is usually controlled by means of insertion of a Foley catheter to measure urinary output, and intravenous therapy with 5% dextrose in water is administered at the rate of 1,000 ml. per hour. If urinary output exceeds 2,000 ml. per hour, Pitressin is usually administered to control diabetes insipidus. Fluid intake must be increased appropriately; however, the patient must be observed closely for water intoxication (headache, nausea, vomiting, excessive perspiration, and altered behavior). All of these are indicative of need for reduction of fluid intake. As soon as the Foley catheter can be removed and the patient is capable, she may begin to keep her own intake and output record.

Diabetes mellitus complicates the care of the patient who must undergo hypophysectomy or bilateral adrenalectomy, since carbohydrate metabolism is altered by these procedures. Thus, the patient must be observed closely in terms of insulin replacement or deferment of use of insulin. Fractional urines should be performed at frequent intervals to determine the need for insulin replacement. It is, therefore, essential that the nurse explain the reasons for change in the amount of insulin administered, especially when the patient has been controlled for many years on a specific dose.

Since hypophysectomy is no longer considered to be an unusual form of therapy, especially for metastatic breast cancer, the nurse must be able to meet the challenge of assisting the patient preoperatively and postoperatively while she is hospitalized and extend her services to home care by referral to the visiting nurse, public health nurse, or other community resources available to the patient and the family.

Taking everything into consideration, immediate goals for the nurse are to help the patient and the family to accept the needed therapy by promoting confidence and understanding of the procedure to be performed. Thinking in terms of long-range goals, the nurse will need to teach the patient and the family the need for continual hormonal therapy, the need for periodic follow-up, and to help them accept and utilize the added lifetime made possible by hypophysectomy.

Even when recurrence appears after hypophysectomy, the patient may still experience remission from chemotherapy with 5-FUDR or other similar agents.

Needless to say, the patient with advanced breast cancer has many opportunities for remission of disease and therefore cannot be considered terminal until all forms of therapy fail to produce remission.

At the time all measures have failed (surgery, irradiation, and chemotherapy), the patient can then be considered to be in the terminal stage of disease. From here on, the nurse can do nothing more than keep the patient as comfortable as possible until death ensues. Maintaining conditions as near normal as possible for the patient and family will undoubtedly help retain morale for all concerned. Allowing the patient to do anything and everything he is capable of doing for himself will avert complete loss of hope.

No other situation can provide a greater challenge to the nurse than caring for the patient with advanced or terminal disease resulting from cancer. The nurse is in the key position to make or break the morale of the patient even in the terminal stage of his illness.

Bibliography

Aldrich, C. K.: The dying patient's grief, J.A.M.A. **184:**329, 1963.
Aring, C. D.: Sympathy and empathy, J.A.M.A. **167:**448, 1958.

Barckley, V.: What can I say to the cancer patient? Nurs. Outlook 6:316, 1958.

Barckley, V.: The crises in cancer, Amer. J. Nurs. 67:278, 1967.

Brauer, P. H.: Should the patient be told the truth? Nurs. Outlook 8:672, 1960.

Cancer manual for public health nurses, Washington, D. C., 1963, U. S. Department of Health, Education, and Welfare, Public Health Service.

Cobb, B.: Emotional problems of adult cancer patients, J. Amer. Geriat. Soc. 7:274, 1959.

Editorial: What man shall live and not see death? Nurs. Outlook 12:23, 1964.

Edwards, L. G.: My most important patient, Amer. J. Nurs. 62:85, March, 1962.

Farberow, N. L.: Taboo topics, New York, 1963, Atherton Press.

Fayer C. A.: Selection of patients with metastatic breast cancer for hypophysectomy, Surg. Clin. N. Amer. 42:701, 1962.

Feifel, H., editor: The meaning of death, New York, 1959, McGraw-Hill Book Co.

Folck, M. M., and Nie, P. J.: Nursing students learn to face death, Nurs. Outlook 7:510, 1959.

Fox, J. E.: Reflections on cancer nursing, Amer. J. Nurs. 66:1317, 1966.

Fuerst, E. V., and Wolff, L.: Fundamentals of nursing, Philadelphia, 1964, J. B. Lippincott Co., chap. 40.

Fulton, R.: Death and the self, J. Religion & Health 3:359, 1964.

Glaser, B., and Strauss, A.: Awareness of dying, Chicago, 1965, Aldine Publishing Co.

Glaser, B., and Strauss, A.: The social loss of dying patients, Amer. J. Nurs. 64:119, June, 1964.

Glaser, B. G., and Strauss, A. L.: Temporal aspects of dying as a non-scheduled status passage, Amer. J. Sociol., June, 1965.

Homberger, F., and Bonner, C. D.: Medical care and rehabilitation of the aged and chronically ill, ed. 2, Boston, 1964, Little, Brown & Co., chap. 3.

Hyde, R. W., and Coggan, N. E.: When nurses have guilt feelings, Amer. J. Nurs. 58:233, 1958.

Ingles, T.: Death on a ward, Nurs. Outlook 12:28, 1964.

Lubic, R. W.: Nursing care after adrenalectomy or hypophysectomy, Amer. J. Nurs. 62:84, April, 1962.

Norris, C. M.: The nurse and the dying patient, Amer. J. Nurs. 55:1214, 1955.

Oken, D.: What to tell cancer patients, J.A.M.A. 175:1120, 1961.

Pearson, O. H.: Adrenalectomy and hypophysectomy, Amer. J. Nurs. 62:80, April, 1962.

Pearson, O. H.: Endocrine consequences of hypophysectomy, Anesthesiology 24:563, 1963.

Quint, J. C., and Strauss, A. L.: Nursing students, assignments, and dying patients, Nurs. Outlook 12:24, 1964.

Ray, B. S., and Pearson, O. H.: Hypophysectomy in treatment of disseminated breast cancer, Surg. Clin. N. Amer. 42:419, 1962.

Schon, M.: Hypophysectomy as a psychological experience. Dis. Nerv. Syst. 20:75, 1963.

Strauss, A. L., Glaser, B. G., and Quint, J. C.: The nonaccountability of terminal care, Hospitals 38:73, 1964.

Taylor, S. G.: Endocrine ablation in disseminated mammary carcinoma, Surg. Gynec. Obstet. 115:443, 1962.

Chapter 15

Community resources for the patient and his family

The family of a cancer patient have heavy financial burdens placed upon them. Not only is the cost of treatment expensive but many other complex problems also arise during the course of the patient's illness. The psychological impact of a diagnosis of cancer can be almost overwhelming.

In many instances, the patient has been the breadwinner of the family, and job security is at stake along with tremendous fears as to how the family will be taken care of. On the other side of the picture is the housewife and mother who has young children in the home to be fed, dressed, and gotten off to school, along with responsibilities for cooking, washing, ironing, and keeping the household in order. Often more traumatic is the diagnosis of cancer in a child or teen-ager. Very likely, the parents may mortgage their home (if they own a house), sell all of their valuables, and actually place themselves in debt to see that everything possible is done for their youngster.

Cancer is no respecter of age, race, sex, or religion. The disease affects the rich or the poor; the young or the old; white, black, or yellow; and Catholic, protestant, or Hebrew. Invariably, many patients and their families are in need of assistance but are reluctant to ask if help is available. At the same time, many nurses may recognize that help is needed by the patient or his family and not know where to turn to provide such assistance.

Needs may be minimal or complex, and the nurse is in a key position to assist the patient and his family to obtain the necessary help, since lack of help may be a major factor in delaying rehabilitation.

The American Cancer Society, Inc., is a national agency, the major purpose of which is to pioneer organizations in cancer control in the United States. It is a voluntary organization of people united in a determination to conquer cancer. The national office is located in New York City. The organization has fifty-eight chartered divisions and 3,081 units.* The National

---

*1967 Cancer facts and figures, New York, 1966, American Cancer Society, Inc., p. 28.

Society is responsible for over-all planning and coordination and provides technical help and materials to divisions and units. The local units, at the grass roots level, provide assistance for the cancer patient and his family to meet the grave problems and heavy financial burdens of this serious illness. The local units provide a variety of services that are available to anyone—information about cancer and cancer detection and facilities for diagnosis may be obtained by calling the local unit, or by visiting in person.

For cancer patients and their families, a telephone call from the family physician or the social worker in the hospital is all that is needed to procure a variety of services. Some services are provided free to all, regardless of financial status, such as information and counseling to help meet the multiple problems resulting from cancer, as well as dressings for the patient whenever necessary.

For the patient who is not eligible for public assistance and is unable to pay, a number of services are offered through the organization. Not all services are available through every unit, since needs vary from one community to another. The nurse should become familiar with the services offered in the community where she works in order to be of assistance to the patient. The various services that may be available include:

1. Visiting nurse service to the patient in the home to provide prescribed nursing care and to teach and/or reinforce teaching of the patient and his family in his care.
2. Care in approved nursing homes when necessary, including drugs and medications.
3. Practical nurses for the patient at home who requires prolonged bedside care.
4. Emergency doctor service to guarantee availability of a physician at all times for patients at home.
5. Oxygen for the patient at home, supplied and delivered by a commercial company but paid for by the local unit.
6. Blood transfusions for patients preoperatively and postoperatively.
7. Cancer drugs, including those for leukemia, are available to patients on doctor's prescription. These include corticosteroids and hormonal substances. Drugs may also be obtained for palliative treatment, to make the patient more comfortable.
8. Radon seeds and radioactive isotopes needed for treatment.
9. Prosthetic equipment for patients requiring braces and artificial parts will be supplied to encourage rehabilitation or for cosmetic purposes.
10. Housecleaners to do periodic heavy cleaning and to help around the house when the services of a homemaker are not necessary.
11. Homemakers who help maintain and preserve family life are available to serve in the home by assuming full or partial management of the household when the mother of a family is ill, or when the patient is alone during the breadwinner's working hours.
12. A loan closet to provide sickroom equipment, hospital beds, wheel chairs, bedding, and other items for the patient's comfort at home.

13. Speech rehabilitation for laryngectomy patients when new speech methods must be learned.
14. Small equipment such as colostomy sets, hot-water bottle, ice bag, basins, catheters, air rings, and a variety of sickroom supplies are provided for patient care.
15. Transportation for the patient who needs to go to the hospital or clinic for treatment and is too ill to go by bus or subway. Volunteers call for the patient and take him home in unmarked station wagons. In some instances, transportation by taxi will be covered.
16. Gifts are sent to patients throughout the year. Bed jackets, slippers, toilet items, games, and so forth are supplied; these have been donated or made by volunteers.
17. The Papanicolaou smear test for uterine cancer is available free to women patients of private physicians if they cannot afford to pay the laboratory charge.

In addition to their patient service program, these units help save lives by bringing cancer education messages into homes, factories, offices, and schools; they keep the physician up-to-date on the newest and best methods of detecting, diagnosing, and treating cancer; and they help support research in hospitals, universities, and laboratories.

While the patient is still hospitalized (and in some cases, even after the patient has gone home), the social worker, who has been apprised of the patient's needs, may contact a number of other agencies or organizations that will provide various forms of assistance for the patient and his family. These may include the Veterans Administration, the Office of Vocational Rehabilitation, the Traveler's Aid Society, the Community Service Society, the local Mental Health Association, the Salvation Army, Social Security Agencies, and so forth. Many times the patient may have other medical problems that complicate his condition, and assistance may be procured from a variety of organizations for these specific conditions—for example, local units of the American Heart Association, the National Arthritis Foundation, the Agency for the Handicapped, the Agency for the Blind, the Tuberculosis Association, Alcoholics Anonymous, and many other agencies that are available in the community.

Many nurses, patients, and families are unaware that frequently help can be obtained through the church or religious affiliation group of which they are members. Thus, the church (or synagogue), the local units of Catholic Charities of the Archdiocese, the Federation of Jewish Philanthropies, or the Federation of Protestant Welfare Agencies can be contacted for assistance.

Still other sources that may be explored for assistance include unions and fraternal organizations, such as the Elks Club and the Shriners. Special interest clubs are often available within a community, such as a local club of the International Association for Laryngectomees (where tracheotomy tubes, laryngectomy tubes, tracheal bibs, and speech lessons may be obtained without cost).

The nurse who is well informed regarding community resources for the cancer patient and his family, can alleviate a number of major emotional and economic problems for them and can hasten and enhance a more speedy recovery and rehabilitation. Sometimes all that is required is a telephone call from the physician, the social worker, or the nurse, and necessary assistance is available. There is really no end to possible resources, and the patient should be provided with anything and everything that will accelerate his recovery or relieve him from constant worry about his family and how they will manage if he is unable to provide for their care.

Chapter 16

Cancer research

Many efforts are being expended throughout the world in cancer research, and some progress in all fields is being made. Experimental research, statistical aspects, clinical aspects, diagnosis, radiotherapy, chemotherapy, and social aspects constitute a seven-pronged attack to solve the cancer problem.*

While cancer is on the increase, more and more people are surviving for longer periods of time without evidence of disease and are living normal lives. Newer developments in cancer treatment are occurring continuously. Surgery is still the most effective method for controlling the disease. Monobloc operations are currently being utilized in treating advanced but localized disease. Hemicorporectomy (or transection) is a surgical procedure that is extremely experimental and can be carried out only in highly specialized cancer centers at the present time. It has been performed only in five or six patients to date; however, the American Cancer Society is of the opinion that it could save many lives. It can be employed for the patient with widespread, but localized, disease within the pelvic area. It involves amputation of the lower half of the body, resulting in a colostomy plus some form of urinary diversion. It is unfortunate that only one patient who has undergone this procedure is living, free of disease, and rehabilitated. Whether such surgery will be continued and gain in popularity remains to be seen.

Another recent advance in this field is the laser device, whose beam is capable of distintegrating the tissue on which it is focused. It is hoped that the laser may eventually be developed to the extent that it will serve as a useful therapeutic tool. Many advances have been made in terms of rehabilitation of the patient who has undergone laryngectomy, radical mastectomy, and certain surgical procedures for cancer of the colon or rectum, by use of prosthetic devices, and so forth. Both modern anesthesia and antibiotics along with perfected surgical techniques have been responsible for lowering mortality rates.

---

*Raven, R. W., editor: Cancer progress 1960, London, 1960, Butterworth & Co., p. xiii.

Considerable hope for future control of advanced cancer is being placed upon chemotherapy, and new compounds are constantly being introduced for clinical use. It is extremely important to know the mechanisms of anti-tumor activity of the chemotherapeutic compounds being utilized. Many problems in this field still exist, and considerable attention is being given to controlling the toxic effects incurred by the use of these agents. In the past ten years, hundreds of thousands of chemical compounds have been tested for activity against experimental tumors. Only a minor number of these drugs have, at present, proved useful in treating human cancer.

In 1962, the American Cancer Society stepped up its campaign against leukemia. Families with a leukemia patient, particularly a child, face many serious difficulties that require the help of friends, neighbors, and skilled counselors to cope with their situation. The most common causes of death among leukemia patients are hemorrhage and infection. Hemorrhage occurs as a result of a thrombocytopenia while infection results from decreased granulocytes in the blood. Progress has been made in solving problems in both of these areas during the past few years.

Platelet transfusions have been found effective in the prevention and control of hemorrhage; however, serious limitations occur that make this procedure extremely difficult—platelets are needed in extremely large quantity, and they must be used within a very few hours after having been withdrawn from a donor. A new method has been devised that has greatly increased the available supply of fresh platelets for transfusion. The advantage of the newly devised procedure permits donors to give platelets as often as twice a week for periods up to 3 months; by conventional methods, blood can be donated only once every 6 to 8 weeks.

The use of platelet transfusions has substantially reduced the frequency of death resulting from hemorrhage, has prolonged the life of the individual, and has permitted the physician to give increased doses of chemotherapeutic agents that under normal conditions depress platelet production. The results, in some instances, have been so dramatic that many patients are given these transfusions as a preventive measure whenever platelet count falls dangerously low.*

From the success achieved with platelet replacement, the National Cancer Institute scientists began working on a test for granulocyte replacement for treatment of infection in acute leukemia patients.* The source of granulocytes was finally found in patients with chronic myelogenous leukemia whose levels of granulocytes are very high in circulating blood. One of the results of this research was that the granulocytes may become transplanted into the recipient and continue to produce mature granulocytes and red cells for varying periods of time.*

The National Cancer Institute is sponsoring the development of a con-

---

*U. S. Department of Health, Education, and Welfare, Public Health Service/National Cancer Institute/National Institutes of Health; Progress against cancer 1966, Washington, D. C., 1967, p. 34.

tinuous flow blood cell separator that utilizes a centrifuge to separate the white cells from the donor's blood and return the other elements back to the donor. The blood will flow in a closed system from a vein in one arm of the donor, through the separator, to a vein in the other arm. It is anticipated that sufficient numbers of granulocytes required for one transfusion will be able to be obtained from the blood of a single donor. With the method currently in use, more than thirty normal donors are needed to obtain an adequate number of granulocytes.

Methods of germ-free isolation technique are being studied as a means of prevention of serious infection in leukemia patients. The patient is placed in a controlled environment unit such as the Life Island (Fig. 6-5, p. 73).

Chromosome studies are being undertaken in an effort to understand the nature of the leukemias. It has been found that in the majority of leukemic patients chromosomal abnormalities are present in their leukemic cells. It has also been observed that this structural abnormality disappears from the bone marrow during the stage of remission only to reappear in relapse. Other chromosome studies are also under investigation to determine whether there is a relationship between mongolism and leukemia, since considerable evidence shows the probability of leukemia occurring in children with mongolism to be 30 to 50 times higher than for the general population.*

A special Virus-Leukemia Program was established about 2 years ago by the National Cancer Institute. The major goals of the program are to identify a human leukemia virus and subsequently develop a vaccine or some other method for prevention or control of the disease. Within the past year, encouraging progress has been made in detection, isolation, characterization, and growth of new viruses recovered from patients with leukemia.

Extensive studies for detection of suspicious masses in the breast are underway through the technique of mammography or examination of the breasts by x-ray. Reports thus far have shown that cancers not detectable by clinical means are being revealed. There is also a possibility that x-ray mammography may be useful in prevention as well as in early detection if certain breast patterns are associated with increased risk to breast cancer development.

An even more recent technique is under investigation for detecting breast cancer in very early stages. This is through the use of infrared thermography. There is considerable evidence that most breast cancers are associated with increased surface temperature and that the degree of increase is related to the patient's prognosis and survival time.

Considerable evidence indicates that Hodgkin's disease, discovered while it is still localized and treated with intensive doses of radiation, can be com-

---

*U. S. Department of Health, Education, and Welfare, Public Health Service/National Cancer Institute/National Institutes of Health; Progress against cancer 1966, Washington, D. C., 1967, p. 3.

Table 16-1. Commonly used radioisotopic compounds*

Radioisotopic compound and symbol	Pharmaceutical name	Physical half-life	Dose (μC)
Thyroid			
Iodine-131 (^{131}I)	Sodium iodide	8.1 days	25-100
Brain			
Radioiodinated serum albumin (RISA) (^{131}I)	Human serum albumin	8.1 days	200-700
Mercury-203-neohydrin (^{203}Hg)	Chlormerodrin	47.9 days	700
Arsenic-74 (^{74}As)	Sodium arsenate	17.5 days	500-1,500
Eye			
Phosphorus-32 (^{32}P)	Sodium phosphate	14.3 days	250-750
Liver			
Colloidal gold-198 (^{198}Au)	Colloidal gold	2.7 days	50-500
Rose bengal-I-131 (tetraiodotetra-chlorfluorescein) (^{131}I)	Rose bengal	8.1 days	50-500
Pancreas			
Selenomethionine-75 (^{75}Se)	Selenomethionine	127 days	150-200

*From Ackerman, N. B.: Use of radioisotopic agents in the diagnosis of cancer, Ca **15**:257, 1965.

Detection method	Rationale	Application
Scintillation scanning at 24 hours	Cancer is rare in "hot" nodules, occurs 3-10% in "warm" nodules and 14-30% in "cold" nodules; some metastatic thyroid cancers concentrate I^{131}, especially after total thyroidectomy	Screening of thyroid nodules; surgery may be indicated for solitary "cold" nodules. Scanning neck or body after thyroidectomy for diagnosis of metastases
Scintillation scanning at 6 to 48 hours	Tumor blood-brain barrier is penetrated more than that of normal brain	Brain tumor diagnosis; retained longer than most of the other compounds
Scintillation scanning at 1 to 4 hours	Same	Brain tumor diagnosis; long half-life, but short retention results in less body radiation than RISA
Coincidence scanning of annihilation photons at 20 minutes to 4 hours	Same	Brain tumor diagnosis; coincidence counting results in high efficiency and low background radioactivity
Eye probe Geiger-Mueller counting directly over eyes at 1 to 48 hours	Increased phosphorus uptake by malignant tumors	Eye tumor diagnosis; accuracy better for melanomas than for retinoblastomas; posterior lesions require introduction of curved probe through incision in Tenon's capsule
Scintillation scanning at 30 minutes to 5 hours	Taken up by reticuloendothelial system of liver; space-occupying lesions, including primary and metastatic cancers, do not concentrate it	Diagnosis of liver tumors; limited to lesions greater than 2 cm. in diameter; does not differentiate between benign and malignant lesions
Scintillation scanning at 20 to 30 minutes	Taken up by polygonal cells of liver; space-occupying lesions, including primary and metastatic cancers, do not concentrate it	Same. Must do study within 2 hours because of rapid excretion, but causes less liver radiation than colloidal gold
Scintillation scanning at 30 minutes to 1 hour	Concentrated by normal pancreas; benign and malignant space-occupying lesions do not concentrate it	Pancreatic disease diagnosis; interpretation difficult due to liver interference and variations in pancreatic size and shape; usually hard to differentiate between benign and malignant lesions

Continued.

Table 16-1. Commonly used radioisotopic compounds—cont'd

Radioisotopic compound and symbol	Pharmaceutical name	Physical half-life	Dose (µC)
Kidney			
Mercury-203-neohydrin (^{203}Hg)	Chlormerodrin	47.9 days	50-200
I-131-hippuran (^{131}I)	Sodium iodohippurate	8.1 days	100-800
Bone			
Strontium-85 (^{85}Sr)	Strontium chloride	65 days	50-100
Strontium-87^m (^{87m}Sr)	Strontium chloride	2.8 hours	100
Calcium-47 (^{47}Ca)	Calcium chloride	4.9 days	50

pletely controlled in about 40% of the patients for periods exceeding 15 years.*

Intensive drug therapy for choriocarcinoma, a rare and highly malignant type of tumor arising from the placenta during or after pregnancy, with methotrexate and actinomycin D has led to complete remission of disease in over 75% of the patients treated. There is good reason to believe that if treated early this tumor can be entirely eradicated.

Encouraging progress is being made in the treatment of Wilms' tumor and retinoblastoma. With Wilms' tumor, combination forms of therapy (radiation therapy with administration of actinomycin D or surgery followed by radiation therapy and actinomycin D) increased life expectancy and produced an apparent cure rate of about 14% in the small sample studied.

Retinoblastoma frequently affects both eyes of the child. Surgery or intensive radiation may save the child's life, but blindness is inevitable. Recent studies indicate that use of smaller amounts of radiation does not decrease

*U. S. Department of Health, Education, and Welfare, Public Health Service/National Cancer Institute/National Institutes of Health; Progress against cancer 1966, Washington, D. C., 1967, p. 51.

Detection method	Rationale	Application
Scintillation scanning at 40 minutes to 4 hours	Diuretic excreted by normal kidney	Renal scanning; more valuable in studying function than in detecting cancer; limited by size of lesion and difficulty in distinguishing between benign and malignant lesions
Scintillation scanning immediately	Excreted by normal kidney	Same; added disadvantage of very rapid excretion by kidneys
Scintillation scanning at 24 to 48 hours	Strontium and calcium compounds localize in actively metabolizing bone and bone tumors	Detection of primary and metastatic bone tumors; problems include high background body radiation and differentiation of benign from malignant lesions
Scintillation scanning at 40 minutes	Same	Same
Scintillation scanning at 1 to 2 days	Same	Same

the survival rate and, more important, does increase the percentage of patients surviving with useful vision.*

Continuing advances in all areas of biomedical science and in health and medical care are contributing to the goals for progress against cancer. Accumulated knowledge concerning DNA and RNA have been helpful in determining how a normal cell can be converted into a malignant one—the genetic code. Success in this area could lead to or reveal the mechanism of action of agents known to be carcinogenic to man.

Cancer chemotherapy has made tremendous strides in producing remission from various forms of cancer, and in the case of choriocarcinoma it may eventually lead to 100% cure.

Through continued education programs for physicians, nurses, and the laity, earlier diagnosis can be anticipated with increased cure rates.

All in all, however, the main hope for a breakthrough in the cancer problem lies in the continued efforts of research.

---

*U. S. Department of Health, Education, and Welfare, Public Health Service/National Cancer Institute/National Institutes of Health; Progress against cancer 1966, Washington, D. C., 1967, p. 56.

Table 16-2. Experimental radioisotopic compounds*

Radioisotopic compound and symbol	Pharmaceutical name	Physical half-life	Dose (μC)
Head and neck tumors			
Thyroid Iodine-125 (^{125})	Sodium iodide	60 days	50-100
Parathyroid Selenomethionine-75 (^{75}Se)	Selenomethionine	127 days	200-250
Cobalt-57-vitamin B$_{12}$ (^{57}Co)	Cyanocobalamin	270 days	18-47
Other head and neck tumors			
Phosphorus-32 (^{32}P)	Sodium phosphate	14.3 days	100-1,000
Phosphorus-32 (^{32}P) and iodine-131 (^{131}I)	Sodium phosphate and sodium iodide	14.3 days and 8.1 days	100 and 50
Brain tumors			
I-131-diiodofluorescein (^{131}I)	Diiodofluorescein	8.1 days	250-1,000
Iodine-131 (^{131}I)	Sodium iodide	8.1 days	300
Phosphorus-32 (^{32}P)	Sodium phosphate	14.3 days	1,000
Potassium-42 (^{42}K)	Potassium chloride	12.5 hours	500-1,000
Copper-64 (^{64}Cu)	Copper versenate Copper phthalocyanine Copper chelate of DPTA	12.8 hours	2,000-3,000
Mercury-197-neohydrin (^{197}Hg)	Chlormerodrin	2.7 days	700
I-131-polyvinylpyrrolidone (PVP) (^{131}P)	Tolpovidone	8.1 days	500
I-131-octoiodofluorescein (^{131}I)	Octoiodofluorescein	8.1 days	200-300

*From Ackerman, N. B.: Use of radioisotopic agents in the diagnosis of cancer, Ca **15:**257, 1965.

Detection method	Rationale	Application
Scintillation scanning at 24 hours	Same as ^{131}I; softer gamma radiation may give improved scans	Screening of thyroid nodules; not yet in widespread use
Scintillation scanning at 2 to 8 hours	Concentrated by parathyroid tissue	Still experimental; used for preop and operative localization of parathyroid adenomas; scans indistinct due to isotope impurities and marrow uptake
Scintillation scanning at 24 hours	Concentrated by parathyroid tissue	Experimental; used for preop and operative localization of parathyroid adenomas; small size of tumors and concurrent uptake by the thyroid are limitations
Geiger-Mueller tube counting at 1 to 48 hours	Increased uptake by active head and neck cancers, including thyroid	Use limited by ^{32}P properties; shallow tissue penetration, low tissue levels, difficulties with inactive tumors and inflammation
Geiger-Mueller tube counting at 24 to 48 hours	High ^{131}I uptake: substernal thyroid; high ^{32}P uptake; lymphoma; low ^{32}P and ^{131}I uptake; cysts and fibromas	Not widely accepted; diagnosis usually made at operation
Scintillation scanning or counting at 15 minutes to 4 hours	Tumor blood-brain barrier is penetrated more than that of normal brain	First agent used for brain tumor diagnosis; rapidly excreted; no longer commonly used
Scintillation scanning or counting at 1 hour	Same	No advantage over RISA; shorter retention in body
Fine Geiger-Mueller probes at operation at 1 to 24 hours	Same	Use limited by shallow penetration
Geiger-Mueller tube counting at 2 to 3 hours	Same	Use limited by high uptake by muscle
Coincidence scanning of annihilation photos immediately to 7 hours	Same	Still experimental; low total body radiation
Scintillation scanning at 1 to 5 hours	Same	Much less body radiation than ^{203}Hg-Neohydrin; possible difficulty in diagnosing deep lesions
Scintillation scanning at 48 hours	Same	Experimental
Scintillation scanning at 5 to 24 hours	Same	Experimental

Continued.

Table 16-2. Experimental radioisotopic compounds—cont'd

Radioisotopic compound and symbol	Pharmaceutical name	Physical half-life	Dose (μC)
Cobalt-57-tetraphenyloporphine-sulfonate (^{57}Ca)		270 days	250-500
I-131-cholografin (^{131}I)	Sodium iodipamide	8.1 days	500-1,000
Fluorine-18-fluoroborate (^{18}F)	Potassium Fluoroborate	1.87 hours	200-3,000
Gallium-68 compounds (^{68}Ga)	Gallium versenate Gallium Phthalocyanate Gallium Protoporphyrin Sodium Galloarsenate	66 minutes	
Technetium-99m (^{99m}Tc)	Technetate	6 hours	10,000
I-124-human globulin (^{124}I)	Human globulin	4-5 days	260-695
I-125-antitumor antibodies (^{125}I)		60 days	200
I-125-macro albumin aggregates (^{125}I)	Human serum albumin	60 days	80-225
I-131 macro albumin aggregates (^{131}I)	Human serum albumin	8.1 days	60-180
Spinal cord			
I-131-diiodofluorescein (^{131}I)	Diiodofluorescein	8.1 days	1,000
Radioiodinated serum albumin (^{131}I)	Human serum albumin	8.1 days	100
Eye tumors			
Mercury-197-neohydrin (^{197}Hg)	Chlormerodrin	2.7 days	1,000
I-125-diiodofluorescein (^{125}I)	Diiodofluorescein	60 days	250-500
Liver tumors			
Rose bengal-I-125 (tetraiodotetra-chlorfluorescein) (^{125}I)	Rose bengal	60 days	150-300

Detection method	Rationale	Application
Scintillation scanning at 24 to 48 hours	Same	Experimental
Scintillation scanning at 3 to 6 hours	Same	Experimental
Coincidence scanning and counting of annihilation photons at 30 minutes to 1 hour	Same	Experimental
Coincidence scanning of annihilation photons at 20 to 60 minutes	Same	Experimental
Scintillation scanning immediately to 3 hours	Same	Experimental; very short physical half-life permits use of very high doses with low resulting tissue radiation; can scan rapidly with high resolution; very promising
Coincidence counting of annihilation photons immediately to 8 days	Same	Experimental
Scintillation scanning in a few days	Used resected gliomas to prepare antibodies	Experimental; for diagnosis of recurrent gliomas
Scintillation scanning immediately	Aggregates are trapped in cerebral capillaries after carotid infection	Experimental
Scintillation scanning immediately	Same	Experimental
Geiger-Mueller counting at 20 minutes	Same as brain	Counting over spine; has not been widely used
Scintillation scanning immediately after infection into subarachnoid space	A "myeloscintigram"; defects in spinal column detected without using a foreign dye substance	Has not been widely used
Scintillation counting and scanning at 24 hours	Increased concentration by eye tumors	Experimental
Scintillation counting at 8 hours	Increased concentration by eye tumors	Experimental; may have special value in diagnosing posterior tumors
Scintillation scanning at 30 minutes	Same as rose bengal-I-131; softer radiation may give greater resolution and less liver radiation	Liver scanning; not yet in wide use

Continued.

Table 16-2. Experimental radioisotopic compounds—cont'd

Radioisotopic compound and symbol	Pharmaceutical name	Physical half-life	Dose (μC)
Colloidal gold-199 (^{199}Au)	Colloidal gold	3.15 days	
I-131-thyroxine (^{131}I)	Thyroxine	8.1 days	40-60
I-131-cholografin (^{131}I)	Sodium iodipamide	8.1 days	150-500
Cobalt-60-vitamin B₁₂ (^{60}Co)	Cyanocobalamin	5.2 years	500-2,000
I-131-macro albumin aggregates (^{131}I)	Human serum albumin	8.1 days	200-300
Molybdenum-99 (^{99}Mo)	Molybdenum	66 hours	50
Colloidal technetium-99m (^{99m}Tc)	Technetate	6 hours	5,000
Rose bengal-I-131 (^{131}I)	Rose bengal	8.1 days	25
Pancreatic tumors			
Manganese-52 (^{52}Mn)	Manganese chloride	6.5 days	100
Manganese-54 (^{54}Mn)	Manganese chloride	310 days	100
Zinc-65 (^{65}Zn)	Zinc chloride Zinc sulfadiazene	250 days	100
Zinc-62 (^{62}Zn)	Zinc chloride	9 hours	
Gastrointestinal tract tumors			
Phosphorus-32 (^{32}P)	Sodium phosphate	14.3 days	500
Phosphorus-32 (^{32}P)	Sodium phosphate	14.3 days	500
Iodine-131 (^{131}I)	Sodium iodide	8.1 days	300-1,00
Phosphorus-32 (^{32}P)	Sodium phosphate	14.3 days	2-20

Detection method	Rationale	Application
Scintillation scanning	Same as colloidal gold-198; softer radiation may give greater resolution and less liver radiation	Still experimental
Scintillation scanning at 6 to 24 hours	Concentrated by the liver; space-occupying lesions do not concentrate it	Experimental
Scintillation scanning at 30 minutes	Same	Experimental
Scintillation counting at 24 to 48 hours	Same	Experimental
Scintillation scanning at 10 to 75 minutes	Colloidal aggregates trapped by normal liver, not by space-occupying lesions	Experimental
Scintillation scanning at 24 hours	Concentrated by enzyme systems of liver cells; space-occupying lesions do not concentrate it	Experimental
Scintillation scanning at 10 minutes	Taken up by reticuloendothelial system of liver, similar to colloidal gold	Experimental; very short half-life permits use of high doses with low resulting tissue radiation; high resolution
Scintillation counting of blood sample at 24 hours	In complete (malignant) obstructive jaundice, clearance of radioactivity in the blood is delayed	Experimental
Scintillation scanning at 1 to 8 hours	Concentrated by normal pancreas	High levels in liver and kidney make it difficult to detect pancreatic tumors
Same	Same	Same
Same	Same	Same
Coincidence scanning of annihilation photons	Same	Same
Geiger-Mueller tube counting at 24 hours	Increased ^{32}P uptake by actively growing cancers	Used experimentally by insertion of small Geiger-Mueller tube into esophagus, stomach, and rectum; limited by difficulty of technique, statistical errors in counting and ^{32}P shortcomings
Intragastric balloon in vivo radioautography at 2 to 18 hours	Same as above; attempt to simplify ^{32}P technique; studies entire organ during test	Experimental; for detection of gastric cancer
Scintillation scanning	Increased uptake reported by gastric cancer	Experimental; contradictory results have been reported
Radioautography of exfoliated cells mixed with ^{32}P	In vitro uptake of ^{32}P by exfoliated cancer cells	Experimental for detection of esophageal cancer

Continued.

Table 16-2. Experimental radioisotopic compounds—cont'd

Radioisotopic compound and symbol	Pharmaceutical name	Physical half-life	Dose (μC)
Urogenital tumors			
Kidney			
I-131-diodrast (^{131}I)	Iodopyracet	8.1 days	480-1,000
Mercury-197-neohydrin (^{197}Hg)	Chlormerodrin	2.7 days	70-200
Bladder			
Phosphorus-32 (^{32}P)	Sodium phosphate	14.3 days	500
Prostate			
Phosphorus-32 (^{32}P)	Sodium phosphate	14.3 days	150-500
Testes			
Phosphorus-32 (^{32}P)	Sodium phosphate	14.3 days	300-500
Cervix and vulva			
Phosphorus-32 (^{32}P)	Sodium phosphate	14.3 days	200-2,000
Skeletal system tumors			
Bone			
Gallium-72 (^{72}Ga)	Gallium citrate	14.3 hours	300-400
Fluorine-18 (^{18}F)	Sodium fluoride	1.87 hours	500-1,000
Cartilage			
Sulphur-35 (^{35}S)	Sodium sulfate	87 days	2,800-6,700
Lung and mediastinal tumors			
Phosphorus-32 (^{32}P)	Sodium phosphate	14.3 days	500-1,000
I-131-macro albumin aggregates (^{131}I)	Human serum albumin	8.1 days	100-300
Radioiodinated serum albumin (RISA) (^{131}I)	Human serum albumin	8.1 days	500

Detection method	Rationale	Application
Scintillation scanning immediately	Radiopaque agent excreted by normal kidneys	Less convenient to use than Neohydrin; very rapid excretion by kidneys
Scintillation scanning at 1 hour	Same as Mercury-203-Neohydrin	Less resulting radiation than Mercury-203-Neohydrin; relatively weak tissue penetration a possible drawback
In vivo radioautography at 2 to 24 hours	Increased ^{32}P uptake by actively growing cancers	Experimental; technically difficult
Intrarectal in vivo radioautography at 24 hours	Same	Experimental
Geiger-Mueller counting at 2 to 24 hours	Same	Not dependable enough for clinical use
Geiger-Mueller counting at 1 to 48 hours	Same	Experimental
Scintillation counting and scanning at 3 to 24 hours	Gallium and fluorine compounds localize in actively metabolizing bone and bone tumors	Experimental
Coincidence scanning of annihilation photons at 1 to 3 hours	Same	Experimental
Geiger-Mueller counting and radioautography of excised tissue at 2 to 11 days	Sulphur is concentrated in actively growing chondrosarcoma	Has been used to distinguish between chondroma and low-grade chondrosarcoma in biopsy material when microscopic appearance was indefinite
Geiger-Mueller tube counting through bronchoscope at 24 hours	Increased ^{32}P uptake by actively growing cancers	Lung tumor diagnosis; limited by difficulty of technique and ^{32}P shortcomings
Scintillation scanning immediately	5-50 μ aggregates are trapped by normal lung; space-occupying lesions do not trap aggregates	Experimental; cannot differentiate benign from malignant lesions
Scintillation scanning at 5 minutes	For mediastinal masses; low radioactivity: tumor; high radioactivity: aneurysm	Has not had wide clinical use

Continued

Table 16-2. Experimental radioisotopic compounds—cont'd

Radioisotopic compound and symbol	Pharmaceutical name	Physical half-life	Dose (μC)
Skin and breast tumors			
Skin			
Phosphorus-32 (^{32}P)	Sodium phosphate	14.3 days	100-500
Phosphorus-32 (^{32}P)	Sodium phosphate	14.3 days	500
Breast			
Phosphorus-32 (^{32}P)	Sodium phosphate	14.3 days	300-500
Phosphorus-32 (^{32}P)	Sodium phosphate	14.3 days	500
Potassium-42 (^{42}K)	Potassium carbonate	12.5 hours	200-750
Miscellaneous tumors			
Iron-59 (^{59}Fe)	Ferrous citrate	45 days	25
I-131-antifibrin antibodies (^{131}I)		8.1 days	400-2,000
I-131-5-iododeoxycytidine (ICdR) (^{131}I)		8.1 days	270-710
Mercury-197-neohydrin (^{197}Hg)	Chlormerodrin	2.7 days	1,000
Cesium-131 (^{131}Cs)	Cesium acetate	9.6 days	134-2,200
S-35-sulfanilic acids of fluorene (^{35}S)		87.1 days	
I-131-aminoacridine (^{131}I)	Quinacrine	8.1 days	

Detection method	Rationale	Application
Geiger-Mueller counting at 1 to 24 hours	Increased uptake of ^{32}P by actively growing cancers	Best results with melanomas; has not received wide acceptance; ease of obtaining biopsies a factor
In vivo radioautography at 2 to 24 hours	Same	In experimental stage for detection of melanomas
Geiger-Mueller counting at 2 to 48 hours	Same	Limited because of false negatives (small, deep, and acellular tumors) and false positives (inflammatory and some benign lesions)
In vivo radioautography at 2 to 24 hours	Same	Experimental
Scintillation counting at 5 to 15 minutes	Increased potassium uptake by actively growing cancers; can detect deep tumors because of gamma emission	Limited because of false negatives (small and acellular cancers) and false positives (high uptake by normal muscle)
Scintillation counting of resected tissue at 2 to 30 days	Increased uptake of iron by various tumors, including esophageal, stomach, colic, and breast	Has not been used clinically; some false positive and false negative results
Scintillation scanning at 1 to 3 days	Increased concentration of fibrin in some tumors	Still experimental; best results with melanomas, sarcomas and some carcinomas; negative results with certain cancers
Scintillation scanning at 1 to 3 hours	Incorporation of halogenated nucleosides into DNA	Experimental; positive results with brain tumors and hepatoma
Scintillation scanning at 24 hours	Probable binding of mercurial compounds to proteins in cancers	Experimental; positive results with eye tumors, squamous cell carcinomas of the skin and nasopharynx, and bone, bowel, and lung tumors
Scintillation scanning and counting at 10 minutes to 3 hours	Greater alkali metal content of tumors	Experimental; positive results with cancers of the breast, cervical nodes, upper $\frac{1}{3}$ of esophagus and lymphomas; negative results with abdominal tumors
Counting of radioactivity in specimens at 6 to 40 hours	Increased concentration and retention of fluorene derivatives in tumor tissue	Studies on experimental animals
Radioautography of specimens at 1 to 5 days	Formation of aminoacridine-DNA-complexes	Studies on experimental animals; positive results with pulmonary, hepatic, and gastric tumors

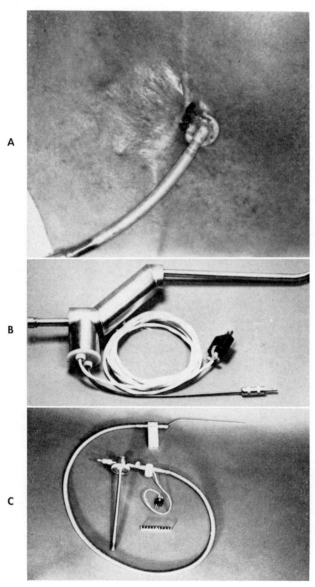

Fig. 16-1. Cryosurgery, latest method for treatment. **A,** Freezing of recurrent breast cancer with modified gynecological probe. **B,** Tonsil probe. **C,** Larynx probe. (Courtesy Dr. W. Cahan, Memorial Hospital, New York, N. Y.)

Glossary

ablative procedures removal of hormone sources that influence the development of cancer.

adenocarcinoma a carcinoma arising in glandular tissue.

adjuvant chemotherapy a combination of surgery and chemotherapy anticancer drugs injected directly into surgical sites or administered intravenously.

Bence-Jones protein test a test upon urine, which when positive may denote a myeloma.

cachexia a state of being cachectic, malnourished to the extent that there is wasting such as occurs in many chronic conditions; an emaciated state.

cancer in situ (intraepithelial or preinvasive carcinoma) a term applied to a lesion confined to the mucosal surface—the cells have not invaded or metastasized.

cancerophobia fear of cancer.

carcinogen a substance that stimulates production of cancer.

carcinoma a malignant epithelial tumor that tends to infiltrate surrounding tissues and give rise to metastases.

carcinomatosis widespread metastatic disease.

castration removal of the testicles in the male, and in the female, the ovaries.

chemotherapy a method of employing certain chemical compounds in the management of malignant lesions and/or their metastases.

cordotomy surgical division of specific tracts of the spinal cord for relief of intractable pain.

curie a unit of measure denoting the rate of radioactive decay.

DNA deoxyribonucleic acid, one of the nucleic acids of the cell that is of particular interest to the cancer investigator since it is involved in the process that converts normal cells into malignant ones.

esophageal speech an acquired technique by which laryngectomees are taught to speak again by swallowing and expelling air through the mouth from the esophagus.

Ewing's sarcoma a malignant tumor of the shaft of a long bone.

exenteration (pelvic) radical surgical procedure wherein the organs, lymph nodes, etc. of the pelvis are excised.

exfoliative cytology study of cells that have been slouged off, or wiped or scraped off, the surface of a body tissue for cancer diagnostic purposes.

Geiger counter an instrument used to detect radioactive particles.

glossectomy surgical removal of the tongue or a major portion thereof.

hypophysectomy removal of the pituitary gland by surgery or by use of radiation.

irradiation the application of x-ray, radium, etc. for therapeutic purposes.

leukemia a fatal cancer of the blood-forming organs characterized by production of abnormal leukocytes.

277

leukoplakia white patches on the tongue or mucous membrane considered to be pre-cancerous lesions.

metastasis the spread of cancer cells from the original site in the body to other sites, resulting in so-called secondary tumors.

millicurie a thousandth of a curie.

myeloma primary malignant tumor of bone marrow.

oncology the study of malignant disease.

osteoporosis a condition in which absorption of lime salts causes bones to become abnormally porous, a loss in bony substances producing brittleness and softness of bones; often seen in people of very advanced age or debility.

osteogenic sarcoma a highly malignant tumor of bone.

Papanicolaou smear a method of collecting and staining cells used in detection of cancer.

palliative treatment therapy that affords relief but not cure.

perfusion the technique of introducing a chemical agent to an isolated part of the circulatory system for limited treatment of a single part or organ of the body.

radionecrosis destruction of tissue as a result of its having been exposed to radiation.

radioresistant tumor resistant to the effects of radiation and therefore not destroyed.

radiosensitive tumor than can be destroyed by radiation therapy.

regional involvement medical term for the stage of cancer when the cells have begun to spread from the original site but are temporarily trapped in a nearby lymph node that retards further spread for a time.

rhabdomyosarcoma a malignant tumor of muscle.

rhizotomy destruction of spinal nerve roots to relieve intractable pain.

sarcoma a form of cancer arising from cells of connective tissue, lymphoid tissue, cartilage, or bone.

scintiscanner a device used to determine the presence of radioactive substances in a given organ or part of the body.

stoma a permanent artificial opening such as a colostomy, ileostomy, or tracheostomy.

teletherapy radiation treatment administered by a radioactive isotope housed in a machine similar to a large x-ray unit (cobalt-60, cesium-137, iridium-192).

Index

A

G

Gallbladder, palpable, in carcinoma of pancreas, 168
Gamma globulin, 60, 62
Ganglioneuroma, 12
Gangrene as mechanism of pain, 19
Gastrectomy
  complications of, 147
  extent of, 146
  indications for, 146
  nursing care in, 147-149
  postoperative care in, 146-149
  transthoracic, 149
Gastric analysis, 142, 145
Gastrointestinal series, 142, 145
Gastrointestinal tract
  accessory structures of, 159-169
  anatomy of 138
  innervation of, 141
  physiology of, 140-141
  symptoms of dysfunction of, 141-142
Gastroscopy, 142
Gastrostomy, 143
Giant cell carcinoma, 120
Giant follicle lymphoma; *see* Lymphosarcoma
Gland; *see* the various glands
Glioblastoma, 12, 95
Glioblastoma multiforme, 96
Gliomas, 12, 95
  in childhood, 108
  types of, 96
Globulin, antihemophilic, 59
Globulin, beta, 60
Globulin, gamma, 60, 62
Globulins, serum, 59
Glucocorticoids, 123, 202
Goiter, definition of, 120
Gonadotropic hormones, 119, 187
Gonads as parent tissue in neoplasm, 12
Granulocytes
  formation of, 62
  function of, 62
  as leukocytes, 61
  replacement of, in leukemia, 260-261
Granuloma, 74; *see also* Hodgkin's disease

H

Haversian systems, 80
Head and neck, cancer of
  postoperative care in, 221-223
  preoperative care in, 215-216, 221
Headache
  in intracranial tumors in childhood, 109
  in secondary polycythemia, 63
  in tumors of brain and spinal cord, 95-96

Heart failure, congestive, 53
Hemangioendothelioma, 12
Hemangioma, 12, 113
Hematemesis in gastrointestinal tract dysfunction, 142
Hematuria
  in carcinoma of kidney, 175
  in carcinoma of prostrate, 190
  in myelocytic leukemia, 66
Hemicorporectomy, 259
Hemipelvectomy, 83, 88
Hemoglobin, 60, 62
Hemophilia, 59
Hemopoiesis, 60-61
Hemoptysis in carcinoma of lungs, 233-234
Hemorrhage
  in cancer of mouth, 215
  in carotid artery rupture, 223
  in leukemia, 105, 260
  after renal surgery, 178
  after surgery for thyroid carcinoma, 121
  as systemic effect of malignant tumors, 17
  after transurethral resection, 192
Hemorrhagic diathesis as symptom of leukemia, 66
Hemothorax after transthoracic gastrectomy, 149
Hemovac, 129
Hepatectomy for carcinoma of liver, 163
Hepatitis, infectious, 60
Hepatoma, primary, 163
Hepatomegaly in myelocytic leukemia, 66
Herpes zoster in leukemia, 67
High-voltage radiation therapy; *see* Radiation therapy
Hirsutism as toxic manifestation of androgen therapy, 53
HN_2; *see* Nitrogen mustards
Hoarseness
  in cancer of larynx, 225
  in cancer of mouth, 215
  as danger signal of cancer, 35
  in thyroid carcinoma, 120
Hodgkin's disease, 74-75, 261, 264
  characteristics of, 74
  incidence of, 74
  nitrogen mustards in treatment of, 50
  survival rate in, 77
  types of, 74
Hodgkin's paragranuloma, 74
Hodgkin's sarcoma, 74
Hormones; *see also* the various hormones
  adrenocortical, 54
  gonadotropic, 187
  secretion of, after pelvic exenteration, 202-203
Horner's syndrome, 227
Hydatidiform mole, 12
Hydration in advanced disease, 248
Hydrochloric acid, 139

Obstruction—cont'd
  in physiology of benign tumors, 13
  tracheal, 223
Occlusion as mechanism of pain, 19
Odors, control of, 247
Office of Vocational Rehabilitation, 257
Oligodendroglioma, 95, 97
Oophorectomy, 193, 250
Operations, monobloc, 259
Oral care; *see* Mouth care
Oral irrigation, 218-219
Orchiectomy, 192
Organs, reproductive; *see* Reproductive organs
Osmolarity of blood serum, 151
Ossification, 79
Osteogenic sarcoma, 12, 80, 82-84, 108
Osteolytic osteogenic sarcoma, 83
Osteoma, 12
Ovarian hormones, 124-125
Ovary
  anatomy and physiology of, 186-187
  carcinoma of, 192-193
    ethylenemines in treatment of, 50
    symptoms of, 193
    treatment of, 193
  cystadenoma of, as precancerous lesion, 13
  tumors of, nitrogen mustards in treatment of, 50
Oxygen therapy, 238
Oxytocin, 120

P

P³²; *see* Radioactive phosphorus
Paget cells, 126
Paget's carcinoma of breast, 125-126
Paget's disease of bone, 13
Pain
  of bone in multiple myeloma, 85
  in cancer
    of large intestine, 152
    of larynx, 226
    of mouth, 215
    of tongue, 217
  in carcinoma
    of kidney, 175
    of liver, 163
    of lungs, 234
    of ovary, 193
    of pancreas, 167
    of prostate, 190
    of stomach, 145
  intractable, 246
  in malignant neoplasm of bone, 82
  after mastectomy, 129
  mechanisms of, 19, 246-247
  in osteogenic sarcoma, 83
  physical effects of, 247
  relief of, in advanced disease, 246-247
  after renal surgery, 178

Pain—cont'd
  in systemic effects of malignant tumors, 17-19
Palliation
  in advanced disease, 248-253
  in carcinoma of ovary, 193
  in carcinoma of prostate, 191, 192
  in Ewing's sarcoma, 85
  in malignant lymphomas, 76
  in multiple myeloma, 86
  in renal neoplasm, 176
Pallor as symptom of leukemia, 66
Pancoast syndrome, 235
Pancreas
  anatomy and physiology of, 167
  carcinoma of
    incidence of, 167
    metastasis of, 168
    preoperative care in, 168
    surgical treatment of, 168-169
    symptoms of, 167
  malignant lesions of, 167
Pancreaticoduodenectomy, 168-169
Pancytopenia
  in chemotherapy in leukemia, 70
  in multiple myeloma, 85
Panhysterectomy, 197
Papanicolaou balloon studies, 142
Papanicolaou test, 37, 193
Papillary adenocarcinomas of thyroid gland, 120
Papillary carcinoma
  of breast, 125
  of kidney pelvis, 175
  of thyroid gland, 121
Papilloma, 12, 152
Paragranuloma, 74; *see also* Hodgkin's disease
Paraldehyde, 98
Paralysis
  of laryngeal nerve after surgery for thyroid carcinoma, 121
  resulting from potassium depletion, 41
Paralytic ileus after pelvic exenteration, 202
Paranoid reactions after cancer surgery, 25
Parasitic action of tumor, 18
Parenchymal tumor of kidney, 175
Parotid gland, 159-161
Pathologic fractures; *see* Fractures, pathologic
Pathology, 10, 13-17
Patient
  communication with
    in preoperative care, 42
    in radiation therapy, 46
  fear of, in leukemia, 68
  informing, in psychological impact of cancer, 22
Pelvic exenteration, 196-208
  artificial menopause after, 203
  discharge from hospital after, 207-208